WOMEN'S
HEALTH

Second Edition

Tolu Oyelowo, DC, PhD
Professor and Chair
Department of Health Promotion
and Associated Clinical Sciences
Northwestern Health Sciences University
Bloomington, Minnesota

Judith Johnson, PhD, RN, FAAN
Consultant
HealthQuest
Editor-in-Chief
Asia-Pacific Journal of Oncology Nursing
Minneapolis, Minnesota

JONES & BARTLETT
L E A R N I N G

World Headquarters
Jones & Bartlett Learning
5 Wall Street
Burlington, MA 01803
978-443-5000
info@jblearning.com
www.jblearning.com

Jones & Bartlett Learning books and products are available through most bookstores and online booksellers. To contact Jones & Bartlett Learning directly, call 800-832-0034, fax 978-443-8000, or visit our website, www.jblearning.com.

Substantial discounts on bulk quantities of Jones & Bartlett Learning publications are available to corporations, professional associations, and other qualified organizations. For details and specific discount information, contact the special sales department at Jones & Bartlett Learning via the above contact information or send an email to specialsales@jblearning.com.

Production Credits

VP, Executive Publisher: David D. Cella
Executive Editor: Amanda Martin
Acquisitions Editor: Teresa Reilly
Editorial Assistant: Emma Huggard
Production Manager: Carolyn Rogers Pershouse
Production Assistant: Molly Hogue
Marketing Communications Manager: Katie Hennessy
Product Fulfillment Manager: Wendy Kilborn
Composition: S4Carlisle Publishing Services

Project Management: S4Carlisle Publishing Services
Cover Design: Kristin E. Parker
Director of Rights & Media: Joanna Gallant
Rights & Media Specialist: Wes DeShano
Media Development Editor: Troy Liston
Cover Image: © tofutyklein/Shutterstock
Printing and Binding: Edwards Brothers Malloy
Cover Printing: Edwards Brothers Malloy

Library of Congress Cataloging-in-Publication Data

Names: Oyelowo, Tolu, author. | Johnson, Judith (Judi) L., author.
Title: A guide to women's health / Tolu A. Oyelowo, Judith (Judi) L. Johnson.
Other titles: Mosby's guide to women's health
Description: Second edition. | Burlington, Massachusetts : Jones & Bartlett
    Learning, [2018] | Preceded by Mosby's guide to women's health / Tolu
    Oyelowo. St. Louis, Mo. : Mosby Elsevier, c2007. | Includes
    bibliographical references and index.
Identifiers: LCCN 2017004819 | ISBN 9781284079616 (pbk. : alk. paper)
Subjects: | MESH: Women's Health | Handbooks
Classification: LCC RA778 | NLM WA 39 | DDC 613/.0424--dc23 LC record available at https://lccn.loc.gov/2017004819

6048

Printed in the United States of America
21 20 19 18 17   10 9 8 7 6 5 4 3 2 1

Dedication

To Our Sons
  and in gratitude to our Heavenly Father

Contents

Contents

Chapter 4: Cardiovascular and Pulmonary Health in Women — 73

Chapter 5: Gastrointestinal Disorders — 105

Chapter 6: Infections and Immune Disorders — 121

VAGINAL INFECTIONS — 122

POSTMENOPAUSAL INFECTIONS — 129

SEXUALLY TRANSMITTED INFECTIONS — 131

Contents

Contents

Contents

Contents

Contents

Contents

Preface

Women make more health-care-related visits than men; however, it is not uncommon for them to receive diagnoses and treatments that are based on medical research that has been done primarily on men. Until recently, medical research largely ignored many health issues important to women, and women have long been underrepresented in clinical trials. As health education programs acknowledge this inequity, more women's health programs are incorporated into curriculum.

Although there are many women's health books and textbooks, most are medical texts designed for the obstetrician or gynecologist and provide far more detail than that needed by the first-contact primary care practitioner. *A Guide to Women's Health, Second Edition* will appeal to practitioners who are seeing patients on a daily basis. Nursing students and nurse practitioners will find this book to be a quick reference for verifying findings and making management decisions. Health and wellness practitioners, including acupuncturists, chiropractors, naturopaths, and therapists, working in integrated health environments will also find this book to be useful.

Introduction

A Guide to Women's Health, Second Edition is a concise, thorough, consistent, and multidisciplinary manual that includes evidence-based conventional, complementary, and alternative care choices for many conditions that affect women. The conditions discussed in this text were chosen either because they are being reported more often in women or because the symptoms reported by women are different from those reported by men.

All chapters from the first edition have been revised to reflect findings from current research and current diagnostic and management approaches. Because of the impact of culture, spirituality, and intimate partner violence on the health of women, chapters on these topics are also included. There is also a chapter that addresses vulnerable populations, such as recent immigrants; lesbian, gay, bisexual, and transgender (LGBT) individuals, older adults, individuals with disabilities and mental illness, and non-English speakers.

An estimated one-third to one-half of women use some form of care that is complementary or alternative to conventional medicine, and approximately 50% disclose their use to their conventional care providers. For this reason, *A Guide to Women's Health, Second Edition* includes evidence-based complementary and integrative care choices for many conditions and uses the following definitions from the National Center for Complementary and Integrative Health:

- Alternative medicine—when a nonmainstream practice is used in place of conventional medicine.
- Complementary medicine—when a nonmainstream practice is used together with conventional medicine.
- Conventional medicine—traditional (mainstream) medicine.

The content is broadly organized into introductory concepts, such as anatomy and physiology; common conditions; and special topics. The discussion for each condition is organized to allow for easy retrieval of information and includes epidemiology, etiology, signs and symptoms, and diagnostic and management considerations. To ensure ease of access by the busy practitioner, management considerations are further organized into conventional, treatments, complementary treatments, and self-care and wellness.

The Appendix includes additional resources, such as descriptions of some of the techniques and procedures described in the manual and links to websites that list current dosages and side effects of many pharmaceuticals and nutraceuticals. The Clinical Pearl features provide the practitioner with brief clinical advice designed to enhance or lend clarity to the information in the body of the text. These clinical observations also fill in the gaps where controlled data do not exist or, as is in the case with some complementary practices, the research is still in its infancy. This pocket-sized manual is an excellent quick reference that is sure to be the go-to guide for the busy practitioner and student.

Reviewers

Rebecca C. Bagley, DNP, CNM
Associate Clinical Professor
Program Director, Nurse-Midwifery Education
East Carolina University, College of Nursing
Greenville, NC

Susan D. Beck, MSN, CNS, RN
Assistant Professor
Bloomsburg University
Bloomsburg, PA

Cara A. Busenhart, PhD, CNM, APRN
Assistant Clinical Professor
Program Director, Nurse-Midwifery Education
University of Kansas School of Nursing
Kansas City, KS

Michelle Collins, PhD, CNM, FACNM
Associate Professor and Director
Nurse-Midwifery Program
Vanderbilt University School of Nursing
Nashville, TN

Dr. Melva Craft-Blacksheare
Assistant Professor
University of Michigan – Flint
Flint, MI

Melicia Escobar, MSN, CNM
Course Coordinator, Course Faculty
Georgetown University
Washington, D.C.

Reviewers

Gay L. Goss, PhD, APRN
Professor
California State University, Dominguez Hills
Carson, CA

Linda A. Graf, RN, CNM, WHNP-C, MSN, DNP
Assistant Clinical Professor
DePaul University School of Nursing
Chicago, IL

Deborah Mandel, PhD, RNC-OB
Assistant Professor
West Chester University
West Chester, PA

Barbara L. Parker, MS, CNM, FNP
Clinical Instructor
University of Kansas Medical Center School of Nursing
Kansas City, KS

Susan Scott Ricci, ARNP, MSN, MEd, CNE
Nursing Faculty
University of Central Florida
Orlando, FL

PART ONE

Normal Anatomy and Physiology Review

The focus of this section is the effect of female gender on human physiology, including the endocrine system, the reproductive tract, and the urinary tract. Other aspects of physiology, such as the cardiovascular system, are integrated into the text of the relative chapter.

CHAPTER 1

Endocrine System

The endocrine and neuroendocrine systems include the hypothalamic–pituitary–adrenal axis, the hypothalamic–pituitary–thyroid axis, and the hypothalamic–pituitary–gonadal axis, complex systems of nerves and organs that secrete hormones into the bloodstream and influence multiple functions. The pineal gland and the gastrointestinal tract are also components of the endocrine system.

Hypothalamus–Pituitary–Thyroid Axis

The hypothalamic–pituitary–thyroid (HPT) axis is a self-regulating system that controls metabolism. In response to low levels of circulating thyroid hormone, the hypothalamus secretes thyrotropin-releasing hormone (TRH), which causes the anterior pituitary to secrete thyroid-stimulating hormone (TSH). TSH stimulates the thyroid gland to synthesize and secrete the thyroid hormones. As the levels of thyroid hormone increase, a negative-feedback mechanism impedes the further release of TRH and TSH.

Hypothalamus–Pituitary–Adrenal Axis

The hypothalamus–pituitary–adrenal (HPA) axis is a self-regulating system that is responsible for regulating stress responses, immune function, digestion, energy expenditure, and several adaptation responses. In response to low levels of corticosteroids or physical or emotional stress, the hypothalamus secretes corticotrophin-releasing factor (CRH). CRH causes the anterior pituitary to secrete several hormones, including adrenocorticotropic hormone (ACTH), which stimulates cortisol release from the adrenal glands.

Hypothalamus–Pituitary–Gonadal Axis

The hypothalamic–pituitary–gonadal (HPG) axis primarily regulates the reproductive system, but it also has a significant influence on the immune system. In response to low levels of estrogen and progesterone, the hypothalamus secretes gonadotropin-releasing hormone (GNRH). GNRH is released in pulses and initiates the release of follicle-stimulating hormone (FSH) and luteinizing hormone (LH) from the anterior pituitary. FSH and LH initiate ovarian follicular development and ovulation and cause the synthesis and release of estrogens, progesterone, and testosterone. As the levels of these three hormones increase, a negative-feedback mechanism impedes the further release of FSH and LH.

Gonadal Hormones

Estrogen

Estrogen is a steroid hormone produced primarily in the ovaries, breasts, and adipose tissue and in smaller quantities in the skin, liver, brain, and intestines. Estrogen has significant effects in the female reproductive system. The three major estrogen derivatives are estrone (E1), estradiol (E2), and estriol (E3). Estrone is the primary form of estrogen after menopause, estradiol is the primary form of estrogen prior to menopause, and estriol is a byproduct of estrogen metabolism that is also produced by the placenta during pregnancy.

Estrogen is synthesized from low-density lipoprotein (LDL) cholesterol in reactions that require transportation of cholesterol across the cellular membrane via a delivery mechanism that is influenced by LH, ACTH, cyclic adenosine monophosphate (AMP), and calcium. Cholesterol is converted to pregnenolone and subsequently to progesterone, androgens, estrogens, and corticosteroids. See Figure 1-1.

Estradiol—Fast Facts

- The most potent of the estrogens occurring naturally in the body
- Primary hormone produced by the ovaries during the reproductive years
- Primary hormone responsible for the menstrual cycle
- Impacts bone, blood vessels, heart, brain, and skin health
- In function intensity, 12 times stronger than estrone and 80 times stronger than estriol
- Responsible for growth and female development
- Increases the amount of fat in subcutaneous tissues, especially the breasts, thighs, and buttocks

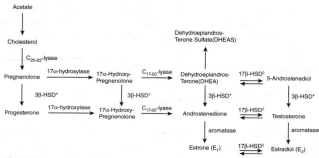

*3β-HSD=3β-hydroxysteroid dehydrogenase-Δ^{5,4}-isomerase
°17β-hydroxysteroid dehydrogenase

Figure 1-1 Steroidogenic pathways

Reproduced from Homburg, R. (2008). The mechanism of ovulation. In *Glob. libr. women's med.*, (ISSN: 1756-2228). Retrieved from http://editorial.glowm.com/?p=glowm.cml/section_view&articleid=289; Homburg, R. (2005). *Ovulation induction and controlled ovarian stimulation: A practical guide.* CRC Press. Reproduced with permission of Taylor & Francis.

- Influences hip-bone formation, resulting in the characteristic female skeletal development
- Can be converted to estrone in the liver, breast, and other peripheral tissues

Estrone—Fast Facts

- Primarily an adrenal-derived estrogen
- Can be converted to estradiol
- Dominates in menopausal women

Estriol—Fast Facts

- A weak estrogen
- Produced in large amounts by the placenta and can be detected by the ninth week of pregnancy
- May be measured in urine
- The most abundant estrogen

Progesterone

Progesterone is a steroid hormone that facilitates female reproductive physiology. It is synthesized in the ovaries and secreted by the corpus luteum following ovulation. Like estrogen, progesterone affects multiple tissues and organs, including the brain, breast, uterus, ovary, and cervix.

Progesterone—Fast Facts

- In the uterus and ovary, progesterone initiates the release of mature oocytes, facilitates implantation of the zygote, and maintains pregnancy by promoting uterine growth and suppressing muscle contractility.
- In the breast, progesterone facilitates glandular development in preparation for milk secretion and the suppression of milk protein synthesis before childbirth.
- In the brain, progesterone mediates signals required for sexually responsive behavior.
- In bone tissue, progesterone modulates bone mass.

The release of progesterone by the corpus luteum is facilitated by LH. The function of LH is mediated by cAMP, FSH, adrenal hormones, prolactin, prostaglandins, and activin. Progesterone is transported through the blood bound to corticosteroid-binding globulin (transcortin). Progesterone's actions and effects are subjected to its nuclear receptor. Progesterone receptors are proteins that are influenced by estrogen to bind progesterone. Progesterone receptors are widely distributed throughout the body and regulate the functions of thyroid hormones, vitamin D, steroids, and retinoids, among others.

Testosterone

Testosterone is an androgen produced primarily by the ovaries but also by the adrenal glands through peripheral conversion of androstenedione to testosterone in adipose tissue. Under the influence of LH, the ovaries secrete 25% of circulating testosterone and 50% of the body's androstenedione. The adrenals secrete another 25% of the body's testosterone.

In healthy women, the majority of testosterone is bound to sex hormone-binding globulin (SHBG), with significantly smaller amounts bound to albumin or circulating freely in the bloodstream.

Androgen receptors have been identified in multiple tissues, including the skin, the brain, the cardiovascular system, adipose tissue, skeletal muscle, and the gut. Testosterone and dihydrotestosterone (DHT) are the only androgens currently known to activate androgen receptors. DHT is more potent than testosterone.

Testosterone—Fast Facts

- Produced peripherally in the skin, liver, adipose tissue, and urogenital system
- Androstenedione and, to some degree, dehydroepiandrosterone (DHEA) are converted to testosterone in the skin.

CLINICAL PEARL

There is no feedback regulatory loop controlling androgen secretion in women. The extent to which a female expresses androgenicity is dependent on the amount of free circulating testosterone.

Adrenal Hormones

The adrenal steroid hormones are the glucocorticoids, cortisol (hydrocortisone), and the mineralocorticoids (aldosterone). They are synthesized from cholesterol and transported through the blood bound to corticosteroid-binding globulin, a carrier protein that is synthesized by the liver. Their actions are dependent on the type of receptor to which they bind.

Glucocorticoids—Fast Facts

- Cause the liver to convert muscle protein and fat to glucose
- Influence the conversion of sugars, fats, and proteins to energy

- Suppress immune responses
- Inhibit swelling and inflammation
- Provide energy needed in response to emotional and physical stress; balance the stress response
- Speed up metabolism
- Influence liver metabolism of stored glucose
- Control temperature (catecholamine-mediated mobilization of free fatty acids for the shivering response; enhanced blood and liver carbohydrate levels during hypothermia)

CLINICAL PEARL

Cortisol is the most abundant and potent of the glucocorticoids. Too much cortisol is a cause of Cushing's syndrome, and too little cortisol is a cause of Addison's disease.

Mineralocorticoids—Fast Facts

- Facilitate sodium retention
- Facilitate potassium and hydrogen excretion
- Maintain water balance

CLINICAL PEARL

Persistently elevated levels of glucocorticoids impede other steroid hormones and can cause infertility.

Excess mineralocorticoid activity may result in systemic edema and elevated blood pressure.

Dehydroepiandrosterone

DHEA is produced primarily by the adrenal glands, with smaller amounts produced by peripheral conversion from ovarian secretions. The ovaries secrete 20% of the body's DHEA. DHEA, dehydroepiandrosterone sulfate (DHEAS), and androstenedione are almost entirely bound to albumin and as such are readily available.

DHEA—Fast Facts

- Converted to androstenedione and subsequently to estrogen and testosterone
- May activate alpha and beta estrogen receptors
- Synthesis may be impacted by chronic stress, causing adrenal depletion as a result of cortisol production

Thyroid Hormones

Thyroid hormones are produced by the thyroid gland under the influence of TSH. They support almost all body systems. Thyroid hormones are made of iodine, which is ingested during daily food and water intake, and thyroglobulin, a substrate made of the amino acid tyrosine. Thyroxin (T4), the most abundant thyroid hormone, is composed of four iodine atoms. Triiodothyronine (T3), the most active form of thyroid hormone, is composed of three iodine atoms. Together, the thyroid hormones regulate growth, control metabolism, and control circadian rhythms.

After thyroid hormones are released into the bloodstream, thyroid transport proteins transport the hormones to a range of target cells. Conversion of T4 to T3 takes place in the target cells. T4 is also converted to various other thyroid hormones. The largest concentrations of thyroid hormone are found in the liver, muscles, and kidneys.

Thyroid Hormones—Fast Facts

- Bind to receptor cells and are activated in peripheral tissue
- May take hours to days to achieve their final effect on cell energy and metabolism
- Necessary for many functions, including the following:
  - Brain development
  - Axial skeleton development

- Metabolism of sugars, fats, and proteins
- Respiratory function
- Immune system function

Insulin

Insulin is a pancreatic hormone that is essential for the regulation of blood glucose. Lack of insulin and the inability to adequately respond to insulin are primary causes of diabetes.

Insulin has a similar function in males and females. However, insulin's ability to regulate blood sugar is significantly more challenging in females than in males because of the influence of female hormones on blood sugar.

Insulin—Fast Facts

- Regulates the body's use of glucose
- Controls blood sugar levels
- Regulates fat storage
- Provides the signals required by the liver, muscles, and fat to take in glucose from the blood
- Signals the liver to take in glucose and store it as glycogen

CHAPTER 2

Reproductive System

Pelvic Neuromusculoskeletal Anatomy (Summarized from Prather, Dugan, Fitzgerald, and Hunt, 2009)

CLINICAL PEARL

Pregnancy places undue stresses on the symphysis pubis.

Pelvic Anatomy—Fast Facts (see Figure 2-1)

- The female pelvis is a bony ring with articulations at the sacroiliac joint in the back and the symphysis pubis in the front.
- The female pelvis is wider in diameter than the male pelvis.
- The sacroiliac joints are weight-bearing joints.
- The symphysis pubis is a cartilaginous joint supported by ligaments.
- The symphysis pubis allows for several types of motion: superior to inferior, anterior to posterior, and slight rotational.
- The fascia and muscles of the pelvic floor support the bladder, uterus, and rectum.
- Fibers from the levator ani originate lateral to the posterior surface of the pubic symphysis and insert on the inner surface of the ischial spine.
- Fibers from the levator ani concurrently attach to the coccyx and anus, and middle fibers insert into the rectum and blend with the fibers of the anal sphincter.
- The anterior fibers of the levator insert into the sides of the vagina.

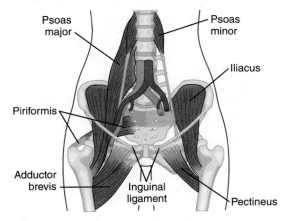

Figure 2-1 Illustration of the pelvis and its muscles

CLINICAL PEARL

The perineal body supports the pelvic floor. Rupture of the perineal body, which can occur during delivery, opens the anterior of the levator ani and can lead to pelvic organ prolapse.

CLINICAL PEARL

The pelvic floor is important in core muscle stabilization. Lax pelvic floor muscles lead to a lax core, which can result in spinal and low back pain.

Pelvic Neurology—Fast Facts

- Innervation of the pelvis is from the lumbar and sacral nerve roots, the lumbosacral plexus, individual peripheral nerves, and the sympathetic chain.

- Motor neurons supplying the external urethral and anal sphincters originate from the nucleus of Onuf.
- The nucleus of Onuf consists of small somatic motor neurons that are located in the ventral horn of the spinal cord at the level of S2.
- The pudendal nerve supplies sensation to the external genitalia.
- The pudendal nerve originates in the sacral plexus and derives its fibers from the second, third, and fourth sacral nerves.
- The pudendal nerve courses between the piriformis and coccygeus muscles, then over the spine of the ischium, and it exits the pelvis through the lower part of the greater sciatic foramen.
- The pelvic autonomous system derives sympathetic innervation from T11, T12, L1, and L2; it derives parasympathetic innervation from the vagus nerve and S1, S2, and S3.
- The levator ani is innervated primarily from the sacral plexus.
- Bladder function requires sympathetic and somatic activity.
- Parasympathetic innervation of the pelvic viscera is from S2–S4.

CLINICAL PEARL

Visceral receptors send afferent impulses via the dorsal horn of the spinal cord. Conditions such as endometriosis and irritable bowel syndrome can predispose to noxious visceral stimulation, which can contribute to persistent muscle contraction of the pelvic floor. A pelvic floor that is never fully relaxed can further cause adaptation responses, such as the recruiting of the psoas and other stabilizing muscles. These mechanisms can result in pelvic and low back pain.

Reproductive Anatomy

Anatomy of the Female Genitalia

The external genitalia are bordered superiorly by the mons pubis, laterally by the labia majora, and inferiorly by the perineum.

- The **mons pubis** (or mons veneris) is the fat pad covering the symphysis pubis (pubic bone), which is the anterior arch of the pelvic bone (see Figure 2-2).
- The **labia majora** are the two lateral borders of the vulva; they consist of skin, sebaceous glands, and adipose tissue and provide cushioning and protection for the sensitive structures encased within the labia minora.
- The **vulva**, also known as the pudendum, includes the labia majora (meaning "large lips"), labia minora (meaning "small lips"), clitoris, urethral and vaginal introitus, fourchette, fossa navicularis, vestibule, vestibular bulb, Skene's glands, Bartholin's glands, perineum, and hymen.
- The **fourchette** is the band of mucous membrane that connects the posterior ends of the labia minora.
- The **labia minora** are the two thin, sensitive internal lips of the vulva that enclose the vestibule at its superior borders and encase the clitoris. The anterior fold of the labia minora forms the prepuce or covering of the clitoris.

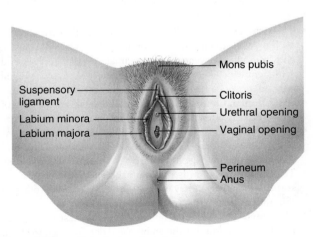

Figure 2-2 Illustration of external genitalia

- The **clitoris** is a small projection of erectile tissue that is homologous to the male penis. It consists of two crura, a body, and a glans. The body consists of two fused corpora cavernosa of approximately 3 cm in length, and it extends from the pubic arch above to the glans below. The two crura are continuations of the corpora cavernosa and attach them to the inferior rami of the pubic bones. The small, rounded glans is the distal end and consists of sensitive erectile tissue.

- The **perineum** is the area below the vagina and above the anus.

- The **anus** is the rectal opening.

- The **hymen** is the thin fibrous tissue that partially covers the vagina, leaving an opening for vaginal or menstrual discharge. It can be stretched or torn by sexual activity and sports activities. The size, shape, and degree of the opening can vary greatly among individuals. This has been known to create challenges within cultural systems that erroneously use the state of the hymen as an assessment of virginity.

The internal genitalia include the two ovaries, two fallopian tubes, uterus, and vagina (see Figure 2-3).

- The **ovaries** are almond-shaped structures that function to produce the ova and the sex steroids. The ovaries during the early reproductive years are approximately 3 to 5 cm long and 1 to 3 cm wide. They shrink with age to the size of a shelled almond and become smaller with the onset of menopause.

- The **fallopian tubes** (also known as the oviducts) are the locus of fertilization and extend from the fundus of the uterus to the ovaries.

- The **fimbriae** (or fringe over the ovary) are fingerlike extensions of the fallopian tube. The fimbriae produce peritoneal fluid and propel the released egg from the ovary into the fallopian tube.

- The **Bartholin's glands** are located on the inferior and lateral surface of the vulva; they open into the vagina and produce a thin mucus that helps to lubricate the vagina.

- The **uterus** is a muscular, hollow, pear-shaped structure that nourishes and supports the embryo and developing fetus from

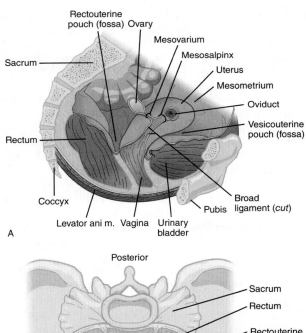

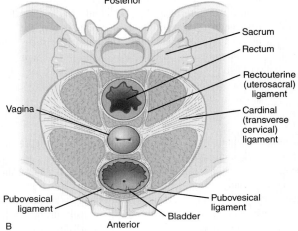

Figure 2-3 Illustration of internal genitalia

the time the fertilized egg is implanted. It is 7 cm long and 5 cm wide, approximately the size of a clenched fist.

- The inner lining of the uterus is the endometrium, which consists of blood-enriched mucous membranes. The middle layer is the myometrium, which functions to induce contractions and consists of smooth muscle. The outer fascia is mostly peritoneum. The peritoneum partly forms the broad ligament, which helps to anchor the uterus to the pelvic wall and pelvic floor.

- The uterus consists of the cervix, the body, and the isthmus (neck). The most superior portion of the body is the fundus. It is situated in the middle of the pelvis, between the sacrum and the symphysis pubis, and is primarily supported by the pelvic diaphragm, two broad ligaments, two round ligaments, and two uterosacral ligaments.

  - The **broad ligaments** connect the lateral borders of the uterus to the pelvis. The **round ligaments** maintain the uterus in the anteverted position and connect the uterus to the pelvis and labia majora. The **uterosacral ligaments** connect the cervix of the uterus to the pelvis and provide stability for the uterus. The **suspensory** (also known as the infundibulopelvic) ligament connects the ovaries to the pelvis. The suspensory ligament is considered to be a component of the broad ligament (see Figure 2-4).

Breast

The **breast** is both a milk-producing organ and an organ of sexual stimulation. It consists of ductal tissue, glandular lobules, and fatty tissue (see Figure 2-5). The tissues of the breast respond to stimuli from the ovarian hormones estrogen and progesterone and the hormones from other endocrine glands. These responses stimulate milk production in the postpartum period, cause swelling and tenderness during the premenstruum period, and can cause aberrations in growth patterns, such as those seen in some malignancies. The brown, pink, or reddish area surrounding the nipple is the

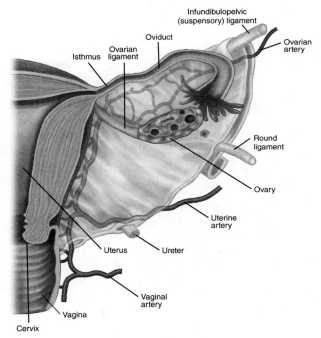

Figure 2-4 Illustration of the uterus and its attachments

areola. The Montgomery glands (or areolar glands) are sebaceous glands that resemble small lumps. Their secretions lubricate the nipple and the areola and thereby prevent cracking
during lactation.

Neuroanatomy

- The endocrine glands are under the influence of the sympathetic, parasympathetic, and central nervous systems. Stimuli
  are mediated through the hypothalamus.

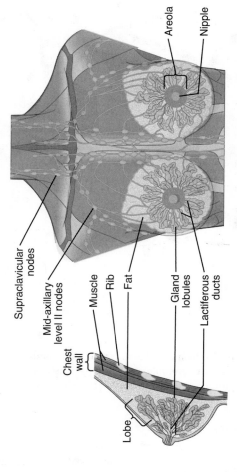

Supraclavicular nodes

Mid-axillary level II nodes

Chest wall

Muscle

Rib

Fat

Gland lobules

Lactiferous ducts

Areola

Nipple

Lobe

Figure 2-5 Anterior and lateral views of the breast

- Vasomotor supply to the hypothalamic area is via the carotid and cavernous plexus from the superior cervical ganglia in front of the second and third cervical vertebrae.
- Endocrine products reach their target areas via blood vessels that are influenced by the vasomotor nerves of the sympathetic nervous system.
- Parasympathetic nerve supply to the uterus is via the inferior mesenteric plexus, with the nerves exiting from the sacral foramen.
- Sympathetic nerve supply to the uterus and ovaries is via the thoracolumbar spine.
- There are no known parasympathetic fibers to the ovaries.
- Sympathetic nerve supply to the breasts is derived from the upper thoracic and midthoracic spines

Arterial and Venous Supply

Ovaries

- Blood supply to the ovaries is derived from the ovarian artery and the ovarian branch of the uterine artery.
- The ovarian artery, ovarian vein, ovarian nerve plexus, and lymphatic vessels are contained in the infundibulopelvic (or suspensory) ligament.
- Venous flow from the left ovarian vein proceeds to the left renal vein. Venous flow from the right ovarian vein proceeds to the right inferior vena cava.

Fallopian Tubes

- Blood supply to the fallopian tubes is via the ovarian and uterine arteries.
- Venous flow from the fallopian tubes proceeds to the ovarian and uterine veins.

Uterus

- Blood supply to the uterus is derived from the ovarian and uterine arteries.

- The uterine artery is derived from the internal iliac artery.
- The uterine venous plexus flows into the uterine vein and subsequently into the internal iliac vein.

Upper Vagina

- The vaginal artery and a branch of the uterine artery supply the upper vaginal vault; the inferior vesicle and middle rectal arteries send branches to the vaginal wall.

Lower Vagina

- The internal pudendal artery supplies the vestibule and the lower vagina.
- Venous return for the upper and lower vagina is via the vaginal plexus and the uterine plexus into the internal iliac vein.

Lymphatics

- The ovaries, fallopian tubes, fundus, and the body of the uterus empty into the preaortic lymph nodes (also known as the deep lumbar nodes).
- The cervix and upper vagina empty into the sacral, hypogastric, and superior iliac glands.
- The vulva and lower vagina empty into the superficial and deep inguinal lymph nodes.

Reproductive Life Cycle

The female reproductive life cycle spans six stages: puberty, menarche, reproductive/childbearing years, perimenopause, menopause, and postmenopause/senescence (see Figure 2-6).

Puberty

- Initiated by gonadotropin-releasing hormone (GNRH) pulses from the hypothalamus, which cause follicle-stimulating hormone (FSH) and luteinizing hormone (LH) from the pituitary to induce secretion of testosterone, which converts to estradiol
- A time of significant physical development and maturation

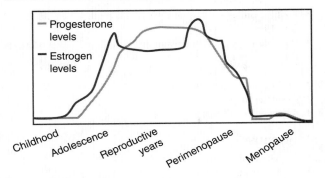

Figure 2-6 Hormones across the life span

Data from CEMCOR Centre for Menstrual Cycle and Ovulation Research. Retrieved from http://www.cemcor.ubc.ca/files/uploads/egg-lessFig1.jpg

- Development of the secondary sexual characteristics, including pubic hair and enlarging breast size
- Onset of menstruation
- Average age: 10 to 15

Menarche
- Onset of menstruation
- Average age: 12 to 13

Childbearing/Reproductive Years
- Influenced by estrogen, progesterone, FSH, LH, prolactin, and human chorionic gonadotrophin
- Average age: 18 to 35

Perimenopause
- Time of transition from the reproductive to the postreproductive years
- Increased variability in the menstrual cycle because the hormonal environment is in transition

- Possible urogenital changes, such as vaginal dryness and menstrual irregularities
- Possible physical changes, such as increased facial hair and thinning scalp hair
- Day 3 FSH of less than 10 mIU/mL
- Longer proliferative phase; estrogen predominant; decline in progesterone levels
- Average age: 35 to 48

Menopause

- Cessation of menses for 12 months
- FSH levels of greater than 40 mIU/mL
- Significant decline in estrogen levels
- Possible urogenital changes: vaginal dryness, vaginal atrophy, and urinary difficulty
- Possible other changes: hot flashes or night sweats, difficulty focusing, decreasing breast size, and other signs of estrogen reduction
- Average age: 51

Postmenopause/Senescence

- Hypoestrogenic endocrine environment
- Health risks: osteoporosis, cardiovascular disease, and cognitive decline
- Average age: typically, 60 and beyond

Menstrual Cycle

The menstrual cycle occurs in four phases:

- Preovulation (proliferative phase)
- Ovulation
- Postovulation (secretory phase)
- Menses

The low levels of estrogen and progesterone that occur during menses trigger the secretions of GNRH from the hypothalamus. GNRH stimulates the anterior pituitary to secrete

FSH, which facilitates the development of the primary follicle in the ovary, estrogen synthesis, and estrogen secretion. Rising levels of estrogen cause the endometrium and breast tissues to proliferate and may contribute to the hypothalamic secretion of GNRH substrates, which facilitate the secretion of LH from the anterior pituitary. The surge of LH is the stimulus for ovulation. The remnant of the follicle, known as the yellow body or the corpus luteum, secretes progesterone and estrogen, which together prepare the endometrial lining for implantation. Progesterone, in particular, causes the endometrium to acquire nutrients that nourish the zygote if implantation occurs (see Figure 2-7).

General Considerations

The length of the menstrual cycle is 22 to 35 days, with most averaging 26 to 28 days.

The duration of the secretory phase is relatively constant, averaging 14 days.

TECHNICAL NOTE

Subtracting 14 days from the length of the menstrual cycle should give an approximate date of ovulation. For example, a woman with a menstrual cycle of 35 days can be expected to ovulate on or around the 21st day; a woman with a menstrual cycle of 23 days can be expected to ovulate on or around the 9th day.

In the absence of fertilization, rising levels of estrogen and progesterone from the corpus luteum have a negative-feedback effect on the anterior pituitary, causing it to "shut off" production of FSH and LH. The result is declining levels of FSH and LH and a subsequent decline in the levels of estrogen and progesterone from the corpus luteum. The blood vessels of the endometrium fail to be nourished; they die and are sloughed off as menstrual blood.

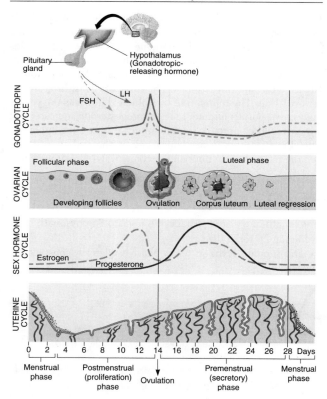

Figure 2-7 Hormone levels during a normal menstrual cycle

If fertilization and subsequent implantation occur, the lining of the uterus changes its morphological structure to become the decidua, which ultimately develops into the placenta. The decidua produces human chorionic gonadotropin (HCG), which nourishes and maintains the corpus luteum. The corpus luteum continues to produce progesterone, which in turn maintains the decidua in a self-propagating cycle. By the 12th week, the placenta has formed and is self-sufficient.

At birth, the ovarian follicles number approximately 600,000. At puberty, that number has declined to approximately 300,000, and by menopause, it has declined to less than 30,000. The presence of large numbers of follicles at the beginning of puberty is essential for normal ovulatory cycles. The full maturation of one dominant follicle depends on the development of the support follicles, which secrete hormones, such as estradiol, inhibin, and androgens, that are necessary for the appropriate functioning of the hypothalamic–pituitary–ovarian–uterine axis.

Summary

- The primary organs involved in the menstrual cycle are the hypothalamus, anterior pituitary, ovaries, and uterus. The hypothalamus produces GNRH, the anterior pituitary produces FSH and LH, and the ovaries produce estrogens and progesterone.
- For most girls, menarche begins at or near age 12, but it can start as early as age 8 and as late as age 16.
- The length of the cycle varies from 22 to 35 days, with an average of 28 days. Cycles occurring at 45-day intervals have been reported.
- Duration of flow varies from 2 to 8 days, with most averaging 4 to 7 days.
- Primary hormones of the first half of the menstrual cycle include FSH from the pituitary gland and estrogen from the ovaries. Primary hormones of the second half of the menstrual cycle include progesterone and estrogen from the ovaries.

TECHNICAL NOTE

The primary ovarian follicles are responsible for the release of the ovum during the normal menstrual cycle while concurrently secreting estrogen and progesterone. During the first half of the cycle, the granulosa cells within the ovarian follicles biosynthesize and secrete estrogen. Following ovulation, the granulosa cells mature to form the corpus luteum, which secretes progesterone and estrogen. Absent fertilization, the corpus luteum continues to enlarge for 10 to 12 days; it then subsequently regresses and ceases to release estrogen and progesterone. Should fertilization occur, the corpus luteum under the influence of HCG continues to grow and secrete its hormones for the first 2 to 3 months of pregnancy; after this, it regresses, and the placenta assumes the role of hormonal biosynthesis.

Breast Development Across the Life Span (see Figure 2-8)

- Fetus: Mammary ridge/milk line develops.
- Newborn: Nipples develop, and development of the duct system is initiated.
- Childhood years: Lobes and mammary glands develop (mammary glands consist of 12 to 24 lobes).
- Puberty: Further development occurs as a result of systemic estrogen. Breasts enlarge as a result of fat accumulation. The duct system develops. The onset of ovulation and menstruation signals the formation of the secretory glands at the ends of the milk ducts. The rate of breast development is highly variable among females.
- Pregnancy: Breasts reach full maturity with pregnancy and lactation.
- Reproductive Years: See "Cyclic Alterations in Breast Tissue."
- Perimenopause: Gradual shrinking of the mammary glands (involution) typically begins around the age of 35.
- Menopause: Estrogen levels decline, connective tissue becomes dehydrated and gradually loses elasticity, glandular tissue declines, and breast tissue shrinks.

Cyclic Alterations in Breast Tissue

The lobules of the breast develop during late puberty and the early reproductive phase and reach full maturity with pregnancy.

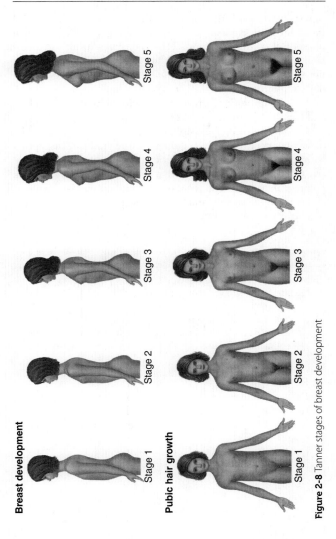

Figure 2-8 Tanner stages of breast development

In response to the normal hormonal fluctuations of the menstrual cycle, breast tissue undergoes mitotic changes in the late luteal phase, followed by apoptosis. These changes result in vulnerability because with each cycle, the cells may deviate from their normal properties, resulting in fibrosis and adenosis with or without symptomatology.

Lobular involution or regression begins around the age of 35 and continues into the postmenopausal phase. During this process, hormone-receptive loose connective tissue is replaced by denser connective tissue, and ductal tissue gradually disappears with aging. Postlactational involution follows weaning; the extensive cell death and remodeling that occur return the breast to its prepregnancy state. The process of involution increases vulnerability to cyst formation and breast cancer; however, completion of lobular involution protects against breast cancer.

CLINICAL PEARL

Physiologic nuances specific to women include the following:
- Gastroparesis—slowed gastric emptying
- Greater immunity against the influenza A virus (the flu) as a result of estrogen's antiviral qualities
- Specific nutritional needs for foods high in vitamins A, B, C, and D; folic acid; calcium; magnesium; and iron because of monthly blood loss

PART TWO

Conditions

Breast Health

Breast conditions are common in women. Estimates are that 90% of women show benign breast tissue changes when examined microscopically. The ultimate goal is to empower women to take control of their breast health by knowing what their breasts look and feel like and to use fundamental health and wellness principles such as diet and exercise to create a healthy environment in the body.

Fibrocystic Breast Changes

Fibrocystic breast changes, including fibrocystic breast disease and cyclic mastalgia, are an exaggeration of the response of breast tissue to changing hormone levels. This is the most common benign condition of the breasts, occurring in as many as half of all American women.

Epidemiology

Fibrocystic breast changes can affect any female during the menstruating years and, in some cases, into menopause. It most commonly occurs in women ages 25 to 40 and affects approximately 50% of women of childbearing age.

Etiology

The cause of fibrocystic breast changes is undetermined. Proposed causes are described in the following subsections.

Focal Tissue Sensitivity

- Focal tissue sensitivity may cause an exaggeration of the normal response of the breasts to fluctuating hormone levels.

Hereditary

- There is some evidence of familial occurrence of fibrocystic breast changes.

Diet

- Dietary modifications have been shown to positively affect some of the symptoms associated with fibrocystic breast changes.

Hormones

- There is some evidence that higher-than-normal estrogen levels alone or in combination with alterations in the ratio of estrogen to progesterone can lead to fibrocystic breast changes.

Alterations in Muscle Tone

- Alterations in muscle tone of the pectoralis and other muscles surrounding and supporting the breast may affect the lymphatic drainage mechanisms in the chest wall. This may result in congestion in the tissues, leading to fibrocystic breast changes.

Postural/Lifestyle Habits

- Rounded shoulders and poor posture are factors that have the potential to interfere with normal lymphatic drainage mechanisms, thereby leading to fibrocystic breast changes.

Signs and Symptoms

- Lumpy breasts
- Breast pain and tenderness
- Swelling of the breast
- One or more soft, moveable lumps in either or both breasts
- Feeling of fullness in the breasts
- Nipple "zingers" or itching
- Breast symptomatology that develops or increases after ovulation and improves following menses
- Breast symptomatology that most commonly occurs in the outer quadrants of the breasts

Diagnosis

Breast Exams

Breast Self-Exams

Women who regularly perform breast self-exams (see Figure 3-1) may note changes in the breasts during the menstrual cycle. The breasts become more lumpy and tender as menses approaches and less lumpy and less tender after menses.

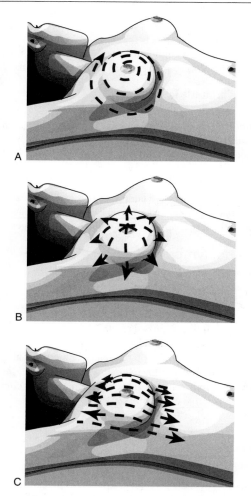

Figure 3-1 Illustration of breast self exam technique. The best time for the breast exam is day 3-5 of the cycle, or on a fixed day every month.

Clinician-administered breast exams may reveal moveable, nonadhered, cyst-like masses with clearly delineated borders.

Needle Biopsy

Fine-needle aspiration of the cyst may be used to both diagnose and treat fibrocystic changes.

Mammography

Mammography may be used to differentially diagnose fibrocystic changes versus changes from breast cancer and other breast disorders.

Tissue Biopsy

Excisional biopsy of breast tissue is used to differentially diagnose fibrocystic changes versus changes from breast cancer and other breast disorders.

Ultrasound

Sonography is used to determine the cystic nature of the lesions.

Magnetic Resonance Imaging

Because magnetic resonance imaging (MRI) elaborates the imaging features of fibrocystic changes, focal mass lesions may be misdiagnosed as malignancy, resulting in false positives.

Management

Conventional

Medications

- Oral contraceptives
- Dopamine agonists (e.g., bromocriptine)
- Synthetic androgens (e.g., danazol)
- Synthetic antiprogestins (e.g., gestrinone)

Procedures

- Needle biopsy and aspiration are procedures that are concurrently diagnostic and curative.

CLINICAL PEARL

Fibrocystic breast changes and *cyclic mastalgia* are terms that are frequently used interchangeably; however, some presentations of fibrocystic breast changes do not involve cyclic pain.

Complementary

Nutraceuticals

- Chasteberry extract
- Eicosapentaenoic acid (EPA) and docosahexaenoic acid (DHA)
- Vitamins B, D, and E
- Magnesium
- Calcium
- Beta-carotene
- Coenzyme Q10 (CoQ10)

TECHNICAL NOTE

Significant statistical evidence validates the use of chasteberry extract (vitex) in cyclic mastalgia. The research evidence for the use of the antioxidants in fibrocystic breast changes is mixed.

Manual Therapy

- Approaches in the comanagement of fibrocystic breast changes include both specific and generalized manipulation of the thoracic and cervicothoracic spine and assessment and management of hypertonicity and trigger points in the muscles of the shoulder and pectoral girdle.

Self-Care and Wellness

- Ensuring good breast support by wearing a well-made, supportive bra to provide symptom relief
- Restricting or eliminating caffeine intake
- Restricting use of alcohol
- Avoiding trans fats and excess salt
- Ensuring several daily servings of fruits and vegetables
- Ensuring diets contains sources of omega-3 fatty acids

- Minimizing exogenous hormones
- Performing monthly breast self-exams
- Exercising, such as adhering to a walking program, being mindful of posture
- Performing pectoralis stretching and strengthening exercises
- Alternating hot and cold packs

Fibroadenoma

Fibroadenoma is a benign, slow-growing tumor of the breast. It is composed of fibrous and glandular tissue.

Epidemiology

- Fibroadenoma occurs in females during their menstruating years and more commonly in younger females age 18 to 30.
- Fibroadenoma is the most common breast tumor seen in adolescent girls.
- Worldwide, fibroadenoma is the most common benign condition of the breast in women under the age of 30.
- Phyllodes tumor is a rare type of large fibroadenoma seen in women over age 40.

Etiology

Etiology is unknown, but proposed causes include the following:

- Increased focal sensitivity to estrogen
- Diets high in consumption of processed fats

Signs and Symptoms

- Round, rubbery, freely movable tumor that is nontender, not attached to the skin, and clearly delineated from the surrounding tissue

41

Diagnosis
- Signs and symptoms
- Needle biopsy
- Mammography
- Ultrasound

Management

Goals of management in the young female include maintaining an acceptable cosmetic outcome, reducing the size of the mass, and preventing growth of the lesion. Once fibroadenoma is confirmed, a wait-and-see approach is appropriate.

Conventional

Medications
- Birth control pills to decrease any associated symptoms

Procedures

Surgical Excision

TECHNICAL NOTE

Criteria for excision of a large mass in an adolescent include the following:
- Diameter greater than 5 cm
- Masses that cause distortion of the breast
- Symptoms associated with breast malignancy

Ultrasound-Guided Vacuum-Assisted Biopsy

Ultrasound-guided vacuum-assisted biopsy is an outpatient procedure that may be used for lesions less than 3 cm in diameter. It requires a local anesthetic. Challenges include the inability to remove the lump completely. Complications include bruising, hematoma, and, rarely, pneumothorax.

CLINICAL PEARL

One-third of excised fibroadenomas recur within 5 years.

Cryoablation (Cryotherapy)

Cryoablation (cryotherapy) is an outpatient procedure that requires a local anesthetic. A cryoprobe is inserted into the core of the lesion, guided by ultrasound. The resulting necrotic tissue shrinks and resolves over a period of up to 12 months. There is a palpable lesion in less than one-third of all patients at 12 months. There is currently no evidence of regeneration of the ablated tissue. Side effects include swelling and ecchymosis.

MRI-Guided Focused Ultrasound

MRI-guided focused ultrasound requires a local anesthetic. In this procedure, focused ultrasound beams tailored to the shape of the lesion are directed into the tissue. High temperatures result in ablation of the tissue. The best results are achieved when the procedure is guided with an MRI. This procedure resolves the lesion in over 75% of cases.

CLINICAL PEARL

Fibroadenomas grow in size during pregnancy.

CLINICAL PEARL

The risk of fibroadenomas becoming malignant is less than 0.5%.

TECHNICAL NOTE

Distinguishing characteristics of large tumors are as follows:

Tumor	Distinguishing Characteristics
Breast abscess	Sudden onset Painful Erythema
Giant lipoma	Soft, moveable, well-defined capsule on ultrasound
Hematoma	Multilobular, sharp margins, heterogeneous echo pattern on ultrasound

(Continues)

Tumor	Distinguishing Characteristics
Fibroadenoma	Slow growth
Giant juvenile fibroadenoma	Adolescent Rapid growth Greater than 5 cm in diameter Associated signs and symptoms that mimic malignancy, including nipple deviation, peau d'orange, vein dilation, and breast distortion and dimpling
Phyllodes tumor	Ages 40–50 Large fibroadenoma

Data from Song, N., Choi, J-Y., Sung, H., Jeon, S., Chung, S., Park, S. K. et al. (2015). Prediction of breast cancer survival using clinical and genetic markers by tumor subtypes. *PLoS ONE, 10*(4): e0122413. doi:10.1371/journal.pone.0122413

Self-Care and Wellness

- Decrease dietary intake of processed fats.
- Perform monthly breast self-exams to watch for any changes in the lump.

Galactorrhea

Galactorrhea is milky discharge from the nipple that is not associated with lactation. It is a symptom, not a disease.

Epidemiology

The actual incidence of galactorrhea is unknown; however, it is estimated that 20% to 25% of women will have an episode of galactorrhea during their lifetime. Galactorrhea most commonly affects women; however, it may affect men and children.

Etiology

- Unknown
- Excessive prolactin secretion
- Pituitary tumors
- Excessive nipple stimulation, such as might occur during exercise and sexual activity

- Pharmaceuticals, including oral contraceptives, antipsychotics, antihypertensives, and antidepressants
- Nutraceuticals, including herbs and nutritional supplements
- Street drugs
- Hypothyroidism
- Kidney disease
- Nerve damage to the chest
- Radiation to the chest

Signs and Symptoms

- Milky discharge from one or both breasts
- Concurrent symptoms:
  - Amenorrhea or oligomenorrhea
  - Headaches or vision problems

Diagnosis

- History and physical exam, including a breast exam
- Hormonal panel to assess levels of prolactin, T4, T3, thyroid-stimulating hormone (TSH) and human chorionic gonadotropin (hCG)
- Cytological assessment of the discharge from the nipple
- Mammography, ultrasound, or MRI of the breast
- MRI of the brain if prolactin levels are significanatly elevated and/or patient has amenorrhea/oligomenorrha with galactorrhea

CLINICAL PEARL

The presence of fat droplets in the nipple discharge confirms galactorrhea.

Stress influences prolactin levels. Blood draw for prolactin should be taken when the patient is in a relaxed state, and not for example, directly following a breast exam.

Management

Conventional

- If treatment is desired, avoid/remove all predisposing factors, including medications.

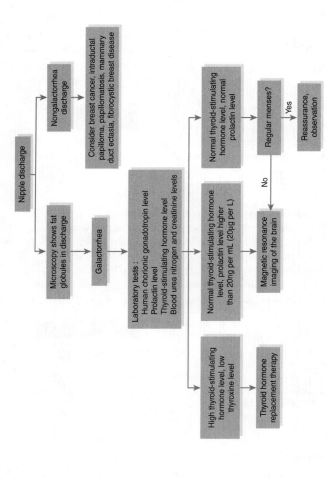

Figure 3-2 Algorithm for evaluation of Galactorrhea

Reproduced from Pena, K., & Rosenfeld, J. (2001). Evaluation and treatment of galactorrhea. *American Family Physician*, 63(9),1763–1771. Retrieved from http://www.aafp.org/afp/2001/0501/p1763.html

- Address all underlying causes, including thyroid and pituitary function.
- Pituitary tumors that don't respond to medication may require surgical excision.

Complementary

- If treatment is desired, avoid/remove all predisposing factors, including nutraceuticals.

Self-Care and Wellness

- Avoid contributing factors, such as nipple friction from running and other forms of exercise.

Breast Cancer

Breast cancer is a malignant neoplasm of the breast. It is classified as in situ if it is limited to the breast and invasive if it has metastasized to the surrounding tissue or a distal site.

> **TECHNICAL NOTE**
>
> Apoptosis, or programmed cell death, is a normal physiological process by which damaged or excessive cells are removed.

> **TECHNICAL NOTE**
>
> Antioxidants prevent oxidative stress. Oxidative stress results in damage to DNA and other molecules. Over time, oxidative stress causes cancer and other diseases.

> **CLINICAL PEARL**
>
> The Breast Cancer Risk Assessment Tool (BCRAT) available on the website of the National Cancer Institute (NCI) provides an estimated risk for women based on factors such as age of menarche, race, and family history of cancer.
>
> The tool may be accessed at http://www.cancer.gov/bcrisktool/.

Epidemiology

Breast cancer affects women of all ages. It is the leading cause of death in women aged 35 to 54 and the second leading cause of cancer death in women of all ages. Currently, one in eight women in the United States will be diagnosed with breast cancer during her lifetime. The majority (75%) of breast cancers occur in women over the age of 50; however, breast cancer has been detected in much younger women.

TECHNICAL NOTE

According to the Centers for Disease Control (CDC), breast cancer has the following characteristics:

- The most common cancer in women, regardless of race or ethnicity
- The most common cause of death from cancer among Hispanic women
- The second most common cause of death from cancer among White, Black, and Asian/Pacific Islander women

Reproduced from Centers for Disease Control and Prevention. (2016). Breast cancer statistics. Retrieved from https://www.cdc.gov/cancer/breast/statistics/index.htm

---

Types of Breast Cancer

There are multiple breast cancer classification systems. Current systems take into consideration such factors as the location of the cancer, the degree of metastasis, the types of receptor cells, genetics, and histopathology.

Histopathology and Location

Ductal carcinoma is the most common of all breast cancers, and ductal carcinoma in situ (DCIS) has the highest cure rate of all the cancers. Ductal carcinoma may be subdivided by growth patterns, such as micropapillary, cribriform, solid, or comedo. The comedo growth pattern is considered the most aggressive.

Ductal carcinoma originates in the epithelial cells lining the ducts. Lobular carcinoma originates in the milk-secreting glands of the breasts.

Breast cancer can also arise from adipose tissue, connective tissue, and the skin.

Receptor Cells

Hormone-receptor-positive cancers, also referred to as estrogen-receptor-positive cancers, are the most common. The majority (~65%) of all estrogen-receptor-positive cancers are also progesterone-receptor-positive cancers. This group is the most amenable to treatment.

Human Epidermal Growth Factor 2 (HER2)

Human epidermal growth factor 2–positive (HER2+) cancers are those with cells producing an overabundance of the HER2 neu protein. This type of cancer is aggressive and fast growing. Five-year survival rates are significantly lower for HER2+ cancers.

Triple Negative

Triple-negative breast cancers are cancers that do not have hormone-receptor-positive cells and do not produce an overabundance of the HER2 neu protein. This group of cancers is frequently associated with genetic factors, such as the BRCA1 and BRCA2 genes.

Genetics

BRCA1 (also known as breast cancer 1, early onset) and BRCA2 (also known as breast cancer 2, early onset) are tumor-suppressor genes that function to prevent abnormal growth and development of cellular tissue. Both BRCA1 and BRCA2 interact with other proteins to repair breaks in damaged DNA resulting from environmental influences, natural causes, iatrogenic causes (e.g., radiation), and the process of cell division. BRCA2 is also thought to have significant involvement in cytokinetic pathways.

BRCA1 regulates the activity of other genes and has a significant influence on embryonic development. BRCA1 mutations have implications for breast cancer, fallopian tube cancer, and pancreatic cancer. BRCA1 mutations change one or more of the amino acids needed for the BRCA1 protein. The resultant protein is unable to repair damaged or mutated DNA. As a result, defects accumulate and divide uncontrollably, forming a tumor. Over 1,000 mutations of BRCA1 have been identified.

Prevalence of *BRCA1* and *BRCA2* Mutations Among U.S. Women with Breast Cancer by Ethnic Group (in alphabetical order)

	BRCA1	**BRCA2**
African-American	1.3%	2.6%
Ashkenazi Jewish	8–10%	1%
Asian-American	0.5%	Data not available
Caucasian (non-Ashkenazi Jewish)	2–3%	2.1%
Hispanic	3.5%	Data not available

Data from Laitman, Y., Simeonov, M., Herskovitz L, et al. (2012). Recurrent germline mutations in BRCA1 and BRCA2 genes in high risk families in Israel. *Breast Cancer Research and Treatment, 133*(3),1153–1157; Malone, K.E., Daling, J.R., Doody, D.R., et al. (2006). Prevalence and predictors of BRCA1 and BRCA2 mutations in a population-based study of breast cancer in white and black American women ages 35 to 64 years. *Cancer Research, 66*(16), 8297–8308; John, E.M., Miron, A., Gong, G., et al. (2007). Prevalence of pathogenic BRCA1 mutation carriers in 5 US racial/ethnic groups. *JAMA, 298*(24), 2869–2876.

BRCA2 mutations allow for the accumulation of defective cells. BRCA2 mutations have implications for ovarian cancer, fallopian tube cancer, melanoma, pancreatic cancer, Fanconi anemia, and breast cancer. Over 800 mutations of BRCA2 have been identified.

Etiology and Risk Factors

- Personal history of breast cancer: Women who have had breast cancer in one breast are more likely to redevelop breast cancer.
- Family history: Of women with breast cancer, 20% have a family history of breast cancer. The primary breast cancer gene is autosomal dominant, with maternal linkage.
- Overweight and obesity: The enzyme aromatase is present in adipose tissue. Common sites for aromatase include the lateral breasts. Aromatase facilitates the conversion of the estrogen derivative estrone to the more potent estradiol. Excessive levels of estradiol may predispose to breast cancer. Postmenopausal breast cancer risk has been shown to increase in women who are overweight or obese.
- Hormonal influences: High or sustained levels of estrogen increase the rate of growth of all cells, including the genetically damaged cells that can cause cancer.

- A long reproductive life (i.e., onset of menarche before age 12 and menopause after age 55) may increase breast cancer risk.
- Nulliparity, not carrying children to term, and delaying pregnancy until after the age of 30 may increase breast cancer risk.
- When used for more than 5 years, hormonal replacement therapy (HRT) may increase breast cancer risk.
- Lifestyle factors such as lack of exercise, poor dietary choices, and excessive consumption of alcohol may increase breast cancer risk.
- Environmental endocrine disruptors may increase breast cancer risk.
- Cultural factors: Caucasian women have the highest risk of breast cancer.
- Mutations of BRCA1 and BRCA2 may increase breast cancer risk.

CLINICAL PEARL

- About 1 in 400 to 1 in 800 U.S. women carry a germ-line mutation for BRCA1 and or BRCA2. Among Ashkenazi jewish women, 1 in 40 have a germ line mutation for BRCA1 and/or BRCA2
- Several other genes have been identified that may also increase breast cancer risk; these include ; *ATM*, *p53*, *CDH1*, *CHEK2*, *PALB2*, *PTEN*, and *STK11*
- Radiation therapy: Repeated chest radiation, as may occur in the management of conditions such as lung cancer, head and neck cancer, and Hodgkin's disease, increases the risk of breast cancer.

CLINICAL PEARL

The younger the age at which radiation treatment was performed, the higher is the lifetime risk of breast cancer
- Medications: Women who used diethylstilbestrol (DES) to prevent a threatened miscarriage and their daughters who were exposed to the drug in utero are at slightly increased risk for breast cancer.

Signs and Symptoms

Often, there are no outward signs of breast cancer. When signs occur, they can include the following:

- A firm, but not rock-hard, mass or lump in one of the breasts, often in the upper or lower outer quadrants, which may have irregular borders and typically is not moveable

- A thickening or "orange-peel" appearance of the breast
- Dilated or aggressive venous patterns on the breast
- A mass in the area of the armpit
- A depression or bulge in the skin of the breast
- Nipple discharge, which often is bloody
- Changes in the nipple, including change in nipple direction, retraction of the nipple, or changes in nipple sensation
- A nonhealing sore on the breast or nipple
- Swelling in the arm or hand
- Back (bone) pain

Diagnosis

- Monthly breast self-examinations and annual expert clinician breast examinations are critical in the early identification of a breast lump.
- Mammography (x-ray of the breast) can be useful in identifying and locating the lump. The procedure involves exposing the breasts to small amounts of radiation. Fine-needle biopsy is used to assess the fluids in the mass.
- Excisional biopsy is used to remove the lump and assess the tissues.
- Laboratory analysis, including complete blood count (CBC) and liver function tests, aids in diagnosis.
- Chest x-ray is performed to rule out other tumors or metastasis.
- Ultrasound can identify masses missed by mammography and differentially diagnose a solid mass versus a fluid-filled mass.
- Pathological review of biopsy, estrogen and progesterone receptor determination, and synthesis-phase (S-phase) determination aid in diagnosis.
- A bone scan should be performed if symptoms suggest bony metastasis, if alkaline phosphatase is elevated, or if widespread disease is suspected.
- Ductal lavage is used to identify cancerous and precancerous cells in the milk ducts of the breast. The procedure involves injecting saline solution into the fluid-producing ducts. The saline solution is suctioned out, along with cells from the

epithelial lining of the ductal system. The fluid is analyzed for normal, atypical, or malignant cells.

- Breast thermography can be used to evaluate the degree of vascular dilation of the breasts. The results are compared with the degree of dilation during lactation, when estrogen levels are elevated. Prolonged exposure to estrogen is a risk factor for breast cancer. The degree of vascular dilation in the breast may provide an assessment of the levels of estrogen in the breast.
  - There is evidence to suggest that the breasts can hold 10 to 50 times more estrogen than the amount identified in a typical blood test. Excess estrogen stimulates breast tissue and dilates blood vessels. Dilated blood vessels are more visible on thermograms than nondilated vessels because they have more blood and heat flowing through them.
- MRI has a higher sensitivity in detection of DCIS and is a preferred method for assessment in women with breast implants. MRI and mammography together have high efficacy in detecting breast cancer lesions in younger women, who typically have more dense breasts.

CLINICAL PEARL

The ductal lavage procedure is suitable for determining preventive therapy in high-risk groups. Factors that affect the accurate cellular analysis of the ductal fluids include medication therapy, chemotherapy, advanced age, prior surgery, prior radiation, and nipple anatomy.

TECHNICAL NOTE

The American Cancer Society recommends a baseline mammogram performed between the ages of 35 and 40 and yearly mammography for all women of age 40 and older.

Data from American Cancer Society. (2015). American Cancer Society recommendations for early breast cancer detection in women without breast symptoms. Retrieved from http://www.cancer.org/cancer/breastcancer/moreinformation /breastcancerearlydetection/breast-cancer-early-detection-acs-recs

The NCI recommends mammogram screening every 1 to 2 years for all women of age 40 and older and sooner for women with a family history of breast cancer; annual mammograms are recommended beginning 10 years earlier than the age at which the relative was diagnosed.

TECHNICAL NOTE

The S phase is the cell cycle during which DNA synthesis occurs. A high S phase is indicative of increased risk of relapse and a poor survival rate.

TECHNICAL NOTE

Breast cancer is the most common cancer in women worldwide and the second leading cause of cancer death in women of all ages. According to the World Health Organization (2014), more than 500,000 women worldwide die of breast cancer. Although breast cancer is thought to be a disease of the developed world, almost 50% of breast cancer cases and 58% of deaths occur in less developed countries.

TECHNICAL NOTE

According to the NCI, the risk of breast cancer for different age categories is as follows:

Age	Risk
30	1 in 227
40	1 in 68
50	1 in 42
60	1 in 28
70	1 in 26
Lifetime	1 in 8

Data from National Cancer Institute. (2012). *Breast cancer risk in American women*. Retrieved from http://www.cancer.gov/cancertopics/types/breast/risk-fact-sheet

CLINICAL PEARL

Mammography remains an effective tool for the early detection of breast cancer in females over the age of 50. In younger females, there is an increased likelihood of false positives because of the increased density of the breast tissue. Thermography, MRI, ultrasound, and ductal lavage may be better screening tools. Breast self-exam continues to be an effective screening tool for women who may find a breast mass before their annual mammogram.

CLINICAL PEARL

A family history of breast or ovarian cancer may not be clinically evident through genetic testing because many women inherit the BRCA mutations from their fathers, not their mothers.

Management

Conventional

Management of breast cancer depends on the type and severity of the breast cancer and can include one or more of the following:

- Lumpectomy
- Mastectomy
- Lymph node resection
- Chemotherapy
- Radiation

In addition, breast cancer management is dependent on the patient's personal and familial history, risk factors, the appearance of the cancer, estrogen and progesterone receptor protein status, HER2 status, and the presence or absence of genes known to cause breast cancer (NCI, 2012).

Mastectomy

The various forms of mastectomy are all performed under general anesthesia and include the following:

- Subcutaneous mastectomy, which involves the removal of the entire breast with the exception of the nipple and areola

- Simple mastectomy, which involves removal of the entire breast, including the nipple and areola, while leaving the axillary or central lymph nodes (those in the armpit and under the arm) intact
- Modified radical mastectomy, which involves removal of the entire breast, including the nipple and areola, and an axillary dissection, which involves removal of the majority of the lymph nodes in the area
- Radical mastectomy, which involves removal of the entire breast and the major muscles of the chest wall (Note: This is an outdated procedure but is nevertheless occasionally performed.)

Lumpectomy

A lumpectomy is performed under local anesthesia, with or without sedatives. An incision is made, and the lump and immediate surrounding tissue are removed and evaluated.

CLINICAL PEARL

Risks associated with lumpectomy include loss of sensation and changes in the size and shape of the breast.

Radiation Therapy

Radiation therapy is directed at the tumor, the breast, the chest wall, or other tissues known or suspected to have residual cancer cells. Where both chemotherapy and radiation therapy are required, chemotherapy will typically precede the radiation therapy. External beam radiation is most common in breast cancer management and is administered every day for 5 days and repeated for up to 6 weeks.

Internal radiation, or brachytherapy, is less common and less effective in breast cancer management. In this procedure, radioactive pellets are inserted around the known cancerous tissue and left in place for a brief period. Treatment occurs twice a day for 5 days.

Chemotherapy

Chemotherapy may be used to help eliminate the remaining cancer cells in the breast or other parts of the body. The drugs used in chemotherapy are administered over several months, may be given orally or intravenously, and are typically dosed cyclically to allow for rest/recovery periods.

Hormone Therapy

Hormone therapies are used as both adjuvant and neoadjuvant therapies in hormone-receptor-positive cancers. Categories include the selective estrogen receptor modulators (SERMs), such as tamoxifen; the antiestrogens, such as Faslodex; the aromatase inhibitors, such as letrozole (Femara); and the luteinizing hormone (LH)–releasing analogs, such as goserelin acetate (Zoladex).

CLINICAL PEARL

SERMs may be antagonistic to estrogen receptor activity in some tissues and simultaneously agonistic in other areas. In postmenopausal women, for example, tamoxifen is antagonistic to estrogen receptor activity in breast tissue and agonist in bone tissue. This means that it simultaneously exhibits properties that both prevent breast cancer and protect bone density. In premenopausal women, however, tamoxifen causes some bone thinning.

Targeted Therapy

Targeted therapy involves treatment with drugs that specifically target the genes in the cells that cause breast cancer. Examples include Herceptin (trastuzumab) and Tykerb (lapatinib), which are used to target HER2 neu protein, which promotes the growth of some cancer cells. These drugs are administered orally or intravenously.

Bone-Directed Therapy

Bone-directed therapies are drugs targeted to manage the consequences of metastasis to bone. These intravenously applied bisphosphonates are purported to strengthen the boney matrices, thereby limiting fracture risk. In addition, drugs such as denosumab may be injected under the skin and are currently being used for patients with osteoporosis caused by early-onset menopause induced by the use of aromatase inhibitors.

Treatment for breast cancer is based on how it is staged (see Table 3-1). The American Joint Commission on Cancer stages breast cancer based on tumor size and nature (T factor), degree of lymph node involvement (N factor), distant metastasis (M factor), and histological/pathological review (P factor). A grading of stage 1, for example, implies that there is a tumor less than 1 cm but greater than 5 mm in diameter; there is some metastasis to the axillary lymph nodes, but there is no distant metastasis.

For more on staging of breast cancer see the Appendix.

Table 3-1 Summary of Treatment Considerations in Breast Cancer

Stage	Treatment Considerations
0	Should treatment be recommended, treatment considerations include lumpectomy or mastectomy with radiation.
1	Lumpectomy and radiation or mastectomy with sentinel and other lymph node removal; chemotherapy, hormone therapy, or both may be recommended following surgery.
2	Lumpectomy and radiation or mastectomy; axillary lymph node dissection (including sentinel node removal); chemotherapy, hormone therapy, or both may be recommended following surgery.
3	Mastectomy, chemotherapy, radiation, hormonal therapy, or some combination may be recommended.
4	Mastectomy, chemotherapy, radiation, hormonal therapy, or some combination may be recommended.

Data from American Cancer Society (2017). *Breast cancer treatment*. Retrieved from https://www.cancer.org/cancer/breast-cancer/treatment.html.

CLINICAL PEARL

According to the NCI (2012), the age of the patient should not be a factor in the selection of breast-conserving treatment versus mastectomy. Treatment with lumpectomy and radiation therapy in women 65 years and older produces rates of survival and freedom from recurrence similar to those of women younger than 65 years of age.

Complementary

Nutraceuticals

- CoQ10
  - Action: CoQ10 is an antioxidant that protects the heart from chemotherapy-induced damage. Low blood levels of CoQ10 have been observed in patients with cancer.
  - Evidence: Multiple studies support CoQ10's cardioprotective effects. There are currently no randomized controlled trials that support CoQ10 as a cancer treatment.
- High-dose vitamin C
  - Action: Vitamin C is an essential nutrient and a cofactor for enzymes, and it is needed for collagen synthesis. It has been shown to improve quality of life in cancer patients, reduce side effects of treatment, decrease cell proliferation in many cancers, and increase radiosensitivity, thereby enhancing radiation therapy. High-dose intravenous vitamin C is well tolerated by patients.
  - Evidence: Multiple studies support the use of vitamin C in cancer treatment. Vitamin C has been shown to improve mortality in patients with breast cancer.
- Omega-3 fatty acids
  - Action: Omega-3 fatty acids dampen inflammation and proliferation in different tissues.
  - Evidence: Multiple lab studies consistently support the efficacy of omega-3 fatty acids in modulating tissue inflammation and proliferation. Results from population-based data remain mixed.
- Calcium D-glucarate
  - Action: Calcium D-glucarate suppresses cell proliferation and inflammation and induces apoptosis. D-glucarate, once converted to D-glucaro-14-lactone, inhibits beta glucuronidase. (Elevated beta glucuronidase activity has been noted in breast and other cancers.)
  - Evidence: No published human research studies have demonstrated the effectiveness of calcium D-glucarate for preventing or treating breast cancer.

- Vitamin E
  - Action: Vitamin E is an antioxidant that protects from free-radical damage.
  - Evidence: Multiple laboratory studies affirm the anticancer properties of vitamin E. Results from population-based data are mixed.
- Vitamin A
  - Action: Vitamin A is an antioxidant that protects from free-radical damage.
  - Evidence: Multiple laboratory studies affirm the anticancer properties of vitamin A. Results from population-based data are mixed.
- Folate (5-methyltetrahydrofolate)
  - Action: Folate is a donor of one-carbon units and is essential for DNA methylation (facilitates the remethylation of homocysteine to methionine), synthesis, and repair.
  - Evidence: Multiple studies have identified folate deficiencies in populations. Results from studies on the effectiveness of folate for preventing or treating breast cancer are inconsistent.
- Vitamin B_6
  - Action: Vitamin B_6 protects from free-radical damage.
  - Evidence: Lab studies support the anticancer effects of vitamin B_6. Data from observational studies and randomized controlled trials are mixed.
- Vitamin D
  - Action: Nuclear vitamin D receptor is thought to modify mammary epithelium. Vitamin D deficiency is observed in breast cancer patients, and low levels of vitamin D increase breast cancer risk.
  - Evidence: Experimental studies suggest protective effects on estrogen-receptor-positive tumors. Results from population-based data are mixed.
- Selenium
  - Action: Selenium is a trace mineral found in the enzyme glutathione peroxidase. Selenium acts as an antioxidant and may lower cancer risk. Selenium has been shown to slow the growth and spread of cancer cells in lab studies.

- Evidence: Multiple population studies and clinical trials have been conducted, with mixed results.

Acupuncture

Acupuncture has demonstrated value in the mitigation of symptoms related to breast cancer treatment, such as fatigue, emesis, bone pain, hot flashes, and depression. Acupuncture may be contraindicated or require special cautions in areas of spinal instability, in areas where there is a significant risk of infection, in patients with coagulopathies, and in patients with extreme needle phobia. Treatment protocols are based on patterns observed with each patient visit.

Herbs

Recommendations for herbs are based on the patient's presentation at each visit and may vary with each consultation, as may the presentation and preparation of the herbs.

Manual Therapies

Manual therapies, including mobilization and passive and active range-of-motion exercises, are employed when upper limb problems follow breast cancer treatment. The best timing for these interventions remains controversial because some patients experience a delay in wound healing with added interventions, whereas others experience increased range of motion in the upper limb when active interventions are employed early.

Massage

In women with breast cancer, massage therapy is shown to help to decrease stress and anxiety, mitigate some depressive symptoms, help with fatigue, and improve quality of life.

Naturopathy

Common naturopathic approaches to breast cancer prevention and management include dietary counseling and supplements, including botanical medicines, antioxidants, vitamins, minerals, amino acids, and proteolytic enzymes.

Self-Care and Wellness

- Maintaining recommended body weight
- Exercising for a minimum of 30 minutes most days of the week (e.g., a daily walking program)
- Breastfeeding
- Having children before age 30
- Avoiding known endocrine disruptors
- Reducing alcohol consumption
- Consuming a diet rich in cruciferous vegetables and other sources of indole 3 carbinol (I3C), thought to influence pathways involved in DNA repair and hormone regulation
  - I3C modulates estrogen metabolism by inhibiting estrogen alpha-receptor activity, inducing phase 1 and phase 2 enzymes, and enhancing 2-OH estrogen. Studies suggest that this may have protective effects for breast cancer. Sources of indole 3-carbinol include the cruciferous vegetables—broccoli, kale, cauliflower, cabbage, brussel sprouts, collard greens, and bok choy.
- Consuming phytoestrogens, such as soy and red clover, which may promote overall hormonal health
  - Note: The effects of ingesting soy vary among individuals. Some individuals experience endocrine-disruptive symptoms following the ingestion of soy. Red clover has been used to stabilize hormonal fluctuations.
- Consuming lignans
  - Diets overloaded with refined foods are often deficient in lignans. Studies demonstrate that women with blood levels of enterolactone above 34 nmol/L had a marked reduction in risk for breast cancers. Once ingested, lignans are converted by the intestinal microflora to enterolactone and enterodiol, which are mammalian lignans.
- Drinking green tea
  - Green tea catechins function in some cancers as a histone deacetylase (HDAC) inhibitor. Epigallocatechin gallate (EGCG), the most abundant catechin in tea, is an androgen antagonist. Preliminary studies affirm the effects of green tea in lowering cancer risk in some high-risk patients.

- Engaging in yoga, meditation, and music therapy, which have demonstrated benefits in reducing stress, reducing anxiety, managing depression, easing fatigue, and improving quality of life

TECHNICAL NOTE

Catechins (antioxidants that protect cells from damage caused by free radicals) make up most of the polyphenols in green tea. Polyphenols are plant chemicals that include catechins.

Histone deacetylase (HDAC) is an enzyme that removes an acetyl group from histones, thereby altering the way the histones bind to DNA. HDAC is found in large quantities in cancer cells.

- Consuming lycopene (found in tomatoes, red peppers, apricots, guava, and watermelon), which has been shown to demethylate DNA in laboratory studies. This suggests that it may have value in mitigating tumorigenic processes. However, results from clinical trials are mixed.
- Modifying exposure to xenoestrogens and exogenous estrogens by eating meats, poultry, and dairy products from nonhormonally fattened livestock, eating organic vegetables, and minimizing the use of high-estrogen hormone replacement therapy

Screening

- Breast self-examinations performed monthly
- Clinician-performed breast exams yearly after age 20

CLINICAL PEARL

According to the NCI (2012), the three most common cancers among women are breast cancer, lung cancer, and colorectal cancer.

Breast cancer is first among women of all races and those of Hispanic origin, and it is the leading cause of death among Hispanic women and the second leading cause of death among White, Black, and Asian/Pacific Islander women (in these groups, and in American Indian/Alaska Native women, lung cancer is first).

Data from Centers for Disease Control and Prevention. (2016). Cancer among women. Retrieved from http://www.cdc.gov/cancer/dcpc/data/women.htm

> **CLINICAL PEARL**
>
> Breast cancer survival rates vary greatly worldwide. The lower survival rates observed in less developed countries is thought to reflect a higher proportion of women presenting with late-stage disease (World Health Organization, 2014).

Prognosis (see Table 3-2)

> **CLINICAL PEARL**
>
> The axillary lymph nodes are the main passageways that breast cancer cells use to reach the rest of the body. Their involvement at any time strongly affects the prognosis.

Prophylactic mastectomy is a choice for women who are at very high risk for breast cancer. Possible candidates for this procedure include women who have removed or will need to have one breast removed because of cancer; women with a strong personal or family history of breast cancer; women who have a mutation in gene p53, BRCA1, or BRCA2; and women who underwent radiation treatment to the chest at an early age. Prophylactic oophorectomy has been shown to significantly lower the risk of breast cancer in women with BRCA2 mutations.

Table 3-2 Breast Cancer Prognosis

Stage at First Diagnosis	5-Year Relative Survival Rate
0	100%
I	100%
II	93%
III	72%
IV	22%

Data from American Cancer Society. (2016). Breast cancer survival rates, by stage. Retrieved from http://www.cancer.org/cancer/breastcancer/detailedguide/breast-cancer-survival-by-stage

CLINICAL PEARL

Late and long-term effects of radiation therapy for breast cancer include the following:
- Changes in the look and feel of the breasts
- Lymphedema
- Pain at the site of the radiation

Late and long-term effects of chemotherapy for breast cancer include the following:
- Infertility/early menopause
- Weight changes (gain/loss)
- Fatigue
- Cognitive changes (chemo-brain)

Late and long-term effects of hormonal therapies for breast cancer include the following:
- Hot flashes
- Vaginal discharge
- Irritation and dryness
- Decreased libido
- Mood swings

Treatment with aromatase inhibitors may cause the following:
- Joint pain
- Muscle pain
- Increased risk of osteoporosis

Late and long-term effects of targeted therapies for breast cancer include the following:
- Fatigue
- Mouth sores
- Bleeding
- High blood pressure
- Diarrhea
- Skin changes
- Blood clots
- Changes in bowel function (constipation/diarrhea)

Side Effects of Breast Cancer Treatment and Management Strategies

The most common side effects of all breast cancer treatments are fatigue, lymphedema, infertility/early menopause, and weight changes.

Fatigue

The type of fatigue experienced by women going through breast cancer treatment may last for weeks to months following completion of treatment and is rarely relieved by rest. At some point, 90% of all women going through breast cancer treatment report some type of fatigue or a feeling of being overwhelmed.

Management

Self-Care and Wellness

- Daily exercise
- Stress management
- Dietary changes: consuming an abundance of fruits and vegetables, remaining well hydrated, and limiting sugars
- Complementary therapies that have been shown to reduce stress and, in turn, reduce fatigue, such as acupuncture, meditation, massage, tai chi, and yoga

Weight Gain

Management

Recommendations are to wait until treatments are completed before addressing weight gain.

Self-Care and Wellness

- Dietary changes: consuming an abundance of fruits and vegetables, remaining well hydrated, and limiting sugars
- Management of fluid retention with a low salt diet, diuretics, use of compression stockings, and avoidance of standing for long periods of time

Menopause and Infertility in Women Desiring Children

For most women, hormonal treatments are not an option. Women desiring children may be counseled to store embryos or freeze unfertilized eggs prior to chemotherapy. For further information, see the chapters on premature ovarian failure (POF) and menopause.

Lymphedema

Lymphedema is swelling of the arm resulting from an accumulation of lymph fluid in the soft tissues of the arm.

Epidemiology

Between 5% and 25% of women develop lymphedema following treatment for breast cancer, including lumpectomy, mastectomy, lymph node dissection, radiation, and chemotherapy.

Etiology

Breast cancer treatment frequently involves removal of a portion of the axillary and surrounding lymph nodes and channels, thereby compromising the lymphatic system. In addition, the compromised immune state following many breast cancer treatments increases the risk of infection. Infection increases blood flow and hence lymphatic flow to the arm.

Risk Factors

- Smoking
- History of diabetes
- Obesity
- Previous surgeries to the arm
- Increase weight gain
- Trauma to the arm
- Heat

Signs and Symptoms

- Swelling of the arm
- Fatigue of the arm
- Sense of heaviness in the arm
- Fluid backup into the surrounding tissues

  Symptoms may last from days to months.

Diagnosis

- History and exam

Management

Conventional

Medications

- Diuretics
- Antibiotics if infection or cellulitis is suspected

Physical Therapy

Physical therapy includes complex decongestive physiotherapy followed by compression bandages. This highly skilled technique involves gentle, stimulating, circular massage of the skin and lymphatic channels in the direction of the shoulder several times a week for several weeks.

Self-Care and Wellness

- Diligent skin care
- Resting of the arm in an elevated position
- Avoidance of the following:
  - Excessive heat to the arm (hot packs, hot weather, hot tubs, hot showers)
  - Use of the affected arm to carry heavy objects, including shoulder bags
  - Clothing that restricts the movement of the arm
  - Blood pressure testing on the affected arm
  - Alcohol use
  - Smoking
- Early treatment of any infection
- Exercise
  - Swimming
  - Mild to moderate range-of-motion exercises with customized bandaging
- Therapeutic aids
  - Compression sleeves
  - Compression bandages
  - Pneumatic pumps
  - Sequential gradient pumps

CLINICAL PEARL

Marriott, Masino, and Casella (2014) recommend the following tips for nurses and others providing support for breast cancer patients:

Support for breast cancer screening

- Encourage breast cancer screening.
- Explain available resources to women who don't have insurance. Many local and national organizations provide programs for women in various at-risk categories. Examples include the Sage Clinics and the CDC-funded National Breast and Cervical Cancer Early Detection Program (NBCCEDP).

Supporting patients during cancer staging workup

- Provide emotional support.
- Help patients get timely medical appointments to promote treatment planning.
- Assist patients in connecting with information resources, such as oncology nurse navigators.
- Help patients identify their concerns and develop a list of questions to ask their physicians.
- Explain how second opinions are obtained.
- Provide education on the various aspects of developing a treatment plan.
- Identify patients who may be at increased risk for genetic or familial-related breast cancers, and encourage them to consult a genetics professional.
- Encourage patients to connect with an accredited breast center.
- Encourage patients to consider clinical trials when choosing treatment.

Supporting patients during treatment

- Network with the treating physician's office to ensure timely communication about any treatment-related side effects the patient may be experiencing.
- Urge patients to communicate their concerns so they can receive appropriate management. Assist patients in understanding the process and it participants. (Treatment may occur over an extended time, with several clinicians involved in the care—these can include the treating physician, oncology nurse, physical or occupational therapist, dietitian, social worker, psychologist, and case manager.)

Supporting patients after treatment

- Coordinate posttreatment care to help ensure the patient's ongoing health and rehabilitation needs are addressed, including the following:
  - Referral to a lymphedema-trained physical therapist
  - Bone-density screening/education on bone health
  - Education on managing side effects, such as hot flashes and sleep problems
  - Screening for long-term psychological problems related to body image and sexuality
  - Referral to patient-oriented websites(see the Appendix)

Modified from Marriott, M., Masino, K., & Casella, G. (2014). CNE: Breast cancer care gets personal. *American Nurse Today, 9*(10).

Mastalgia

Mastalgia is breast pain in women that may be mild, moderate, or severe. It may be cyclical, intermittent, or constant and most commonly occurs during the reproductive phase.

CLINICAL PEARL

Synonymous terms for *mastalgia* include *mastodynia* and *mammalgia*.

Epidemiology

Most women who experience mastalgia are in their 20s, 30s, and 40s; however, mastalgia sometimes does occur in the menopausal and postmenopausal phases. An estimated 40% to 70% of all women experience some form of mastalgia.

Etiology

- Unknown
- Female reproductive hormones
- Prostaglandin imbalances, such as an overabundance of the inflammatory prostaglandins
- Medications, including contraceptives, hormonal replacement therapies, and selective serotonin reuptake inhibitors (SSRIs)

- Breast morphology, including cysts, size, and possible scar tissue
- Referred pain from trigger points in the chest and surrounding muscles

Signs and Symptoms
- Breast pain that has following characteristics:
  - Cyclical, intermittent or constant
  - Mild, moderate, or severe
  - Localized or diffuse
  - Bilateral or unilateral

Diagnosis
- Clinician-performed breast exam
- Ultrasound or mammography
- Biopsy if lumps or cysts are noted

Management
Conventional
Medications
- Assessment and adjustment of hormonal medications, especially contraceptives and hormonal replacement therapies
- Symptom-specific medications, including bromocriptine, danazol, nonsteroidal anti-inflammatory drugs (NSAIDs), and tamoxifen

Complementary
- Nutraceuticals, including the following:
  - Evening primrose oil
  - Borage oil
  - Vitamin E
  - EPA/DHA
  - Chasteberry

TECHNICAL NOTE

✗ Cyclic mastalgia worsens as menses approaches and improves following the onset of menses, most commonly affects both breasts, and is frequently accompanied by breast swelling and lumps.

✗ Noncyclic mastalgia appears to be unrelated to the menstrual cycle. It most commonly affects one breast and more commonly affects menopausal women.

Self-Care and Wellness

- Wear a well-fitting bra.
- Adapt exercises to stretch and strengthen the shoulder girdle.

Cardiovascular and Pulmonary Health in Women

Cardiovascular diseases include those diseases affecting the cardiovascular system, primarily cardiac disease, peripheral arterial disease varicosities, and vascular diseases of the kidney and brain. The causes of cardiovascular disease are diverse, but atherosclerosis and hypertension are the most common. Also, aging brings a number of physiological and morphological changes that alter cardiovascular function and lead to increased risk of cardiovascular disease, even in healthy, asymptomatic individuals. The most common cardiovascular diseases seen in women are arrhythmias, hypertension, heart attack, varicose veins, and stroke.

CLINICAL PEARL

- Heart disease is the number one cause of death worldwide,
- Approximately 20% of the U.S. population will experience a cardiovascular event, regardless of their efforts to comply with all preventative measures.
- Close to 80% of strokes and heart attacks could be prevented through lifestyle factors, such as diet and exercise, and with medications.

Arrhythmias

Arrhythmias are abnormal rhythms of the heart caused by problems with the heart's electrical system and can reflect either tachycardia or bradycardia. Arrhythmias have the following characteristics:

- Occur in the atria or the ventricles
- Occur at any age
- May be life threatening and cause a stroke or sudden cardiac arrest
- Lack of blood flow that impedes blood flow to vital organs, resulting in damage to the brain, heart, or other organs

Common forms include supraventricular arrhythmia, ventricular arrhythmia, and bradyarrhythmia.

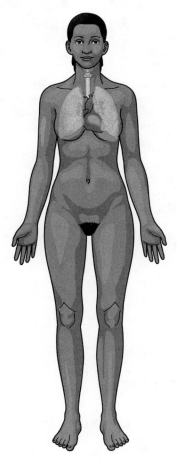

Figure 4-1 Normal cardiopulmonary anatomy/physiology

> **CLINICAL PEARL**
>
> The most common arrhythmia in adults is atrial fibrillation, which is a supraventricular arrhythmia.

Epidemiology

Arrhythmias are more common in women approaching menopause and in any individual whose heart has been compromised by earlier illnesses or as a result of a valvular disorder or an abnormality in the structure of a heart vessel, such as the aorta.

Signs and Symptoms

Often, there are no signs, but signs and symptoms include the following:

- Anxiety
- Weakness
- Dizziness/light-headedness/fainting
- Sweating
- Shortness of breath/chest pain

Diagnosis

- Electrocardiogram
- Holter monitor
- Event monitor
- Stress test
- Echocardiogram
- Cardiac catheterization
- Electrophysiology study (EPS)
- Head-up tilt-table test

Management

Sometimes, no treatment is needed.

Conventional Therapies

Medications

Treatment is recommended when activities of daily living (ADLs) are compromised, symptoms increase in frequency and severity, and there is concern for progression to a more serious and potentially lethal arrhythmia.

Conventional therapies include the following:

- Antiarrhythmic medications
  - Amiodarone (Cordarone)
  - Flecainide (Tambocor)
  - Procainamide (Procanbid)
  - Sotalol (Betapace)

In addition, other types of drugs can be used to treat arrhythmias, including the following:

- Beta blockers, such as metoprolol or Toprol XL, which reduce the heart's workload and the heart rate
- Calcium channel blockers, such as verapamil or Calan, which also reduce the heart rate
- Blood-thinning medications
  - Coumadin
  - Pradaxa
  - Xarelto
  - Eliquis
  - Lovenox
  - Fragmin
  - Lupirudin

Procedures

- Cardioversion
- Catheter ablation
- Pacemaker
- Implantable cardioverter defibrillator
- Maze procedure
- Coronary bypass surgery

Complementary

- Acupuncture has been shown to reduce heart rates in certain arrhythmias.

Self-Care and Wellness

- A heart-healthy diet with moderate intake of caffeine drinks
- Regular exercise
- Avoidance of cigarette smoke
- Limited intake of alcohol
- Maintenance of a healthy weight
- Vagal maneuvers, including holding the breath and straining, dunking the face in ice water, or coughing
- Stress reduction through yoga, meditation, and relaxation techniques
- Religious and spiritual practices

CLINICAL PEARL

There is emerging evidence that omega-3 fatty acids may be helpful in preventing and treating some arrhythmias.

CLINICAL PEARL

Palpitations are the most common arrhythmia and typically do not need treatment.

Hypertension (High Blood Pressure)

High blood pressure arises from the heart pumping blood into arteries narrowed by atherosclerosis. Untreated hypertension can lead to heart disease, kidney problems, stroke, diabetes, and other medical conditions. The two main types of hypertension are essential hypertension, which has no known cause and accounts for 95% of all cases, and secondary hypertension, in which there is a known cause, such as kidney abnormalities or narrowing of the arteries.

Epidemiology

Hypertension is more common in women over the age of 65; however, anyone can develop hypertension. High-risk populations include Africans, African Americans, smokers, people who

Table 4-1 Table on Normal Ranges for BP and pre-Htn–htn and htn in Diabetics

Blood Pressure Calculation	Systolic Blood Pressure (SBP), mm Hg	Diastolic Blood Pressure (DBP), mm Hg
Normal	<120	and <80
Prehypertension	120–139	or 80–89
Stage 1 hypertension	140–159	or 90–99
Stage 2 hypertension	≥160	or ≥100

Reproduced from Chobanian, A.V., Bakris, G.L., Black, H.R., Cushman, W.C., Green, L.A., Izzo, J.L. Jr., et al. (2003). Seventh report of the Joint National Committee on Prevention, Detection, Evaluation, and Treatment of High Blood Pressure. *Hypertension, 42*(6):1206–52.

are overweight, people who overuse alcohol, and individuals with a family history of high blood pressure.

Etiology

- Hereditary/family history
- Advancing age, which causes decreased flexibility in the arteries (Rates of hypertension increase exponentially in women over age 65.)
- Noncompliance with taking medications in right amount and on schedule and with other physician orders such as low salt intake and regular exercise
- Lack of physical activity
- High salt intake
- Excessive use of alcohol
- Hormone replacement therapy, birth control pills, and pregnancy/preeclampsia
- Stress
- Sleep apnea
- Both tobacco use and secondary smoke

Signs and Symptoms

Approximately one-third of all individuals with hypertension have no symptoms, but sign and symptoms include the following:

- Blurred vision and other vision anomalies
- Shortness of breath

- Chest pain
- Headache, moderate to severe
- Persistent fatigue
- Irregularities in heartbeat
- Hematuria
- Pounding in the ears, chest, or neck

Diagnosis

- Medical history that includes a family history of hypertension
- Two or more blood pressures greater than 130/90 taken 2 minutes apart
- 12-lead EKG
- Urinalysis
- Blood analysis, including fasting blood glucose, hematocrit, serum sodium, potassium, creatinine, calcium, and lipid profile

Management

Conventional

Medications

Medications include thiazides and other diuretics, beta blockers, angiotensin-converting enzyme (ACE) inhibitors, calcium channel blockers, angiotensin receptor blockers, and combinations of these drugs. Only one of these drugs may be prescribed at a time, but they often are ordered in combination. Many of these drugs should not be abruptly discontinued.

Complementary

- Relaxation and stress management techniques, such as biofeedback and massage
- Nutraceuticals (see the Technical Note)
- Acupuncture
- Manipulation—specifically, the National Upper Cervical Chiropractic Association (NUCCA) manipulation technique (see the Technical Note)

Self-Care and Wellness

- Patient and family education
- Lifestyle modifications, such as weight loss, limiting use of sodium and alcohol, exercising for at least 30 minutes daily, avoiding tobacco, and relaxation and stress management
- Risk assessment
- Management of blood pressure

  Note: The American Heart Association, in 2016, set the new normal for blood pressure at under 120/80.

- Relaxation and stress management techniques, such as tai chi, yoga, and hypnotherapy

TECHNICAL NOTE

In a pilot study, restoration of atlas alignment using the NUCCA technique was associated with marked and sustained reductions in blood pressure similar to the use of two-drug combination therapy. Randomized controlled trials are under way.

TECHNICAL NOTE

Studies are under way to elucidate the effects of numerous nutraceuticals on high blood pressure, including potassium, L-arginine, vitamin C, cocoa flavonoids, beetroot juice, coenzyme Q10, controlled-release melatonin, and aged garlic extract. The risk–benefit ratio and effects of long-term use are undetermined.

CLINICAL PEARL

The Mediterranean diet and the dietary approaches to stop hypertension (DASH) diet have demonstrated efficacy in reducing hypertension.

Myocardial Infarction (MI)/Heart Attack

A heart attack is a consequence of atherosclerotic narrowing of the arteries that limits oxygen supply to the heart, resulting in heart muscle damage or death.

Epidemiology

- Women over the age of 55 (and men over the age of 45)

Etiology

- Smoking and long-term exposure to secondhand smoke
- High blood pressure, which accelerates atherosclerosis
- Hypercholesterolemia
  - This includes low density lipoprotein (LDL) levels higher than 100 mg/dl and high-denisty lipoprotein levels (HDLs) less than 40 mb/dl and cholesterol over 200. There is shift toward reviewing ratios of LDL and HDL rather than total cholesterol. A high level of triglycerides is also considered a risk factor for heart attack.
- Uncontrolled diabetes
- Family history of heart attack or stroke
- Inactive lifestyle, which contributes to hypercholesterolemia and obesity
- Overweight and/or obesity
- Stress
- Illegal drug use.
  - Use of stimulant drugs, such as cocaine or amphetamines, can trigger a spasm of the coronary arteries that can cause a heart attack.
- A history of preeclampsia

TECHNICAL NOTE

Cholesterol is needed for a variety of functions, one of which is to help make the many hormones of the body. Cholesterol is not soluble in the blood; to reach the various target organs, it is bound to a protein, forming a lipoprotein. LDL is the form in which cholesterol travels away from the liver to the various target organs, including the heart. HDL is the form in which cholesterol is removed from target organs and blood vessels and transported back to the liver, where it is prepared for excretion. HDL helps to keep cholesterol from building up in the walls of the arteries.

The greater the levels of a certain LDL in the bloodstream, the greater is the risk of heart disease; the greater the levels of HDL in the blood, the lower is the risk of heart disease.

Estrogen raises HDL levels and lowers LDL levels. Estrogen also helps to prevent oxidation, making the LDLs less harmful to the blood vessels.

Smoke damages the interior walls of arteries, allowing deposits of cholesterol and other substances to collect and slow the blood flow. Smoking also increases the risk of clot formation.

Signs and Symptoms

Symptoms common to women include the following:

- Chest pain or discomfort (angina) described as an uncomfortable pressure, squeezing, or fullness in the center of the chest that can last for several minutes or diminish and subsequently recur
- Pain in one or both arms or the jaw
- Neck or shoulder pain
- Abdominal discomfort
- Shortness of breath
- Nausea and vomiting
- Sweating
- Light-headedness
- Sleep disturbances
- Extreme fatigue

Diagnosis

- Electrocardiogram (EKG) to monitor heart rate and rhythm and detect degree of damage to the heart muscle
- Cardiac enzyme assessment to determine degree of heart muscle damage and location of the damage
- Echocardiography (ECHO) imaging of the heart to assess for injury of the valves and ejection fraction
- Cardiac catheterization to visualize the blocked artery and provide insight into treatment measures

83

Management

Conventional

Acute

The primary goal is to restore blood flow to the heart quickly. Treatment may include the following:

- Aspirin to prevent further clotting
- Nitroglycerin to improve blood flow by relaxing the vascular smooth muscle
- Oxygen therapy for shortness of breath

Medications

- Beta blockers reduce the heart's workload by slowing the heart rate, which in turn reduces oxygen requirements, thus relieving the angina.
- ACE inhibitors lower blood pressure and reduce the strain on the heart by preventing an enzyme in the body from producing angiotensin II, a substance that narrows blood vessels and releases hormones that can raise blood pressure.
- Anticoagulants prevent blood clots from getting larger or forming in the heart or circulatory system.
- Statins are used to treat hypercholesterolemia.

CLINICAL PEARL

Many of the conventional medications must be given within the first few hours of experiencing the heart attack.

Procedures

- Coronary angioplasty, also known as percutaneous coronary intervention (PCI), is used to open the blocked coronary arteries. A stent may be placed in the artery to keep it open.
- Coronary artery bypass grafting (CABG) is a procedure in which a healthy artery or vein is taken from a part of the patient's body (the internal mammary from the chest or the saphenous vein from the leg) and grafted to the blocked

coronary artery to establish a new route for the blood to flow to the heart muscle.

Complementary

Nutraceuticals

- Vitamin C and the carotenoids, which are found mainly in fruits and vegetables, such as green and red peppers, broccoli, brussel sprouts, leafy greens, tomatoes, strawberries and oranges, which help to keep cholesterol and fat deposits from being deposited in the blood vessels
- Antioxidants, which help to prevent cholesterol from damaging the linings of the arteries
- Folate, which helps to decrease homocysteine levels
- Counseling to address fears and reduce stress

Self-Care and Wellness

- Manage obesity. Fatty tissue, like other tissue in the body, needs oxygen and nutrients. As weight increases, the amount of fat tissue increase, and the demand for oxygen and nutrients increases. This means the amount of blood circulating throughout the body also increases, which leads to added pressure on the arterial walls. Excess weight is often associated with an increased heart rate and a reduced capacity of the blood vessels to support blood. Excess weight can also lead to diabetes, high cholesterol, and high blood pressure, all of which increase the likelihood of heart disease.
- Ensure yearly screening, or more often if previous heart problems or family history.
- Ensure regular blood pressure checks and lipid tests. If B/P is above normal, then it should be taken daily and recorded.
- Adopt a heart-healthy diet that includes vegetables, fruits, whole grains, lean meats, and fish or poultry.
- Increase physical activity to at least 30 minutes a day or 1 hour 3 or 4 days a week.

- Avoid cigarette smoke.
- Limit alcohol to one or two drinks a day.
- Engage in tai chi or yoga.

CLINICAL PEARL

The Recommended Daily Allowance (RDA) for vitamin C is 75 mg for females and 90 mg for males. The American Journal of Clinical Nutrition (Hathcock et al., 2005) has stated that vitamin C is safe at dosages up to 2,000 mg daily. Many authorities recommend higher dosages of vitamin C because of its role in multiple biosynthetic functions. Vitamin C in excess can cause loose stools or diarrhea.

TECHNICAL NOTE

Homocysteine is an amino acid normally found in the blood, and elevated levels of homocysteine are a risk factor for coronary heart disease and stroke. Elevated homocysteine levels may also impair endothelial vasomotor function, further affecting the ease with which blood flows through blood vessels. High levels of homocysteine may damage coronary arteries and make it easier for platelet aggregation to occur, predisposing to heart attack and stroke.

A deficiency of folate, vitamin B_{12}, or vitamin B_6 may increase blood levels of homocysteine. Folate supplementation has been shown to decrease homocysteine levels and to improve endothelial function. Spinach, turnip greens, and other green leafy vegetables and citrus fruits, dried beans, and peas are all natural sources of folate.

- Omega-3 fatty acids may decrease the risk of heart attack by providing protection against arrhythmia and lowering blood pressure levels. Omega-3 fatty acids can be found in fish, fish oils, flaxseed oil, and borage oil.

TECHNICAL NOTE

Lipid profiles should be performed for the first time around age 20 and repeated every 5 years if within normal ranges. The lipid profile includes cholesterol and triglyceride (HDL and LDL) levels.

CLINICAL PEARL

Total cholesterol levels over 200 but less than 240 may not be of high risk if LDL levels are low and HDL levels are high. Women in the peri-menopause frequently have slightly elevated total cholesterol levels and desirable HDL and LDL levels.

HDL levels of 60 mg/dL or higher may protect against heart disease.

HDL cholesterol levels of 40 mg/dL (1.04 mmol/L) or lower may increase the risk of developing heart disease, especially in the presence of high total cholesterol.

Very high cholesterol and triglyceride levels may be caused by inherited forms of elevated cholesterol (hypercholesterolemia or hyperlipidemia).

CLINICAL PEARL

- Heart disease claims more women's lives than all cancers combined.
- Death from cardiovascular diseases is not decreasing at the same rate in women as it is in men.
- More women die the first year after their heart attacks than men.
- Of American women, one in five has some form of heart disease.
- Heart disease is the leading cause of death in older women worldwide, regardless of race.

Cerebral Vascular Accident

A cerebral vascular accident (CVA), also known as a stroke, is a medical emergency. It occurs when a blood vessel in the brain bursts or when a blockage develops that cuts off the blood supply to the brain. If blood flow is cut off for longer than a few seconds, the brain cannot get nutrients and oxygen. Without treatment, cells in the brain quickly begin to die. In 85% of cases, this loss of brain function is a result of ischemia. Hemorrhages cause approximately 10% to 12% of strokes. The remaining causes of stroke are rare (see the Technical Note). A transient ischemic attack (TIA), in which blood flow to part of the brain stops for a short period of time, often occurs before a full-blown stroke. It serves as a warning sign and requires immediate attention. TIA symptoms occur rapidly and last a relatively short time. Most TIAs last less than 5 minutes. About one-third of individuals who have a TIA will have a stroke within the year.

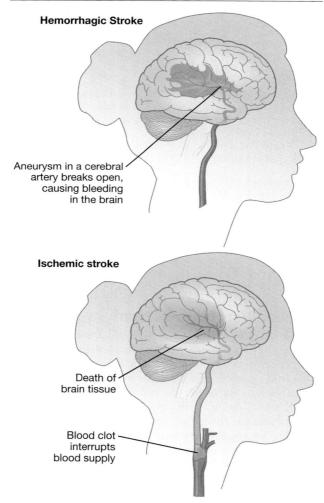

Figure 4-2 Types of stroke

Epidemiology

More women than men have strokes each year, in part because women live longer. African Americans are more affected by stroke than any other racial group in America. Approximately 800,000 people in the United States have a stroke every year, with about three in four being first-time strokes. Stroke is a leading cause of long-term disability and the leading preventable cause of disability.

Etiology

Ischemic strokes are caused by blood clots occluding the blood vessels to the brain, which may occur in two ways:

- Thrombotic strokes occur when a clot forms in a cerebral artery that is already very narrow.
- Embolic strokes (cerebral embolisms) occur when a clot breaks off from some other part of the body and travels to the brain. Ischemic strokes may also be caused by plaque, which can clog arteries.

An ischemic stroke can develop bleeding and become a hemorrhagic stroke.

Hemorrhagic strokes occur when a blood vessel in part of the brain becomes weak and breaks open, causing blood to leak into the brain. This is likely a result of defects in the blood vessels, such as aneurysm or a AVM. Hemorrhagic strokes may also occur as a result of anticoagulants. Very high blood pressure may also cause blood vessels to break, leading to hemorrhagic stroke.

Signs and Symptoms

- Sudden numbness, tingling, weakness, or loss of movement in the face, arm, or leg, especially on only one side of the body.
- Sudden vision changes
- Sudden trouble speaking
- Sudden confusion or trouble understanding simple statements
- Sudden problems with walking or balance
- A sudden, severe headache that is different from past headaches
- Sudden bladder or bowel incontinence
- Loss of balance or coordination

Should any of the signs and symptoms be present, getting to an emergency room as quickly as possible is essential.

Diagnosis

- History and physical examination
- Assessment of vital signs and patient wakefulness
- Neurologic examination using the standardized stroke scale
- Computed tomography (CT) alone or in combination with magnetic resonsnce imaging (MRI)

There is urgency to make the diagnosis and determine whether treatment with thrombolytic medications to "reverse" the stroke is a possibility. The time frame to intervene is narrow and may be as short as 3 to 4 ½ hours after onset of symptoms.

Management

Conventional

Ischemic Stroke

- Medications
  - Injection of tissue plasminogen activator (tPA) within 4 hours of symptom onset to break up blood clots in the arteries of the brain.
  - Antiplatelet medicine, such as aspirin, within 48 hours of symptom onset
  - Anticoagulants (blood thinners) to keep blood clots from getting larger and prevent new blood clots from forming
- Medical procedures
  - Carotid endarterectomy or carotid artery PCI, commonly called an angioplasty, to open blocked carotid arteries if warranted

Researchers are testing other treatments for ischemic stroke, such as intraarterial thrombolysis and mechanical clot (embolus) removal in cerebral ischemia (MERCI).

Hemorrhagic Stroke
- Medication
- Surgical procedures: aneurysm clipping, coil embolization, and arteriovenous malformation (AVM) repair

> **TECHNICAL NOTE**
>
> A CT scan is used to differentiate an ischemic from a hemorrhagic stroke and to look for bleeding or masses in the brain. In certain circumstances, an MRI of the brain may be indicated.

> **TECHNICAL NOTE**
>
> In acute stroke, blood tests and CT scans of the head are ordered to plan treatment.

Self-Care and Wellness
- Management of contributing factors with diet and exercise
- Management of hypertension
- Rehabilitation

> **CLINICAL PEARL**
>
> The focus of rehabilitation is carefully directed, well-focused, repetitive practice. It is a lifelong process.

> **CLINICAL PEARL**
>
> Stroke causes five types of disabilities:
> - Paralysis or problems controlling movement, such as walking
> - Sensory disturbances, including pain
> - Problems using or understanding language
> - Problems with thinking and memory
> - Emotional disturbances

CLINICAL PEARL

Stroke survivors will see their biggest improvements in the first year. However, they will often continue to have small gains long after formal rehabilitation is completed if they faithfully adhere to a home program of exercise and activity.

TECHNICAL NOTE

Stroke studies under way include the following:

- Examination of the brain's response and adaption to determine whether rehabilitative techniques, such as constraint-induced movement therapy and transcranial magnetic stimulation, can stimulate brain plasticity and improve motor function
- Implantation of neural stem cells to determine whether these cells may be able to replace the cells that died as a result of a stroke

CLINICAL PEARL

According to the National Stroke Association (2016):

- Ten percent of stroke survivors recover almost completely.
- Twenty-five percent recover with minor impairments.
- Forty percent experience moderate to severe impairments that require special care.
- Ten percent require care in a nursing home or other long-term facility.
- Fifteen percent die shortly after the stroke.

Reproduced from National Stroke Association. (2016). Rehabilitation therapy after a stroke. Retrieved from http://www.stroke.org/we-can-help/stroke-survivors /just-experienced-stroke/rehab

CLINICAL PEARL

There is considerable evidence that hypovitaminosis D is associated with increased risk for cardiovascular disease, although the mechanisms still remain largely unclear. It is also unclear whether this increase in risk can be reversed by through supplement use.

Varicose Veins

Varicose veins are enlarged, swollen, and twisting veins, frequently the result of faulty valves in the vein. Although they can be found anywhere in the human body, varicose veins are most often in the legs and feet, especially the calves.

CLINICAL PEARL

Varicose means "enlarged or swollen."

CLINICAL PEARL

Spider veins are similar to varicose veins, but they're smaller. They are found closer to the skin's surface and are often blue or dark purple in color.

Epidemiology

The National Institute of Health (2016) estimates that 33% of U.S. women have varicose veins.

Etiology

Veins have one-way valves that prevent blood from flowing backward. When these valves fail, blood begins to collect in the vein rather than continuing toward the heart. Also, muscle contractions in the lower legs act as pumps, and elastic vein walls help the blood return to the heart. In the aging process, the walls of the veins lose elasticity, which impedes the flow of blood. Conditions such as pregnancy and obesity press down on the pelvis, causing pressure on the woman's pelvis and legs. The veins that are pushing the blood flow from the legs must push the blood upward against gravity. This results in varicose veins, more often affecting the legs.

Risk factors include the following:

- Aging: As individuals age, their veins lose elasticity, which causes them to stretch, allowing blood to pool in the veins, resulting in them becoming enlarged and varicose.
- Pregnancy: During pregnancy, the uterus enlarges, putting pressure on the legs and pelvis.

- Gender: Women are more likely to develop the condition.
- Obesity: Being overweight puts added pressure on the veins.
- Standing or sitting for long periods: Blood will not flow well if a person is stationary for long periods.
- Heredity is also a factor.
- Use of birth control pills can increase risk.
- Postmenopausal hormonal replacement can increase risk.
- History of blood clots can increase risk.
- Conditions that cause increased pressure in the abdomen, such as tumors, constipation, and externally worn garments such as girdles, can increase risk.

Signs and Symptoms

- Veins that are dark blue and are twisted or bulging in appearance
- Achy or heavy feeling in the legs
- Burning, throbbing, and swelling in lower legs
- Increased pain after sitting or standing for a long period
- Itching around one or more of the veins
- Bleeding from the varicose veins
- A painful cord in the vein, with red color of the skin

CLINICAL PEARL

Color changes, hardening of the vein, inflammation of the skin, and skin ulcers near the ankle are serious symptoms that require medical intervention.

Diagnosis

- Physical exam of legs and pelvis and self-reported description of pain and aching in legs
- Family history
- Ultrasound to further evaluate the involved veins
- Angiogram (a dye injected and x-ray taken) to evaluate blood flow

Management

Conventional

Procedures

- Sclerotherapy is a procedure in which the physician injects small- and medium-sized varicose veins with a solution that scars and closes those veins.
- Foam sclerotherapy of large veins is a newer treatment in which an injection of a large vein with a foam solution closes the vein and seals it.
- Laser surgeries direct strong bursts of light to the vein, making it slowly fade and disappear. No incisions or needles are used.
- In catheter-assisted procedures using radiofrequency or laser energy, a thin catheter is inserted into an enlarged vein, and the tip of the catheter is heated using either radiofrequency or laser energy. As the catheter is pulled out, the heat destroys the vein by causing it to collapse and seal shut. This technique is more often used for large veins.
- High ligation and vein stripping involve tying off a vein where it joins a deep vein, followed by removal of the vein through small incisions.
- Ambulatory phlebectomy uses a series of tiny skin punctures to remove smaller varicose veins.
- Endoscopic vein surgery is done in advanced cases that involve leg ulcers.

Complementary

Nutraceuticals

- Coenzyme Q10 (CoQ10) can aid circulation and tissue oxygenation.
- Omega-3 oils may help with elasticity of the blood vessels.
- For chronic venous insufficiency, the following herbs have been anecdotally reported to improve symptoms:
  - Butcher's broom
  - Sweet clover

- Grape (leaves, sap, seed, and fruit)
- Horse chestnut

Self-Care and Wellness

- Exercise
- Elevating the legs
- Wearing compression stockings
- Low-calorie diet if overweight

Chronic Obstructive Pulmonary Disease

Chronic obstructive pulmonary disease (COPD) is a progressive disease characterized by airflow limitation. It includes emphysema and/or chronic bronchitis. COPD is the third leading cause of death in the United States.

- Emphysema is characterized by damage to the alveoli that causes diminished exchange of gases
- Chronic bronchitis is a consequence and cause of irritated and inflamed airways. The lining thickens, mucus builds up, and breathing is compromised.

Epidemiology

The World Health Organization (WHO, 2016) estimates that 65 million people worldwide (including 7 million women in the United States) have COPD.

Etiology

- Smoking or secondhand smoke
- Indoor air pollution
- Long-term exposure to environmental toxins
- Preterm birth/neonatal chronic lung disease
- Alpha-1 antitrypsin deficiency, a genetic disorder

Signs and Symptoms

- Shortness of breath, especially with activity
- Noisy breathing with wheezing, whistling, gurgling, or rattling sounds
- Persistent cough
- Sleep disturbances and anxiety
- Chest breathing
- Generalized fatigue
- Blue or gray tint to lips or fingernails
- Rapid heartbeat
- Loss of appetite
- Morning headaches
- Edema of ankles or legs
- Abdominal swelling and pain
- Frequent respiratory infections

Diagnosis

- Spirometry
- Chest x-ray
- CT scan
- Arterial blood gas analysis

Management

A team of professionals is required to manage symptoms and improve quality of life. The team includes primary care physicians, pulmonologists, nurse specialists, and social workers.

Conventional

Medications

- Bronchodilators
- Steroids
- Symptom-specific medications as needed for infections, anxiety, and smoking cessation
- Opioids

Procedures

- Oxygen therapy
- Surgery (bullectomy, lung volume reduction, lung transplant)

Self-Care and Wellness

- Avoidance of environmental pollutants
- Exercise adjusted to limits of COPD
- Maintenance of a healthy weight
- Pulmonary rehabilitation (disease education, adapted exercise program, nutritional counseling, psychological support, what constitutes a crisis and need for emergency intervention, support groups and other resources)
- Immunization against influenza and pneumonia

CLINICAL PEARL

Females with COPD are often misdiagnosed with asthma.

CLINICAL PEARL

The American Lung Association (2013) postulates that women are biologically more susceptible to COPD because women tend to develop the disease at a younger age, endure more comorbidity (e.g., depression), and have an overall lower quality of life in comparison with men.

Data from American Lung Association. (2013). Taking her breath away: The rise of COPD in women. Retrieved from http://www.lung.org/our-initiatives/research/lung-health-disparities/the-rise-of-copd-in-women.html

Pulmonary Embolism

Pulmonary embolism (PE) is a blockage in one of the pulmonary arteries in the lungs. It is most often caused by blood clots that travel to the lungs from the legs. Occasionally, they travel from other parts of the body. A pulmonary embolism usually occurs in conjunction with deep venous thrombosis (DVT).

Epidemiology

According to the Centers for Disease Control (2012), the incidence of venous thromboembolism (VTE), which includes PE and DVT, is 117 cases per 100,000 person-years. It contributes to 5% to 10% of deaths in hospitalized patients, making it one of the leading causes of preventable hospital deaths. It is estimated that over 50,000 Americans die every year as a result of a PE.

Etiology

PE is a common complication of hospitalization. Women are especially vulnerable following gynecological surgeries, during pregnancy, and with use of high-estrogen birth control pills or hormonal replacement therapy. Risk factors include advanced age, prolonged immobility, surgery, trauma, malignancy, pregnancy, estrogen therapy, congestive heart failure, and inherited or acquired defects in blood coagulation factors.

Signs and Symptoms

- Shortness of breath that is worse with activity
- Unresolving chest pain
- Cough with blood stained sputum
- Leg pain or swelling
- Cyanosis
- Fever
- Excessive sweating
- Rapid or irregular heartbeat
- Dizziness or light-headedness

Diagnosis

- History and exam that elicit symptoms
- Blood analysis of substance D dimer
- Duplex ultrasonography
- Chest x-ray to rule out other lung pathology
- Pulmonary angiogram
- MRI or CT scan

Management

Conventional

Medications

Medicines can help prevent repeated episodes of PE by preventing new blood clots from forming or preventing existing clots from getting larger. Convention medicines include the following:

- Anticoagulants: Heparin augments the activity of antithrombin III and prevents the conversion of fibrinogen to fibrin. After initial dosing with heparin, other anticoagulants are used for maintenance. These drugs include enoxaparin (Lovenox), dalteparin (Fragmin), and tinzaparin (Innohep).
- Thrombolytics: Thrombolysis is indicated for stabilizing patients with PE. These drugs include alteplase, reteplase, urokinase, and streptokinase.

Surgery

- Catheterization

Self-Care and Wellness

- Avoiding prolonged sitting
- Remaining well hydrated
- Wearing support stockings
- Engaging in regular exercise

Lung Cancer

Lung cancer is the uncontrolled growth of abnormal cells and can occur in one or both lungs. The abnormal cells divide rapidly and form tumors. Primary lung cancer originates in the lungs, whereas secondary lung cancer starts elsewhere and metastasizes to the lungs via the lymphatic system. The two main types of primary lung cancer are non-small-cell lung cancer (NSCLC), which accounts for 80% of lung cancers, and small-cell lung cancer, which is responsible for the remaining 20%.

CLINICAL PEARL

Scientists from King's College London (National Health Service (NHS), 2012) have reported that over the next three decades, rates of lung cancer in females will increase 35 times faster than rates for lung cancer in males. In the United Kingdom, female lung cancer deaths will increase to 95,000 annually in 2040 from 26,000 in 2010—an increase of more than 350%. Male annual lung cancer deaths will increase by 8% over the same period, to 42,000 in 2040 from 39,000 in 2010. The main reason for the increase is the longer life span. The older a person is, the higher is the risk of cancer, including lung cancer.

Epidemiology

American Cancer Society (2016) gave data that says in women, the incidence over the past 37 years has risen by 98%, whereas the incidence in men over the same time period has declined. Non-Caucasian people are more likely to develop and die from lung cancer.

CLINICAL PEARL

According to the American Cancer Society (2016), lung cancer currently accounts for 14% of all newly diagnosed cancers in the United States. More patients die annually from lung cancer than prostate, breast, and colon cancers combined. A woman's lifetime risk of developing lung cancer in the United States is 1 in 16, and the risk is higher for smokers.

Data from American Cancer Society. (2016). Key statistics for lung cancer. Retrieved from http://www.cancer.org/cancer/lungcancer-non-smallcell/detailedguide /non-small-cell-lung-cancer-key-statistics

Etiology

Inhaling carcinogenic substances such as cigarette and cigar smoke causes gene cell mutations, resulting in cells that are unable to correct DNA damage.

Risk factors for lung cancer include the following:

- Exposure to radon gas: This naturally occurring gas accounts for 12% of lung cancer cases in the United States.
- Passive smoking: Nonsmokers who reside with a smoker have a 24% increase in risk for developing lung cancer when compared with other nonsmokers.

- Asbestos: Asbestos was historically used as thermal and acoustic insulation material. Microscopic fibers that break loose from the material are released into the air and inhaled. Following exposure, asbestos fibers can persist in lung tissue for a lifetime. Both lung cancer and mesothelioma have been linked to asbestos exposure.
- Genetic susceptibility: Lung cancer is more likely to occur in both smoking and nonsmoking relatives of people with a history of lung cancer.
- Air pollution: An estimated 2,000 lung cancer deaths per year are attributable to breathing polluted air, in part caused by vehicles, industry, and power plants.

CLINICAL PEARL

High-dose supplementation with beta-carotene increases the risk for lung cancer.

CLINICAL PEARL

Arsenic in drinking water in areas of the world where the water supply is not regulated increases lung cancer risk.

Signs and Symptoms

Symptoms of lung cancer often go unnoticed until it is in an advanced stage and difficult to cure. The most common symptoms are as follows:

- Cough that does not go away and/or continually gets worse
- Chest pain that worsens with deep breathing, coughing, or laughing
- Hoarseness
- Loss of appetite
- Cachexia
- Weight loss
- Change in color (bloody or rust colored) or volume of sputum
- Stridor sounds when breathing
- Dyspnea
- Neck or facial swelling

- General weakness and fatigue
- Headaches
- Bone or joint pain
- Recurrent infections of lungs and bronchi

CLINICAL PEARL

Apical cancers of the lungs may damage nerves that pass from the upper chest into the neck and cause severe shoulder pain and Horner's syndrome. Symptoms of Horner's syndrome include the following:
- Drooping or weakness of one eyelid
- Having a smaller pupil in the affected eye
- Reduced or absent sweating on the affected side of the face

---

Diagnosis

- Blood tests, including protein biomarkers associated with the presence of a cancerous tumor in the lung
- Bronchoscopy
- Fine-needle biopsy of the lung with a microscopic exam of the cells
- Thoracentesis alone or in combination with thoracotomy to obtain fluid and lung tissue for microscopic exam
- Bone-marrow aspiration and biopsy
- Imaging tests such as CT, MRI, positron emission tomography (PET), and bone scans to determine the size and location of the tumor and if and where it has metastasized

Management

Conventional

- Surgical resection of tumor and adjacent nodes
- Radiation therapy
- Chemotherapy
- Targeted therapy to address specific genes, proteins, or the tissue affected by cancer
- Management of side effects of treatment

Note: For some patients, resection alone is sufficient, whereas others are recommended to also receive chemotherapy, targeted therapies, radiation, or some combination of the three modalities.

Complementary

- Hypnosis for symptom management
- Biofeedback and autogenic training to manage the pain, symptoms, and stress
- Art and music therapy
- Yoga to improve mood and quality of life

Self-Care and Wellness

- Cessation of smoking and avoidance of secondhand smoke
- Energy conservation
- Good nutrition, with emphasis on protein intake
- Daily planned exercise program
- Relaxation
- Meditation
- Guided imagery—visualizing something positive and helping the body accept the treatments
- Self-expression in words through writing or humor

TECHNICAL NOTE

Emerging treatments for lung cancer include the following:
- Ablation therapies, such as radiofrequency ablation and cryotherapy, that eliminate cancer cells without surgery. Ablation uses imaging guidance to place a needle electrode through the skin into a tumor within the chest. High-frequency electrical currents are passed through the electrode, creating heat that destroys the cancer cells. Cryothrapy freezes the lung cancer cells to kill them.
- Photodynamic therapy which uses photosensitizizng drugs along with light to kill cancer cells.
- Vaccine therapy—vaccines that target specific proteins identified in lung cancer

CHAPTER 5

Gastrointestinal Disorders

Gastroesophageal Reflux Disease

Gastroesophageal reflux disease (GERD), also known as acid reflux, is a chronic condition of the lower esophagus and stomach that occurs when contents of the stomach reflux back into the esophagus.

Epidemiology

Approximately 14% of all adult women suffer from GERD.

Etiology

Control of the transport of food from the esophagus to the stomach is regulated by the lower esophageal sphincter. Inadequate functioning of the sphincter allows the stomach's acidic contents to regurgitate back into the esophagus. Causes of lower esophageal sphincter anomalies include hiatal hernias and general sphincter weakening, sometimes as a result of smoking.

Other causes of GERD include the following:

- Pregnancy
- Diet
- Obesity
- Chronic, persistent cough
- Excessive physical exertion
- Iatrogenic causes (e.g., heartburn is a side effect of some medications)

TECHNICAL NOTE

Current understanding implicates *Helicobacter pylori* infection as a cause of GERD. *H. pylori* can cause low-grade inflammation and lead to ulcers in the stomach.

CLINICAL PEARL

Some anecdotal evidence supports the proposed theory that GERD is in part caused by the stomach producing too little acid.

Signs and Symptoms

- Acid indigestion
- Burning pain in the chest
- Pain in the neck
- Pain in the throat

Diagnoses

- Esophageal pH monitoring to measure the quantity of acid in the esophagus over a 24- to 48-hour period
- Endoscopy if symptoms are moderate or severe to examine for esophagitis, esophageal strictures, and Barret's esophagus
- Manometry to assess the function of the lower esophageal sphincter and the need for surgery

TECHNICAL NOTE

Conventional and alternative medicine sources differ dramatically in the understanding of and approach to managing GERD. Whereas the conventional medicine literature espouses high acid levels as the cause of GERD, alternative medicine sources espouse abnormal gut health as a result of the wrong balance of the gut flora as a primary cause of GERD.

Management

Conventional

Medications

- H2 blockers to decrease stomach acid, including the following:
  - Cimetidine (Tagamet)
  - Famotidine (Pepcid)
  - Ranitidine (Zantac)

CLINICAL PEARL

Research evidence suggests that suppression of stomach acid, although helpful for symptomatology, does not address the underlying causes of GERD.

CLINICAL PEARL

Proton pump inhibitors are recommended primarily for severe GERD with bleeding ulcers.

Complementary

Acupuncture

Some studies suggest that acupuncture may provide some benefit for GERD.

Nutraceuticals

Small-scale studies and anecdotal reports suggest that the following may decrease symptoms of GERD:
- Probiotics
- Melatonin

Self-Care and Wellness

Conventional Approaches
- Eating smaller meal portions
- Avoiding known triggers, including cigarette smoke, some citrus fruits, alcohol, fatty foods, and tomatoes
- Eating a few hours before bedtime
- Managing weight
- Sleeping with the head and upper back elevated

Complementary and Alternative Approaches
- Eating whole foods
- Eating unprocessed foods
- Enhancing gut health via the following:
  - Fermented vegetables
  - Cultured dairy products, including yogurt, sour cream, and kefir

- Fish, such as mackerel
- Himalayan (and other) sea salts with high chloride content to increase the production of hydrochloric acid
- Gut stimulants, such as cabbage

Hiatal Hernia

Hiatal hernias occur when parts of the stomach herniate through the diaphragm.

Epidemiology

The incidence of hiatal hernia is thought to be significantly underreported; however, estimates are similar to those for GERD. Approximately 14% of all women and 40% of obese women have some form of hiatal hernia.

Etiology

The cause is unknown but may include anything that places pressure on the diaphragm and surrounding tissue, such as pregnancy, persistent coughing or straining, and obesity. In addition, laxity associated with age may cause a predisposition to hiatal hernias.

Signs and Symptoms

- Sometimes none
- Heartburn
- Chest pain
- Belching/burping
- Difficulty swallowing
- Excessive feelings of fullness following a meal

Diagnosis

- Blood analysis (complete blood count [CBC]) to rule out anemia
- Barium swallow to visualize the stomach, esophagus, and duodenum on x-ray

- Endoscopy to check for inflammation
- Manometry to assess function of the lower esophageal sphincter and assess for the need for surgery

Management

Medications

- Antacids, such as Maalox, Tums, and Rolaids
- H2 receptor blockers, such as cimetidine (Tagamet) and famotidine (Pepcid AC), to decrease acid production
- Proton pump inhibitors, such as omeprazole (Prilosec OTC), to block acid production and heal the esophagus

Surgery is rarely performed in severe cases.

Complementary

- The hiatal hernia maneuver, as performed by many chiropractors (see the Appendix)

Self-Care and Wellness

- Eat smaller meals.
- Minimize heavy lifting, straining, and bending over.
- Improve seated and standing posture; avoid slouching.
- Sleep on an incline, with the head of the bed raised 4 to 6 inches on blocks.
- Choose activities that involve standing rather than sitting or reclining.
- Avoid meals within 2 hours of bedtime.
- The following exercise is anecdotally reported to provide some patients with relief: After drinking a small glass of warm water, stand on the toes, and then drop down to the heels, with the arms above the head. The exercise is repeated 10 times every morning on arising.

TECHNICAL NOTE

Hiatal hernias may be classified as follows:

Type 1	Sliding Hiatal Hernia (Concentric/Axial)	Accounts for 95% of all hiatal hernias Correlated with GERD
Type 2	Paraesophageal hernia	Gastric fundus herniates Accounts for 5% of all hiatal hernias
Type 3	Combination of type 1 and type 2	Rare
Type 4	Herniation of other abdominal organs, such as the spleen or colon	Very rare

Irritable Bowel Syndrome

Irritable bowel syndrome (IBS) is a disorder of the large intestine. It is characterized by changes in stool frequency, abdominal pain, cramping, and bloating or distension. Although IBS is considered a chronic condition, epidemiologic data suggest that symptoms may subside over time.

Epidemiology

Reported IBS symptoms are two to three times higher in women than in men. Globally, the prevalence of IBS is 67% higher in women than in men. Of patients who report with IBS, 50% are under 35 years of age; prevalence is 25% lower in people over age 50. Less than half of patients with IBS seek medical attention.

Etiology

- Unknown
- Food allergies/sensitivities
- Fluctuating hormones

- Stress
- Prior illness of the gut

Signs and Symptoms

- Abdominal pain relieved by defecation
- Frequent stools
- Constipation
- Altered stool frequency
- Bloating
- Passing mucus during a bowel movement
- Symptoms for more than 6 months

Diagnosis

- Symptoms (see Table 5-1)
- Sigmoidoscopy
- Colonoscopy
- Imaging of the abdomen, including x-rays, computed tomography (CT) scans, and barium studies
- Blood tests to rule out other diseases, such as celiac disease
- Assessment for lactose intolerance
- Stool analysis

Management

Conventional

Medications

- Antidiarrheals, such as loperamide (Imodium)
- Antispasmodics, such as dicyclomine (Bentyl)
- Antibiotics, such as rifaximin (Xifaxan)
- Antidepressants, including the tricyclics, such as Amitriptyline (Elavil); the selective serotonin reuptake inhibitors (SSRIs), such as fluoxetine (Prozac); and the serotonin–norepinephrine reuptake inhibitors (SNRIs), such as duloxetine (Cymbalta)
- Fiber supplements, including psyllium (e.g., Metamucil)
- Medications to relax the colon, such as alosetron (Lotronex)
- Other symptom-specific medications

Table 5-1 Manning Criteria—Two or More Symptoms Suggest IBS

Onset of pain linked to more frequent bowel movements
Looser stools associated with onset of pain
Pain relieved by passage of stool
Noticeable abdominal bloating
Sensation of incomplete evacuation more than 25% of the time
Diarrhea with mucus more than 25% of the time

Data from Manning, A.P., Thompson, W.G., Heaton, K.W., & Morris, A.F. (1978). Towards positive diagnosis of the irritable bowel. *British Medical Journal, 2*(6138):653–654.

Complementary

- Acupuncture: Several research studies suggest that acupuncture is a valuable therapy for relieving the symptoms of IBS.
- Therapies aimed at regulating the nervous system: Therapies such as Logan Basic and spinal touch (see the Appendix) are anecdotally reported to relieve the symptoms of IBS
- Herbs: Numerous herbs have been identified in multiple studies as improving some of the symptoms of IBS. They include the following:
  - Single herbs:
    - Essential oil of *Mentha piperita*
    - *Cynara scolymus*
    - *Curcuma longa* extract
    - *Maranta arundinacea*
  - Herbal preparations:
    - Carmint
    - STW 5
    - Padma Lax

Self-Care and Wellness

Diet

- Remove lactose-containing foods from the diet if lactose intolerance is contributing to the symptoms.

- Remove gluten-containing foods from the diet if gluten sensitivity or celiac disease is contributing to the symptoms.
- Complete a food diary to assess for other foods that may aggravate symptoms.
- Try food-elimination diets to assess for other foods that may aggravate symptoms.
- Eat at regular intervals.
- Ensure adequate hydration.
- Exercise regularly.

Constipation

Constipation is a condition in which there is difficulty emptying the bowel, usually associated with hardened feces.

Epidemiology

Depending on the definition of constipation, prevalence rates range from 2% to 28%. Constipation is twice as common in women as in men.

Etiology

- Inadequate dietary fiber
- Perceived and real difficulties in defecation, including limited urge to defecate
- Impaired colonic motor activity
- Dysfunction of the pelvic floor
- Dysfunction of the anal sphincter
- Medications, including antacids, psychoactive medications, opioids, and numerous others, that impair defecation
- Endocrine and metabolic disorders, such as hypothyroidism, parathyroidism, and diabetes
- Pregnancy
- Gastrointestinal conditions, such as Crohn's
- Neurologic conditions, including multiple sclerosis and Parkinson's
- Structural abnormalities

Signs and Symptoms

- Lumpy or hard stools
- Less than three bowel movements every week
- The need to manually remove stools
- Significant straining to have bowel movements
- Incomplete emptying of stools

Diagnosis

- Colonoscopy
- Sigmoidoscopy
- Colonic transit studies
- Defecography (x-ray study of the rectum during defecation)
- Anorectal manometry (evaluation of the anal sphincter)

Management

Conventional

- Fiber and bulking agents to increase stool weight, such as psyllium, polycarbophils, and methylcellulose
- Laxatives
  - Saline laxatives, including mineral oil, glycerin, and docusate (oral or rectal)
  - Osmotics, such as magnesium citrate and MiraLax (polyethylene glycol 3350)
  - Stimulants, such as cascara, used with caution
- Motility agents, such as Tegaserod (Zelnorm)
- Physical therapy—pelvic floor training and biofeedback
- Surgery in severe cases

Complementary

- Spinal manipulation: Multiple studies using chiropractic adjustments delivered through various chiropractic technique systems (e.g., activator, diversified, Thompson, Gonstead) suggest improved symptoms in patients with constipation and other gastrointestinal (GI) symptoms.

- Acupuncture: Multiple studies using acupuncture and electroacupuncture suggest improved symptoms following treatment in patients with constipation.

Self-Care and Wellness
- Increasing fiber and water intake
- Engaging in daily exercise
- Paying attention to the urge

Diarrhea

Diarrhea is the passing of three or more loose stools per day or more frequent passage of stools than is normal for the individual.

Epidemiology

The epidemiology of diarrhea in women remains unclear; estimates are that approximately 9% of the general population has some experience with diarrhea. Diarrhea is an identified manifestation of IBS, a condition that predominates.

Etiology

- Infection in the intestinal tract
- Contaminated water sources
- Poor personal hygiene
- Food prepared or stored in unhygienic conditions
- IBS
- Stress
- Family violence
- Antibiotics
- Hormones
  - Estrogen, progesterone, docosahexaenoic acid (DHEA), and cortisol have all been implicated in either slowing or increasing gut transit time.

Signs and Symptoms

- Loose, watery, frequent stools
- Signs of dehydration
- Abdominal pain

Diagnosis

- History and exam (including blood pressure to assess for dehydration; abdominal examination)
- Review of medications
- Stool testing for mucus, blood, and pathogens
- Laboratory analysis for dehydration, altered blood chemistries, and antibody tests for parasites or celiac disease

Management

Conventional

- Rehydration (water, salt, sugar/juices)
- Zinc supplements (may reduce the duration of diarrhea by as much 25%)
- Nutrient-rich foods
- Medication adjustment
- Intravenous rehydration if necessary

Complementary

- Assessment for and removal of all food allergens
- Probiotics
- Green tea
- Pomegranate extract

Self-Care and Wellness

- Avoid caffeine and alcohol.
- Avoid foods with high sensitivity risk, including dairy products and spicy foods.
- Practice good hygiene habits.

Other management strategies include those described earlier for IBS.

> **CLINICAL PEARL**
>
> The most severe threat posed by diarrhea is dehydration.

> **CLINICAL PEARL**
>
> According to the World Health Organization (2013) diarrheal disease is the second leading cause of death in children under 5 years old and is responsible for the deaths of 760,000 children every year.

Colorectal Cancer

Colorectal cancer is cancer of the large intestine and rectum.

Epidemiology

Colorectal cancer is the second most common cancer in U.S. women of Hispanic, American Indian/Alaska Native or Asian/Pacific Islander descent and the third most common cancer in U.S. Caucasian and African American women. It is most commonly diagnosed in women after age 50.

> **CLINICAL PEARL**
>
> Deaths from colorectal cancer rank third, after lung and breast cancer, for women.

Etiology

- Unknown
- Gene mutations and other hereditary factors
- Diet
  - Diets that are high in fat and low in fiber have been associated with colorectal cancer.

Signs and Symptoms

- Rectal bleeding
- Rectal pain
- Altered bowel patterns that persist

Table 5-2 Staging for Colorectal Cancer

Stage	Cancer Distribution
1	Involves the mucosa of the colon and rectum
2	Involves the colon and rectum; doesn't involve lymph nodes
3	Involves local lymph nodes
4	Involves distal sites

Data from AJCC.

- Abdominal bloating
- Abdominal pain
- Signs of anemia, including fatigue and generalized pallor
- Weight loss

Diagnosis

- History and exam
- Colonoscopy
- Blood analysis for carcinoembryonic antigen
- Abdominal CT scans

Management

Conventional

Conventional management is dependent on staging (see Table 5-2) and might include the following:

- Surgery
- Chemotherapy
- Radiation therapy

Self-Care and Wellness

- Exercise—as recommended by the National Cancer Institute (NCI, 2010), thirty minutes a day for most days of the week; avoiding exercises that increase intra-abdominal pressure
- Diet that is low in red and processed meat
- High-fiber foods, such as split peas, lentils, and black beans
- Colonoscopy every 5 years after age 50

CHAPTER 6

Infections and Immune Disorders

VAGINAL INFECTIONS

General Considerations
Bacterial Vaginosis
Candidiasis (Yeast Infection)

POSTMENOPAUSAL INFECTIONS

Postmenopausal Bladder Infections/
    Urinary Tract Infections

SEXUALLY TRANSMITTED INFECTIONS

Pubic Lice (Phthiriasis)
Trichomonas Vaginitis (Trichomoniasis)
Gonorrhea
Syphilis
Human Papillomavirus
Human Immunodeficiency Virus
Hepatitis B Virus
Hepatitis C
Chlamydia
Herpes

AUTOIMMUNE DISORDERS

Lupus

ASTHMA AND ALLERGY

Food Allergy

VAGINAL INFECTIONS

General Considerations

The pH of the vaginal tract is normally slightly acidic at 3.8 to 4.2. Factors that create a shift in the pH can lead to vaginal infections. These factors include the following:

- Douching
- Diabetes
- Antibiotics
- Hormonal birth control methods
- Decreased immunity
- Pregnancy

TECHNICAL NOTE

Local endogenous flora such as *Lactobacillus* maintain the acidic environment of the vagina by converting sugars to lactic acid. Antibiotics and douching interfere with this process by destroying the endogenous bacteria. Systemic conditions such as diabetes contribute by altering the sugar content of the cells. For this reason, dietary habits and insulin resistance inadvertently contribute to vaginal infections.

Bacterial Vaginosis

Bacterial vaginosis (BV) is a condition in which the normal balance of bacteria in the vagina is disrupted, and overgrowth of certain bacteria occurs. BV can be transmitted sexually and is considered a sexually transmitted infection; however, it can also occur in the absence of sexual contact.

Epidemiology

BV primarily affects women who are sexually active; however, it is unclear what role sexual activity plays in the development of BV.

BV is the most frequently diagnosed symptomatic vaginitis in U.S. women. BV affects 29% of all women aged 14 to 49. Of women who are affected with BV, 19% are not sexually active, and 25% are pregnant. (Masese et al., 2014).

CLINICAL PEARL

The prevalence of BV increases based on lifetime number of sexual partners.

Etiology

Previously referred to as *hemophilus vaginitis, nonspecific vaginitis*, and *corynebacterium vaginale*, BV is a symbiotic infection in the vaginal tract caused by abnormal proliferation of *Gardnerella vaginalis* and microbes such as *Bacteroides, Prevotella, Peptococci* (peptostreptococcus), *Mobiluncus*, and *Mycoplasma hominis*.

Risk factors for BV include having multiple sex partners or a new sexual relationship, repeated douching, oral-genital sexual activity, previous history of sexually transmitted infections, use of intrauterine devices (IUDs), and pregnancy.

CLINICAL PEARL

A change in partner is strongly associated with relapse of BV.

Signs and Symptoms

- Burning and itching of the external genitalia
- Vaginal discharge with the following characteristics:
  - Profuse
  - Grayish or white
  - Foul-smelling; may have a fishy odor that is worse after intercourse

Diagnosis

- Amsel's diagnostic criteria (Amsel et al., 1983; Mohammadzadeh et al., 2015)—clinical criteria requiring three of the following:
  - Homogeneous, thin, white or yellow discharge that smoothly coats the vaginal walls
  - Clue cells (vaginal epithelial cells with a stippled appearance caused by adherent coccobacilli) on microscopic examination
  - pH of vaginal fluid greater than 4.5
  - Fishy odor of vaginal discharge before or after addition of 10% KOH (whiff test)
- Gram stain

Management

Conventional

Medications

- Oral metronidazole (for 7 days)
- Oral clindamycin
- Oral tinidazole
- Vaginal metronidazole gel or clindamycin cream

CLINICAL PEARL

BV in pregnancy has been associated with preterm labor, premature rupture of membranes, and infection of the amniotic fluid.

TECHNICAL NOTE

The CDC (2016a) does not recommend treating male sexual partners. Although it is recognized that 90% of male sexual partners of women with BV also culture positive for *Gardnerella* vaginosis, treatment of male partners does not appear to reduce the rate of recurrence. Condom use does reduce the rate of recurrence. Female sex partners should be treated.

Complementary

Nutraceuticals

- Oral garlic tablets

CLINICAL PEARL

In randomized control trials, the therapeutic effects of garlic on BV were similar to those of metronidazole and resulted in fewer side effects.

CLINICAL PEARL

Vaginal clindamycin ovules weaken latex or rubber products, including condoms and diaphragms. Use of such products within 72 hours following treatment with clindamycin ovules is not recommended.

CLINICAL PEARL

Alcohol consumption should be avoided during treatment with tinidazole and for 72 hours following treatment.

TECHNICAL NOTE

Studies are ongoing to determine the efficacy of intravaginal *Lactobacillus* for the treatment of BV.

Candidiasis (Yeast Infection)

Candidiasis, also known as vulvovaginal candidiasis (VVC), is an infection caused by the fungi *Candida albicans*, *Candida tropicalis*, and *Candida globrata*. *Candida* species are part of the normal endogenous flora; infection is caused by systemic and local overgrowth.

Candidiasis is not a sexually transmitted disease; however, in refractory cases, treatment of the partner may be needed.

Epidemiology

All women can develop candidiasis. Some estimates suggest that 75% of women will have an episode of candidiasis at least once, and 40% will have recurrent infections.

Etiology

Candidiasis is caused by alterations in the vaginal milieu as a result of predisposing factors such as the following:

- Pregnancy
- Systemic antibiotics
- Some contraceptives
- Use of corticosteroids
- Decreased immunity, as seen in the following:
  - Patients with AIDS
  - Patients born significantly premature
  - Patients on chemotherapeutic or radiation therapy
- Poorly managed diabetes
- Frequent douching
- Improper sanitary habits

Signs and Symptoms

- The presence of vaginal discharge that is white, has a curdlike/cottage-cheese appearance, and adheres to the vaginal wall (Note: Attempts to remove the white coating may leave a hemorrhagic area.)
- Intense pruritus
- Dysuria
- Dyspareunia
- Burning and or inflammation of the vulvar and vaginal surfaces

The classic presentation is vulvovaginitis and intense pruritus accompanied by whitish discharge.

Diagnosis

- Pelvic exam—vaginal discharge that is white, thick, cottage-cheese-like in appearance, and adheres to the vaginal surface
- DNA hybridization probe test, such as Affirm VP III
- Wet-mount preparation
  - The discharge is mixed with 10% KOH potassium hydroxide or saline solution to lyse the white and red blood cells and epithelial cells. The hyphae, psuedohyphae, or budding yeast cells are viewed under a microscope.
- Fungal cultures in recurrent or resistant cases

Management

Management of VVC is dependent on its classification: complicated or uncomplicated (see Table 6-1).

Conventional

Uncomplicated VVC

- Over-the-counter vaginal creams, such as clotrimazole (Gyne-Lotrimin) and miconazole (Monistat)
- Prescription medications, such as terconazole vaginal cream, terconazole suppository, and miconazole single-dose treatment
- Oral medications, including one-dose fluconazole (Diflucan) and 3-day itraconazole (Sporanox, Onmel)

Table 6-1 Classification of Vulvovaginal Candidiasis (VVC)

Uncomplicated	Complicated
Sporadic or infrequent VVC	Recurrent VVC
Mild to moderate VVC	Severe VVC
Etiologic agent: *Candida albicans*	Non–*Candida albicans* candidiasis
Nonimmunocompromised female	Female with uncontrolled diabetes, immunosuppression, or debilitation

Modified from Centers for Disease Control and Prevention. (2015). Vulvovaginal candidiasis. Retrieved from http://www.cdc.gov/std/tg2015/candidiasis.htm

> **TECHNICAL NOTE**
>
> Uncomplicated VVC responds to all azole treatments, including oral and vaginal therapies.

Complicated or Resistant VVC (Four or More Episodes per Year)

- Topical therapy for 7 to 14 days or oral dose of fluconazole repeated in 72 hours, followed by suppressive therapy with clotrimazole vaginal suppository, fluconazole, or other maintenance regimens

Non–Candida albicans VVC

The optimal treatment for non–*Candida albicans* VVC is unknown. Recommendations include 7 to 14 of nonfluconazole therapy or boric acid in gelatin capsule vaginally daily for 2 weeks.

> **TECHNICAL NOTE**
>
> Topical agents only are recommended in pregnancy. Fluconazole is contraindicated in pregnancy.

Complementary

Nutraceuticals

- Probiotics: Supplementation with live *Lactobacillus acidophilus* cultures and Ultra Bifidus
- Supplementation with caprylic acid (Caprystatin), a naturally occurring nystatin

Traditional Chinese Medicine

- The Chinese herb Xian He Cao is anecdotally reported to improve candidal infections when rubbed on a tampon or cotton ball and inserted into the vagina overnight.

Self-Care and Wellness

- The vaginal area should be kept clean and ventilated.
- Wipe from front to back following bowel movements.

- Urinate before and after intercourse.
- Avoid unnecessary douching.
- Avoid intercourse while the infection is active.
- Avoid chemical irritants.
- Get adequate rest.
- Avoid potentially immunosuppressive agents, such as alcohol, drugs, caffeine, and cigarette smoke.
- Drink pure, unsweetened cranberry juice.

Diet
- Boost the immune system with a diet that contains immune-supporting vitamins and minerals and natural yogurt with live cultures of *L. acidophilus*.
  - Vitamins include vitamins B_2, B_5, and C, found in whole grains, eggs, fish, poultry, spinach and leafy other vegetables, citrus fruits, and berries; vitamin A, found in brightly colored fruits and vegetables; and vitamin E, found in nuts and wheat germ.
  - Minerals include selenium, found in nuts and whole grains, and zinc, found in large quantities in eggs, seafood, whole grains, and legumes.
- Avoid sugars, artificial sweeteners, and high-sugar fruit juices.

TECHNICAL NOTE

Extract from the bark of *Curatella americana* L. *Dilleniaceae* has demonstrated effects similar to those of fluconazole and nystatin on some *Candida* species.

POSTMENOPAUSAL INFECTIONS

Postmenopausal Bladder Infections/ Urinary Tract Infections

Urinary tract infections (UTIs) in the postmenopause phase are a common finding. Studies suggest that as many as 40% of postmenopausal women with a diagnosis of UTI do not have bacteria in the urine. When present, the bacteria most commonly identified is *Escherichia coli*. *E. coli* normally inhabits the small intestine, but it causes infection when it spreads to the urinary tract.

Epidemiology

Bladder infections afflict 10% to 20% of women in the postmenopause phase. It is the most common bacterial infection in postmenopausal women.

Etiology

- Unknown
- Estrogen deficiency
- Altered elasticity and resultant incomplete emptying of the bladder

Signs and Symptoms

- Burning pain on urination
- Increased urinary frequency and urgency
- Turbid, foul-smelling urine
- Lower abdominal pain

Diagnoses

- Urinalysis

Management

Conventional

- Antibiotics: If and when *E. coli* is identified in the urinalysis, a low dose of trimethoprim/sulfamethoxazole is commonly ordered. (Note: The risk of antibiotic resistance is high.)
- Topical estrogens or an estradiol vaginal ring every 3 months may be ordered. (Note: Contraindications to the use of the ring may include a history of breast or uterine cancer.)

Complementary

- Drinking pure, unsweetened blueberry juice
- Drinking pure, unsweetened cranberry juices
- Taking probiotics
  - *Lactobacillus* is known to have effects similar to those of low-dose antibiotics, without the risk of resistance.

Self-Care and Wellness

- Urinating after intercourse
- Eliminating food allergens
- Enhancing urine flow by drinking adequate amounts of water
- Avoiding soft drinks and concentrated fruit drinks
- Drinking pure cranberry and blueberry juices to help prevent bacterial adherence to the endothelial cells of the bladder
- Using probiotics to balance the endogenous flora

SEXUALLY TRANSMITTED INFECTIONS

Pubic Lice (Phthiriasis)

Pubic lice are approximately 1 to 2 mm in length and are typically found attached to hair in the pubic area but have also been observed on the eyebrows, eyelashes, armpits, and anywhere where there is coarse hair.

Epidemiology

Pubic lice are not a reportable condition in the United States. Estimates are that pubic lice infest 2% to 10% of the population worldwide. According to Planned Parenthood (2017) estimates, there are 3 million cases of pubic lice in the United States each year.

Etiology

Pubic lice are spread primarily through sexual contact and also by close personal contact or contact with articles such as clothing and bed linen. Pubic lice do not transmit disease; however, secondary bacterial infections can occur from scratching of the skin.

Signs and Symptoms

- Intense itching in the genitals or anus
- Lice in the pubic hair
- Mild fever
- Generalized malaise
- Irritability

Diagnosis

Diagnosis is by observation, which may require a magnifying lens.

CLINICAL PEARL

Clinicians are encouraged to check a person diagnosed with pubic lice for other sexually transmitted diseases.

Management

Conventional

- Over-the-counter (OTC) lotions or mousses containing 1% permethrin, pyrethrins, or piperonyl butoxide
- Prescription Lindane shampoo (Note: Side effects include stinging, burning, redness, skin rash, itching, dryness of the skin, swelling of the face and throat, severe dizziness, and drowsiness.)
- Prescription malathion (Ovide) lotion (Note: Side effects include scalp irritation and second-degree chemical burn.)
- Topical ivermectin

Self-Care and Wellness

- The infested areas should be washed and dried, then saturated with a lice-killing solution, following which, the lice may be removed by brushing with a fine brush or a fine-toothed comb.
- Sexual contact should be avoided.

- Ideally replace (buy new) underclothing.
- Wash clothing, bedding, and other products used by the infected individual with hot water.
- Seal any items that cannot be washed in a plastic bag for 2 weeks.

> **CLINICAL PEARL**
>
> Lindane is contraindicated during pregnancy and lactation.

> **CLINICAL PEARL**
>
> Sex partners of the affected individual should be informed that they are at risk, and affected individuals should be treated.

Trichomonas Vaginitis (Trichomoniasis)

Trichomonas vaginitis, also known as trich, is a sexually transmitted disease caused by the flagellated protozoan *Trichomonas vaginalis*.

Epidemiology

Trich primarily affects sexually active women of reproductive age. Trich affects 3% of women in the United States between the ages of 14 and 49.

Etiology

Trich is caused by infection with *T. vaginalis*, which does not survive in the normally low acidic pH of the vaginal vault. However, with a shift in the pH—as occurs during menses, times of stress, and in the presence of other organisms such as streptococcal bacteria—infection may occur.

Signs and Symptoms

Signs and symptoms typically occur following menses and include the following:

- Vaginal discharge with the following characteristics:
  - Profuse
  - Malodorous

- Yellowish, green, or gray in color
- Frothy or bubbly
- Red and sore vaginal opening
- Itching and burning
- Dysuria
- Dyspareunia
- Strawberry appearance of the cervix in approximately 10% of cases

In extreme cases, the entire vulvar area, the inside of the thighs, and the anus may be affected.

CLINICAL PEARL

Of women affected by trich, 1% have no history of sexual intercourse, and 85% of women who are found to have trich have no symptoms.

TECHNICAL NOTE

Up to 53% of women with HIV infection also are infected with *T. vaginalis*.

Diagnoses

- Nucleic acid amplified test (NAAT) (high sensitivity)
- Wet-mount microscopy (poor sensitivity)
- Methods to detect RNA, including the APTIMA *T. vaginalis* assay
- Antigen detection tests, such as the OSOM Trichomonas Rapid Test
- DNA hybridization probe test, such as Affirm VP III
- Vaginal pH greater than 5

CLINICAL PEARL

The OSOM Trichomonas Rapid Test provides results within 10 minutes and may soon be available for self-testing.

> **CLINICAL PEARL**
>
> The Affirm VP III evaluates for *T. vaginalis*, *G. vaginalis*, and *C. albicans*.

Management

Conventional

Medications

- A single oral dose of metronidazole or tinidazole has a 98% cure rate.
- The CDC currently advises that women can be treated with 2 g metronidazole in a single dose at any stage of pregnancy.

Adjunctive Management

- Treat the sexual partner.
- Advise on the use of condoms.
- Counsel to keep the vulvar area dry.

> **CLINICAL PEARL**
>
> *T. vaginalis* infection in pregnant women is associated with premature rupture of membranes, preterm delivery, and delivery of a low-birthweight infant.

> **CLINICAL PEARL**
>
> Metronidazole crosses the placenta; however, studies show no positive or negative association between metronidazole use during pregnancy and adverse outcomes of pregnancy.
>
> Metronidazole is secreted in breastmilk; following maternal treatment with metronidazole, patients should defer breastfeeding for 12 to 24 hours.

> **CLINICAL PEARL**
>
> Tinidazole should be avoided in pregnant women, and breastfeeding should be deferred for 72 hours following a single 2-g dose of tinidazole.

Gonorrhea

Gonorrhea is a sexually transmitted infection caused by the bacteria *Neisseria gonorrhea* that affects the reproductive tract, rectum, mouth, throat, and eyes.

Epidemiology

Gonorrhea is most common among young women aged 15 to 24. The incidence of gonorrhea is declining in women, but the infection currently afflicts about 300,000 people (men and women) in the United States.

Etiology

- Sexual contact with an infected individual

Signs and Symptoms

- Often, no symptoms
- Symptoms that may mimic a bladder infection or other UTI
- Painful or burning sensation when urinating
- Increased urinary frequency
- Increased vaginal discharge
- Spotting or bleeding between cycles or after intercourse
- Rectal discharge, bleeding, itching, soreness
- Painful bowel movements
- Dyspareunia
- Fever
- Yellow or green vaginal discharge
- Vulvar swelling
- Vomiting
- Abdominal or pelvic pain
- Light sensitivity
- Joint pain

CLINICAL PEARL

According to the CDC (2016h), four out of every five women with gonorrhea are symptom-free.

Data from Centers for Disease Control and Prevention. (2016). *Gonorrhea—CDC fact sheet*. Retrieved from https://www.cdc.gov/std/gonorrhea/stdfact-gonorrhea.htm

Diagnoses

- Microbiologic assessment of urine
- Endocervical and vaginal swabs

Management

Conventional

Dual therapy with a cephalosporin plus either azithromycin or doxycycline

Prevention

- Abstinence
- Consistent use of latex condoms

CLINICAL PEARL

Gonorrhea can be passed from mother to baby during delivery. Babies infected with gonorrhea are at risk for prematurity and stillbirth, and they may experience blindness and blood and joint infections.

Syphilis

Syphilis is a sexually transmitted infection caused by the bacteria *Treponema pallidum*. Syphilis is categorized into stages: primary, secondary, latent, and late.

Epidemiology

The incidence of syphilis is declining in women, but the infection currently afflicts approximately 100,000 men and women in the United States.

Etiology

- Syphilis is contracted through sexual contact with an infected individual.
- Syphilis is spread by direct contact with a syphilitic sore, commonly on the genitals.

- There are rare incidences of syphilis spread as a consequence of kissing.
- Syphilis can become dormant and reside in the human body for decades.

Signs and Symptoms

Primary

- Painless sore or chancre on the genitals or other mucosal surface that resolves in a few weeks

Secondary

- Genital sores that look like warts
- Reddish-brown, rough rash that appears on the entire body, including the palms and soles
- Generalized myalgia
- Fever, sore throat, and headaches
- Lymphadenopathy
- Weight loss
- Generalized fatigue

CLINICAL PEARL

Symptoms of secondary syphilis may spontaneously resolve; however, secondary syphilis should still be treated to prevent progression to latent syphilis.

Latent

- No symptoms
- Pathogen remains latent
- May advance to late or tertiary syphilis

Tertiary

Symptoms occur 10 to 30 years following the onset of infection and afflict approximately 30% of individuals with untreated syphilis. Symptoms include the following:

- Dementia
- Blindness

- Cardiovascular damage
- Liver damage
- Neuromusculoskeletal complaints
- Tabes dorsalis (syphilitic myelopathy)—loss of coordination of movement
- General paresis

Diagnosis

Serologic Evaluation

- Nontreponemal assays, such as the rapid plasma reagin, detect antibodies to nonspecific antigens, such as cardiolipin, which is produced in most patients with syphilis.
- Treponemal serology assays, such as the fluorescent treponemal antibody or enzyme immunoassays, detect antibodies against specific antigens from *T. pallidum*.
- A spinal tap may be ordered to evaluate the cerebrospinal fluid.

CLINICAL PEARL

Nontreponemal serology tests will revert to normal following successful treatment; thus, they are used to monitor response to therapy. Treponemal serology tests remain positive for several years following treatment.

Management

Conventional

- Single-dose penicillin for primary syphilis; multiple doses for secondary, tertiary, and latent syphilis

Prevention

- Abstinence
- Consistent use of latex condoms

CLINICAL PEARL

Syphilis can be passed from mother to baby in utero and during delivery. Babies infected with syphilis may appear asymptomatic; however, they are at risk for low birthweight, stillbirth, cataracts, seizures, teeth deformities, saddle nose (nasal bone collapse), and deafness.

CLINICAL PEARL

It is important that clinicians are cognizant of the appropriate penicillin preparation because *T. pallidum* can reside in sites not penetrable by all penicillin preparations.

CLINICAL PEARL

According to the CDC (2016) parenteral penicillin G is the only therapy with documented efficacy for syphilis during pregnancy.

Data from Centers for Disease Control and Prevention. (2016). Syphilis during pregnancy. Retrieved from https://www.cdc.gov/std/tg2015/syphilis-pregnancy.htm

Human Papillomavirus

Human papillomavirus (HPV) is a group of about 150 viruses, each of which has been assigned a number indicating its type. Of the 150 identified strains, approximately 40 are associated with genital HPV infections. Some types of HPV cause cervical cancer, others manifest with warts, and some are asymptomatic. Most HPV infections are self-limiting and have no harmful effects. HPV-16 and HPV-18 are associated with genital cancers; HPV-6 and HPV-11 cause genital warts. HPV is the most common sexually transmitted infection.

Epidemiology

The prevalence of HPV in women aged 14 to 59 in the United States is 27%. According to the CDC, most sexually active individuals will become infected at least once.

In the United States, it is estimated that 79 million people are currently infected, and there are 14 million new HPV infections diagnosed every year, with half of these in individuals aged 15 to 24.

> **CLINICAL PEARL**
>
> HPV is believed to be responsible for nearly all cases of cervical cancer. HPV types 16 and 18 are linked to 70% of all cervical cancers, 90% of anal cancers, and 71% of vulvar and vaginal cancers.

Etiology

HPV is transmitted by skin-to-skin contact.

Signs and Symptoms

- In most cases, there are no signs or symptoms.
- The presence of a lesion is the most common symptom.

> **CLINICAL PEARL**
>
> Persistent oncogenic HPV infection is the strongest risk factor for the development of HPV-related genital cancers.

Prevention

- Abstinence
- Use of latex condoms with all sexual activity
- Vaccination
  - There are currently many HPV vaccines available. The two most common are Cervarix, a bivalent vaccine that prevents infection with HPV types 16 and 18, and Gardasil, a quadrivalent vaccine that prevents infection with HPV types 6, 11, 16, and 18.

> **CLINICAL PEARL**
>
> HPV vaccines are administered as a two or three-dose series of injections. The same vaccine product should be used for the entire series. The CDC recommends a two dose series (at least six months apart) for younger girls (age 11 and 12); and a three dose series for girls age 15 through 26) (CDC, 2016b).

CLINICAL PEARL

The vaccine is recommended for boys between the ages of 11 and 21.

CLINICAL PEARL

HPV vaccination may be a risk factor for premature ovarian failure (POF) in adolescence.

CLINICAL PEARL

HPV vaccination is not recommended for pregnant women.

Management

- Subclinical genital HPV spontaneously resolves and does not require treatment.
- Screening for cervical cancer is guided by the recommendations for Pap smear from the American Cancer Society (see the Clinical Pearl).

CLINICAL PEARL

The U.S. Preventive Services Task Force (2012), and the CDC (2015a) provide the following screening recommendations for cervical cancer.
- Routine cervical screening should be performed starting at age 21 years and continue through age 65 years to prevent invasive cervical cancer.
- Pap testing is recommended every 3 years from ages 21 to 29 years.
- During age 30 to 65 years, women should either receive a Pap test every 3 years or a Pap test plus HPV test every 5 years; co-testing can be done by either collecting one swab for the Pap test and another for the HPV test or by using the remaining liquid cytology material for the HPV test. Because of the high negative predictive value of two tests, women who test negative for both the HPV and the Pap test should not be screened again for 5 years.

- Cervical screening programs should screen women who have received HPV vaccination in the same manner as unvaccinated women.
- Women who are at high risk for cervical cancer may need more frequent screening.
- All major medical organizations concur that no Pap testing is recommended before age 21 years.

Data from AJCC.

CLINICAL PEARL

The HPV DNA test (cobas HPV test) is a first-line primary screening test for use in women age 25 and older. This test detects HPV types 16 and 18. First-line HPV testing is currently not a component of cervical cancer screening guidelines.

Human Immunodeficiency Virus

Human immunodeficiency virus (HIV) is a viral infection that can be transmitted through sexual contact, through blood, or from mother to child during pregnancy, childbirth, or breastfeeding. According to the CDC (2016f) HIV commonly begins with a brief acute retroviral syndrome; transitions to a multiyear chronic illness that progressively depletes CD4 T lymphocytes, which are critical for the maintenance of effective immune function; and ends with symptomatic, life-threatening immunodeficiency. The late stage of infection, known as acquired immunodeficiency syndrome (AIDS), develops over months to years. Absent treatment, most people with HIV will die from AIDS. With early and ongoing treatment, the majority will survive.

CLINICAL PEARL

The trajectory from HIV to AIDS spans an average of 11 years.

Epidemiology

Over 1 million people in the United States have HIV infection, and 16% are unaware of their infection. In 2014, women made up 19% (8,328) of the estimated 44,073 new HIV diagnoses in the United States. Of these, 87% (7,242) were attributed to heterosexual sex, and 13% (1,045) were attributed to injection drug use. Among all women diagnosed with HIV in 2014, an estimated 62% (5,128) were African American, 18% (1,483) were White, and 16% (1,350) were Hispanic/Latina. Women accounted for 25% (5,168) of the estimated 20,792 AIDS diagnoses among adults and adolescents in 2014 and represented 20% (246,372) of the estimated 1,210,835 cumulative AIDS diagnoses in the United States from the beginning of the epidemic through the end of 2014 (CDC, 2016g).

Etiology

- Sexual contact with an infected individual
- Infected blood from shared needles or an accidental needlestick
- Mother-to-fetus transmission in utero, during delivery, or via breastfeeding

Signs and Symptoms

- Gastrointestinal (GI) symptoms, such as stomach cramps, nausea, vomiting, and diarrhea
- Lymphadenopathy
- Fever, headaches, muscle pain, joint pain
- Sore throat
- Skin rash
- Weight loss

Diagnoses

HIV-1 and HIV-2 Antibody and Antigen Evaluation

- Serologic tests that detect antibodies against HIV-1 and HIV-2
- Virologic tests that detect HIV antigens or RNA

CLINICAL PEARL

HIV concentrations are extremely high in plasma and genital secretions following initial infection; therefore, diagnosing HIV infection during the acute phase of the disease is particularly important because people with acute HIV infection are highly infectious.

CLINICAL PEARL

Tests for HIV antibodies are often negative during the acute phase of the infection, causing individuals to mistakenly believe they are uninfected and unknowingly continue to engage in behaviors associated with HIV transmission. Of persons with acute HIV infection, 50% to 90% are symptomatic.

Management

Early diagnosis of HIV infection and linkage to care are essential to management. Linkage to care includes the following:

- Immediate referral to a health-care provider or facility experienced in caring for HIV-infected patients
- Education and referral for support services
- Counseling for alcohol and drug addiction and other potential mental health problems

Hepatitis B Virus

Hepatitis B is a liver infection caused by the hepatitis B virus (HBV). Hepatitis B is transmitted via blood, semen, or other bodily fluids.

Epidemiology

In the United States, 0.1% to 0.5% of the population are chronic carriers. HBV remains endemic in developing regions. An estimated 1 million people in the United states are chronically infected with hepatitis B. Hepatitis B affects men at twice the rate in women.

CLINICAL PEARL

Hepatitis B remains infectious for at least 7 days on environmental surfaces and is transmissible in the absence of visible blood.

Etiology

- Sexual contact
- Sharing of needles, syringes, or other drug-injection equipment
- Mother-to-baby transmission at birth
- Contact with open sores
- Sharing of toothbrushes or razors with an infected individual

CLINICAL PEARL

For some people, hepatitis B is an acute, or short-term, illness; for others, it can become a long-term, chronic infection. The risk for chronic infection is related to age at infection: approximately 90% of infected infants become chronically infected compared with 2% to 6% of adults. Chronic Hepatitis B can lead to serious health issues, such as cirrhosis or liver cancer.

CLINICAL PEARL

HBV can survive outside the body for at least 7 days and still be capable of causing infection.

CLINICAL PEARL

Infected blood spills should be cleaned using a 1:10 dilution of 1 part household bleach to 10 parts water. Gloves should be used when cleaning up any blood spills.

Signs and Symptoms

- Age specific
- Often asymptomatic

- Fever
- Fatigue
- Loss of appetite
- Nausea, vomiting
- Abdominal pain, joint pain
- Dark urine
- Clay-colored feces
- Jaundice
- Chronic hepatitis
- Liver cancer

Diagnoses

- Blood analysis for hepatitis B surface antigen, hepatitis B surface antibody, and hepatitis B core antibody

Management

- Referral to a hepatologist
- Adjustment of medications that may be hepatotoxic
- Avoidance of alcohol

Acute

- Supportive care—no available medications

Chronic

- Medications
  - Interferons (Peginterferon alfa 2a [Pegasys]) are used to inhibit viral replication in infected cells.
  - Antihepadnaviral reverse transcriptase inhibitors, such as tenofovir disoproxil fumarate (Viread), have antiviral capacity.
- Monitoring for liver damage
- Monitoring for hepatocellular cancer

Prevention

- Vaccination

Hepatitis C

Hepatitis C is a disease caused by a virus that infects the liver. The hepatitis C virus can cause both acute and chronic hepatitis infection. Hepatitis C is a bloodborne virus with a 2- to 6-week incubation period

Epidemiology

According to the CDC (2016e) 2.7 million people in the United States have hepatitis C, and more than half are unaware that they have it. Estimates of the incidence in women vary; however, the highest rates (41 per 100,000) are in women aged 25 to 29.

Etiology

Risk Factors

- Injected drug use
- HIV
- Children born to moms who test positive
- People who have had tattoos or piercings
- People who have had transfusions

Signs and Symptoms

Individuals may be asymptomatic or have symptoms specific to acute or chronic infection.

Acute

- Fever
- Nausea
- Decreased appetite
- Fatigue

Chronic

- Cirrhosis
- Hepatocellular carcinoma

Diagnosis
- Screening for anti-HCV antibody
- Liver biopsy—assessment for liver damage (fibrosis and cirrhosis)

Management
Conventional
Antiviral Drugs—Direct Antiviral Agents (DAAs)

- Medications
  - Interferons (Peginterferon alfa 2a [Pegasys]) are used to inhibit viral replication in infected cells.
  - Antihepadnaviral reverse transcriptase inhibitors, such as tenofovir disoproxil fumarate (Viread), have antiviral capacity.
- Liver transplantation

Chlamydia

Chlamydia is a sexually transmitted bacterial infection caused by *Chlamydia trachomatis*.

Etiology
Chlamydia is transmitted through sexual contact with an infected person.

Epidemiology
Chlamydial infection is the most frequently reported infectious disease in the United States. It primarily affects women under the age of 25. The CDC (2016c) estimates that chlamydia affects 5% of all sexually active women aged 14 to 24 in the United States.

Signs and Symptoms

- Abnormal vaginal discharge
- Dyspareunia
- Dysmenorrhea
- Vulvovaginal itching and burning
- Pain with urination
- Hematuria
- Fever
- Abdominal pain
- Spotting

Diagnoses

- Analysis of first-catch urine
- Swab specimens from the endocervix or vagina
- Liquid-based cytology specimens collected for Pap smears

Management

Medication

- Antibiotic therapy: Azithromycin and doxycycline cure chlamydia in up to 95% to 100% of cases (depending on severity, hospitalization may be warranted).
- Partners should be treated.

CLINICAL PEARL

C. trachomatis infection in women can cause pelvic inflammatory disease (PID), ectopic pregnancy, and infertility.

Prevention

- Abstinence
- Use of condoms
- Annual screening of all sexually active women under 25 years of age

- Annual screening of older women at increased risk for infection (e.g., those who have a new sex partner, more than one sex partner, a sex partner with concurrent partners, or a sex partner who has a sexually transmitted infection)

Herpes

Herpes is an infection caused by the herpes simplex virus. The herpes simplex virus (HSV) is an enveloped DNA-containing virus that is subgrouped into two varieties. HSV-1 is usually associated with oronasal infections (i.e., cold sores), and HSV-2 usually causes infections of the vulva, vagina, cervix, and anus. Either type may be found in either location of the body.

HSV is a highly contagious sexually transmitted infection. The infected partners may or may not have active lesions and may be asymptomatic, yet they may be actively shedding viral particles prior to the outbreak of the vesicle. Many individuals describe a prodromal phase of malaise, fever, tingling of the vulvar skin, and inguinal adenopathy prior to the outbreak of a vesicle. Following infection, the incubation period is 2 to 7 days before the onset of a primary herpes infection. Vesicles develop on the vulva and rupture after several days, leaving shallow ulcers that are often painful.

During the primary infection, the ulcers persist for 1 to 2 weeks, then heal spontaneously. The ulcers may develop a secondary bacterial infection, which causes more pain and delays healing. Viral shedding may persist for 2 to 3 weeks after complete resolution of the lesions.

The genital herpes virus is latent and resides in the dorsal root ganglia of S2, S3, and S4 and within the autonomic nerves along the uterosacral ligaments. Recurrences appear to be associated with stress, emotional upheaval, and immunosuppressive states. Symptoms of recurrent infection are usually milder.

Complications include the following:

- HSV-2 has been associated with increased HIV viral load but has not been conclusively shown to accelerate HIV disease progression.
- HSV-2 during pregnancy increases the risk of neonatal infection and neurologic injury, with significant fetal morbidity and mortality. During early pregnancy, HSV-2 increases the risk for spontaneous abortion in some women.

CLINICAL PEARL

The risk of neonatal HSV transmission at the time of delivery increases significantly if the mother has a first episode genital HSV-2 and does not elect to have a cesarean section.

CLINICAL PEARL

The majority of HSV-2 transmission to the neonate occurs in asymptomatic women.

CLINICAL PEARL

Prior research evidence demonstrated a cause-and-effect relationship between HSV-2 and invasive cervical carcinoma. More recent studies are less conclusive.

Current research affirms a close correlation between HPV and cervical cancer and an association between HSV-2 alone or HSV-2 and HPV coinfection with cervical cancer.

Epidemiology

Any sexually active female can contract HSV. An estimated 65% of people in the United States and 90% of people worldwide are seropositive for HSV types 1 and 2. According to CDC (2010) estimates, 25% of women in the United States are seropositive for HSV-2 antibodies.

Etiology

- Infection with HSV

Signs and Symptoms

- Small blisters at the site of infection 3 to 4 days following the infection
- Lesions that may tingle, itch, burn, break, ooze, or scab over
- Abnormal bleeding
- Vaginal pain
- Dysuria
- Dyspareunia
- Leukorrhea
- Inguinal adenopathy
- Concurrent symptoms such as fever, malaise, headache, myalgia, and diffuse low back pain
- Possible urethral or vaginal discharge

Diagnoses

- Viral inclusion bodies (giant cells) recognized on cytologic (pap) smear
- The herpes virus culture, ideally obtained from the vesicles rather than the crusted ulcers
- HSV DNA (HSV polymerase chain reaction [PCR]) testing
  - This is done only if the culture is negative but herpes remains suspected or if the patient has received prior treatment for herpes. Samples are taken from the blister, blood, or other fluids, such as spinal fluid.
- HSV antibody testing
  - Serologic tests for viral-type antibodies may be used to determine past exposure. HSV IgM antibody production begins several days after a primary infection and is detectable for several weeks. HSV IgG antibody production begins following IgM production and remains forever.

Management

There is no known cure for herpes. Management is directed at symptomatic relief and shortening the period of the outbreak.

Conventional

Medications

Antiviral medications come in varying doses based on intended use—first-time outbreak, recurrent outbreak, or suppression—and include the following:

- Valacyclovir (Valtrex)
- Famciclovir (Famvir)
- Acyclovir (Zovirax)
  - All are designed to reduce the duration of viral shedding, the time of healing, the duration of symptoms, and the clinical course of the disease. Low-quality evidence suggests that these antivirals further decrease the number of herpes events when compared with placebos.

CLINICAL PEARL

The benefits of topical application of acyclovir are equivocal.

CLINICAL PEARL

Intravenous acyclovir is reserved for patients with severe systemic infections.

CLINICAL PEARL

When the first infection is in the first trimester of pregnancy, there is an increased risk of spontaneous abortion. When the first infection is in the third trimester of pregnancy, the risk is highest (at 30%–50%) for neonatal infection.

Recommended Doses of Antiviral Medications for Herpes in Pregnancy

Pregnancy	First Episode			Recurrent Episodes		
	Antiviral Drug	Recommended Daily Dosage	Length of Therapy	Antiviral Drug	Recommended Daily Dosage	Length of Therapy
Episodic treatment	Acyclovir	Orally: 5 × 200 mg	10 days	Acyclovir	Orally: 5 × 200 mg	5 days
	Valacyclovir	Orally: 2 × 500 mg	10 days	Valacyclovir	Orally: 2 × 500 mg	5 days
Suppressive treatment	Acyclovir	Orally: 3 × 400 mg		Acyclovir	Orally: 3 × 400 mg	
	Valacyclovir	Orally: 2 × 250 mg	From week 36 until delivery	Valacyclovir	Orally: 2 × 250 mg	From week 36 until delivery

Reproduced from Straface, G., Selmin, A., Zanardo, V., De Santis, M., Ercoli, A., Scambia, G. (2012). Herpes simplex virus infection in pregnancy. *Infectious Diseases in Obstetrics and Gynecology*, 2012:385697. doi:10.1155/2012/385697.

Complementary

Nutraceuticals

- Proper ratios of lysine and arginine

CLINICAL PEARL

In laboratory studies, the amino acid arginine was shown to inactivate HSV-2.

Self-Care and Wellness

- Regular Pap smears
- Stress reduction and management
- Cold compresses of aluminum acetate (Burrow's solution), which has been anecdotally reported to provide some relief
- Sitz baths
- Easing the pain of urination by directing the stream away from the lesions with a rolled tissue or urinating while pouring warm water over the area

AUTOIMMUNE DISORDERS

Autoimmune disorders are a group of almost 100 known disorders of autoimmunity. In these disorders, the immune system becomes misdirected and attacks the organs it was designed to protect. Autoimmune disorders affect almost all organ systems.

Some of the more common autoimmune disorders are Graves's disease, Hashimoto's thyroiditis, rheumatoid arthritis, and systemic lupus erythematosus (SLE, lupus).

Epidemiology

Autoimmune disorders disproportionately affect women; 75% of all people living with autoimmune disorders are women.

Etiology

- Unknown
- Genetic predisposition

- Environmental factors
- Suspected triggers in some women include the following:
  - Viruses
  - Infections, including chlamydia
  - Certain drugs/medications
  - Nutrient depletion, such as lack of iodine in Graves's disease

Signs and Symptoms

The signs and symptoms vary depending on the disorder. Symptoms are wide and varied and might include the following:

- Joint pain
- Muscle pain
- Weight loss
- Endocrine anomalies
- Visual disturbances
- Generalized fatigue

Diagnoses

- History and physical exam, which may elicit:
  - Family history of an autoimmune disorder
  - Multiple signs and symptoms that are inconsistent with any one condition
- Blood testing, including complete blood count (CBC), erythrocyte sedimentation rate (ESR), and C-reactive protein (CRP)
- Autoantibody testing
- Antinuclear antibody (ANA) testing

Management

Conventional

- Medications
  - Pain relievers
  - Anti-inflammatory drugs
  - Immunosuppressive agents

- Hormone replacement therapy
- Rehabilitation modalities, including physical therapy
- Counseling for stress and depression

Complementary
- Manual therapies
- Massage therapy
- Acupuncture
- Nutraceuticals

Self-Care and Wellness
- Diet and exercise
- Rest
- Stress management
- Avoidance of known triggers

Lupus

SLE is a chronic autoimmune disorder that primarily affects women. It follows a relapsing and remitting course and affects multiple systems.

Epidemiology

Of all patients with lupus, 80% to 90% are women. The onset of lupus is frequently during the reproductive phase.

Etiology

The cause of lupus is unknown. Proposed causes include the following:

- Environmental factors, such as ultraviolet light from sunlight and fluorescent light bulb
- Reaction to medications, particularly sulfa drugs, penicillin, and tetracycline
- Epstein-Barr virus
- Hormones
  - Lupus symptoms are worse during estrogen peaks.

- Genetics
  - Lupus does appear in families; however, there is no clear genetic link.

> **CLINICAL PEARL**
>
> The risk for heart attack in women with lupus aged 35 to 44 is 50 times greater than in healthy controls.

> **CLINICAL PEARL**
>
> Lupus is more common in African Americans, Hispanics, Native Americans, Pacific Islanders, and Asians.

Signs and Symptoms

- Fatigue
- Fever
- Weight loss
- Pain in the joints
- Musculoskeletal pain
- Swollen and discolored nailbeds
- Persistently swollen lymph nodes
- Raynaud's phenomenon
- Thinning hair
- Pathology of the skin, joints, and internal organs
- Pathology of the heart, lungs, and kidneys
- Butterfly rash on the face
- Photosensitivity
- Swollen hands, wrists, knees, and feet

Diagnoses

- Antiphospholipid antibody and low complement
- ANA, which is positive in 95% of lupus patients but also positive in other inflammatory disorders
- Evaluation for proteinuria and thrombocytopenia when the ANA is positive

---

CLINICAL PEARL

SLE should be suspected in any female of childbearing age who presents with the triad of fever, joint pain, and rash.

CLINICAL PEARL

According to the American College of Rheumatology (2015), SLE is the likely diagnosis whenever 4 of the following 11 symptoms are present:

- Serositis
- Oral ulcers
- Arthritis
- Photosensitivity
- Blood disorders
- Renal involvement
- Antinuclear antibodies
- Immunologic phenomena
- Neurologic disorder
- Malar rash
- Discoid rash

Data from American College of Rheumatology. (2015). Lupus: Fast facts. Retrieved from http://www.rheumatology.org/I-Am-A/Patient-Caregiver/Diseases-Conditions/Lupus

Management

The goals of management are to control symptoms, manage flare-ups, and mitigate long-term risks.

Conventional

Medications are targeted at specific symptoms and include the following:

- Steroids, such as prednisone, prednisolone, and methylprednisolone (Medrol), for inflammation
- Antimalarials, such as hydroxychloroquine (Plaquenil) and chloroquine (Aralen), for joint pain, ulcers, and rashes
- Topical ointments, such as tacrolimus (Protopic), pimecrolimus (Elidel), and thalidomide (Thalomid), for skin rash

- Nonsteroidal anti-inflammatory drugs (NSAIDs), such as ibuprofen (Motrin), for sore joints and inflammation and fever
- Immunosuppressant medications, such as azathioprine (Imuran)

Complementary

Nutraceuticals

- Whole plant extracts of *Harpagophytum procumbens* (devil's claw), which contains flavonoids, glycosides, sugars, phytosterols, and aromatic acids
- *Zingiberaceae officinale* (ginger), which contains volatile oils, oleoresin, linoleic acid, magnesium, phosphorus, and potassium
- *Boswellia serrate* (Indian olibanum), which contains boswellic acids
- *Curcuma longa* (turmeric), which contains curcumin
- *Ananas comosus* (bromelain), which contains proteolytic enzymes
- Dehydroepiandrosterone (DHEA) for arthritic symptoms
- Pomegranate and green tea, for which preclinical evidence of efficacy exists

CLINICAL PEARL

DHEA may lower the levels of high-density lipoprotein (HDL) cholesterol in patients with lupus.

CLINICAL PEARL

Bromelain is obtained from the stems and immature fruits of the pineapple plant.

Self-Care and Wellness

- Manage stress.
- Avoid cigarette smoke.
- Exercise regularly.
- Cover up when outside in the sun.
- Pomegranate and green tea are anecdotally reported to relieve the pain and symptoms of inflammation.

> ### CLINICAL PEARL
>
> Comorbidities caused by lupus include pericarditis and other cardiovascular diseases, kidney failure, pleuritis, depression, and anxiety. Management of patients with lupus requires a community of health practitioners.

ASTHMA AND ALLERGY

Asthma is a chronic lung disorder that manifests with repeated episodes of shortness of breath, wheezing, chest tightness, and coughing. Allergic reactions and/or hypersensitivity cause inflammation, bronchial swelling, and narrowed airways. Symptoms may range from mild to life-threatening.

Epidemiology

Approximately 1 in 20 people has chronic asthma. Prior to puberty, asthma affects more boys than girls. Around puberty, asthma prevalence appears to be about the same for boys and girls. Retrospective studies suggest that asthma is more common in women than in men throughout adulthood. In general, the lifetime likelihood of developing asthma is about 10.5% greater in women than men, and women make up 65% of asthma-related deaths.

Etiology

The main causes of asthma and allergy can be categorized into three groups: immunologic, genetic, and environmental mechanisms. Specific to women, fluctuating hormone levels especially estrogen levels, induce an inflammatory response that can bring on asthma symptoms.

Studies suggest that estrogen fluctuations may have as much of an effect on asthma symptoms as allergies and hay fever. Pregnancy, menopause, and monthly menstrual cycling may place women at an increased risk for asthma symptoms.

Causes of adult-onset asthma include workplace exposure, cigarette smoke, and marijuana use.

Among the occupations identified as risk factors for asthma are the following:

- Car painting (isocyanates)
- Hairdressing (various chemicals)
- Domestic and commercial cleaning (cleaning solutions)
- Health-care professions (latex)
- Baking (flour dust)

Signs and Symptoms

- Shortness of breath
- Chest tightness
- Coughing
- Wheezing

Diagnoses

- Peak flow meter
- Spirometry
- Chest x-ray
- Provocative testing for exercise-induced asthma
- Allergy screening

Food sensitivities, such as lactose intolerance, may heighten asthma symptoms.

Management

Conventional

Medications

- Beta-adrenergic inhalers, such as albuterol, that function as long-term bronchodilators (Note: Albuterol is also available as a nebulizer.)
- Oral steroids, including prednisone and solumedrol

- Oral bronchodilators, such as theophylline
- Immunomodulators, such as Xolair (a one-time injection)
- Inhaled corticosteroids, such as Flovent, QVAR, and Pulmicort.
- Leukotriene modifiers, such Singulair
- Estrogen replacement therapy (ERT)

CLINICAL PEARL

Most hospitalizations for asthma in women occur right before menses when estrogen levels are at their lowest.

Complementary Therapies

Nutraceuticals

- The polyunsaturated fatty acids are substrates for inflammatory mediators, the omega-3 and omega-6 fatty acids
- Pycnogenol, a bioflavonoid extracted from pine bark, has anti-inflammatory and antiviral properties.

Acupuncture

- Studies suggest that acupuncture may provide short-term relief for asthma patients by improving pulmonary function and reducing the levels of interleukin and immunoglobulin E.

Manual Therapies

- Small-scale studies suggest that manipulative therapy leads to a significantly greater reduction in the symptoms of asthma.

Self-Care and Wellness

- Avoid known allergens/triggers.
- Avoid known allergens right before the onset of menses.
- Use maintenance medication daily as prescribed; use rescue inhaler only when needed.
- Use air conditioning to reduce airborne allergens and lower humidity.
- Reduce indoor allergens, including pet dander, dust, and mold.
- Engage in regular exercise.

- Perform hyperventilation-reduction breathing exercise twice daily. The exercise involves breathing slower and more shallowly with a capnometer to provide feedback on CO_2 levels.
- Practice yoga.
- Follow a healthy diet.

CLINICAL PEARL

The National Center for Complementary and Integrative Health (2015) states that practicing yoga (and other forms of regular exercise) might confer health benefits, such as reducing heart rate and blood pressure, and may also help alleviate anxiety and depression. The center also notes that a few individual trials have reported positive effects of breathing exercises performed in yoga or other interventions.

CLINICAL PEARL

Pregnant women should be encouraged to take their maintenance medications. An asthma attack during pregnancy places both mother and fetus at risk for hypoxia.

TECHNICAL NOTE

Asthma classification is as follows:

Classification	Signs and Symptoms
Mild intermittent	Mild symptoms up to 2 days a week and up to 2 nights a month
Mild persistent	Symptoms more than twice a week but no more than once in a single day
Moderate persistent	Symptoms once a day and more than 1 night a week
Severe persistent	Symptoms throughout the day on most days and frequently at night

Data from National Asthma Education and Prevention Program, Third Expert Panel on the Diagnosis and Management of Asthma, & National Heart, Lung, and Blood Institute. (2007). Guidelines for the diagnosis and management of asthma. (NIH Publication No. 08-5846). Bethesda, MD: NHLBI; Pollart, S. M., & Elward, K. S. (2009). Overview of changes to asthma guidelines: Diagnosis and screening. American Family Physician, 79(9), 761–767.

Food Allergy

A food allergy is an abnormal response to a food that is triggered by the body's immune system. A food allergy is different from a food intolerance/sensitivity because allergies trigger the immune system, whereas intolerances and sensitivities are primarily a problem with digestion.

Epidemiology

According to the CDC(2015b, 2016i) 4% of adults and 4% to 6% of children suffer from a food allergy.

Etiology

The cause of food allergies is unknown. Factors that may influence food allergies include the following:

- Ancestry
- Genetics
- Environmental factors
- Stressors

Signs and Symptoms

Reactions to foods occurring immediately after ingesting the food include the following:

- Vomiting
- Abdominal pain and cramping
- Urticaria
- Respiratory symptoms, including shortness of breath, wheezing, coughing, and cyanosis
- Cardiovascular symptoms
- Dizziness
- Light-headedness
- Fainting
- Dysphagia
- Anaphylaxis

Diagnosis

- Detailed history (including a food diary review)
- Physical exam
- Blood test for immunoglobulin E
- Skin-prick test
- Oral food challenge test
- Elimination diet

CLINICAL PEARL

The foods that most commonly cause food allergies are peanuts, tree nuts, shellfish, eggs, and milk.

CLINICAL PEARL

Oral allergy syndrome (itchy mouth and throat after eating a raw or uncooked fruit or vegetables) is a reaction to pollen; it can be resolved by heating the food.

CLINICAL PEARL

The most common food allergens in adults are as follows:
- Fruit and vegetable pollen (oral allergy syndrome)
- Peanuts and tree nuts
- Fish and shellfish

Management

Conventional

- Medications
  - Antihistamines, such as diphenhydramine (Benadryl) and cetirizine (Zyrtec), for mild reactions
  - Epinephrine (EpiPen or Adrenaclick) for serious reactions
- Development of a Food Allergy and Anaphylaxis Emergency Care Plan in collaboration with the patient

Self-Care and Wellness

- Adhere to strict avoidance of the problem food(s).
- Check all labels.
- Use caution when eating out.
- Wear emergency medical identification.
- Take medications at the first sign of a reaction.
- Keep an epinephrine injection (EpiPen) on hand for prompt treatment of anaphylaxis.
- Develop a Food Allergy and Anaphylaxis Emergency Care Plan (see the Appendix).

CHAPTER 7

Managing Fertility, Pregnancy, and Menopause

Constipation
Itching from Episiotomy Stitches
Loss of Bladder Sensitivity
Nipple Pain
Sore Perineum
Vaginal Drainage
Weight Loss

LONGER-TERM POSTPARTUM CONCERNS

Diabetes
Postpartum Depression

LACTATION

Dyad Bonding
Achieving Good Latch
Effective Feeding
Mastitis

PREGNANCY LOSS

Spontaneous Abortion (Miscarriage)
Induced Abortion
Stillbirth

CONTRACEPTION

Contraceptive methods should be considered by any female of childbearing age who wishes to engage in sexual activity but does not desire pregnancy. All methods come with some risk, compromise, and responsibility. The only foolproof, risk-free method is abstinence. Approximately 90% of sexually active women who do not use any form of contraception become pregnant within 1 year.

Primary considerations in the choice of contraception method include the following:

- Frequency of administration: How often does the patient want to think about contraception?
- Cost: How much is the patient willing or able to spend on contraception?
- Hormones: Does the patient have a preference for hormonal or nonhormonal methods?
- Effectiveness: Both theoretical and in terms of correct use
- Safety: Sexually transmitted infection (STI) risks and concerns
- Personal values and beliefs, including religious and spiritual practices

Contraceptive Methods

Barrier Methods

Cervical Cap

The cervical cap is a silicone based "cap" that is inserted vaginally and covers the cervix. It may be inserted up to 6 hours before intercourse and may remain in place for up to 48 hours. The cervical cap is best suited for the nonparous female and should be used with a spermicide.

Advantages
- May be inserted several hours prior to intercourse
- Inexpensive once fitted
- Portable
- No systemic hormones

Disadvantages

- Some women have allergies to silicone or spermicide.
- Insertion and removal pose challenges for some women.
- Vaginal irritation may result.
- The cap may become dislodged during sexual activity.

Cervical Sponge

The cervical sponge is a round foam sponge with a large dimple in the center. It contains a spermicide that is activated by water. The sponge may be inserted up to 24 hours prior to intercourse, and must it be left in place for a minimum of 6 hours following intercourse.

Advantages

- No systemic hormones
- Inexpensive
- Portable

Disadvantages

- Allergic reaction to the spermicide and other materials found in the sponge, including polyurethane and sulfa
- Higher failure rates in parous women

CLINICAL PEARL

The American College of Obstetricians and Gynecologists (2014) reported a few cases of toxic shock syndrome in women who used the sponge.

Male and Female Condoms

Male and female condoms come in latex and nonlatex varieties. They act as a physical barrier both to semen and sexually transmitted infections. Male condoms fit over the penis; female condoms have a closed ring on one end and are inserted into the vagina. Female condoms may also cover the vulva.

Advantages

- Added protection from STIs
- Multiple options, including spermicide-coated, spermicide-free, latex, and nonlatex condoms
- Easily accessible
- Inexpensive
- No prescription or clinician visit necessary

Disadvantages

- Female condoms can be awkward to insert.
- Each act of intercourse requires a new condom.
- Wearing a condom may reduce sensitivity.

TECHNICAL NOTE

Nonlatex condoms are typically made from lambskin or polyurethane.

CLINICAL PEARL

Lambskin condoms do not prevent the transmission of STIs, including HIV.

Diaphragm

A diaphragm is made of silicone and is inserted so as to cover the upper vaginal vault and prevent sperm from entering the cervical os. It is used with a spermicide. The diaphragm may be inserted any time prior to intercourse but must be retained for a minimum of 6 hours and up to 24 hours after intercourse.

Advantages
- Inexpensive
- Portable
- Decreases the risk of pelvic inflammatory disease

Disadvantages
- Each act of intercourse requires additional spermicide.
- Women may have allergies to silicone or spermicide.
- Some women report increased urinary tract infections.

Oral Contraceptives

The many oral contraceptives fall into two main categories: those that contain a combination of estrogen and progesterone and those that contain progesterone only. Estrogen–progesterone combinations limit follicular development, blunt ovulation, thicken the cervical mucus, and may regulate the menstrual cycle. Progesterone-only methods thicken the cervical mucus, thereby retarding sperm motility, and blunt the surge in luteinizing hormone (LH) that triggers ovulation.

Estrogen–Progesterone Combinations

Estrogen–progesterone combinations are available in 28-day and 21-day packs. Twenty-one-day packs contain 21 days of active pills. Twenty-eight-day packs contain 21 days of active pills and 7 inactive pills. Menstruation occurs during the fourth week. The birth control pill Seasonale comes in packs with 11 weeks of hormones and 1 week of inactive pills, resulting in four menses per year. Seasonique comes in packs of 11 weeks of hormones and 1 week of low-dose ethinyl estradiol, also resulting in four menses per year. Packs of both Seasonale and Seasonique contain 91 days of pills and 7 reminder pills.

Advantages
- Convenient and effective
- Does not interfere with sexual spontaneity

- Lighter and, in some cases, fewer periods
- Reduced incidence of endometrial cancer
- Reduced incidence of ovarian cysts and ovarian cancer
- Reduced incidence of acne in some women

CLINICAL PEARL

Estrogen–progesterone combination oral contraceptives significantly reduce the risk of endometrial cancer when used for a minimum of 5 years. This effect is sustained for a minimum of 30 years after contraceptive use ceases and is not dependent on estrogen dosage or individual female characteristics such as age at menarche, ethnic origin, and alcohol use.

TECHNICAL NOTE

Researchers noted that in high-income countries, 10 years of oral contraceptive use reduced the absolute risk of endometrial cancer in women younger than 75 years of age from 2.3 to 1.3 per 100 women (Nelson, 2015).

TECHNICAL NOTE

Estrogens increase the liver's ability to manufacture clotting factors.

Disadvantages
- Decreased libido
- Side effects such as nausea, vomiting, acne, headaches, weight changes, headaches, depression, and sore breasts
- No protection against STIs
- Increased risk of breast and cervical cancers

Contraindications
- Smokers over the age of 35 because "the pill" accelerates the incidence of cardiovascular events such as hypertension, deep venous thrombosis, and pulmonary embolism

- Personal history of cardiovascular events, liver disease, and diabetes because synthetic hormones can be toxic to the liver and disrupt the delicate hormonal balance in diabetes

CLINICAL PEARL

Some users of Seasonale and Seasonique may experience chest pain and jaundice. In addition, Seasonal and Seasonique may be contraindicated in women with a history of reproductive cancers.

CLINICAL PEARL

Some combination pills contain ethinyl estradiol and drospirenone, a progestin derived from spironolactone (also known as Aldactone). Drospirenone may increase potassium levels and cause heart disease and may be contraindicated in individuals with a history of adrenal, kidney, or liver disease. These combination pills, sold under such brand names as YAZ, Gianvi, YASMIN, Ocella, Syeda, Zarah, Beyaz, and Safyral, may be recommended in patients for whom acne and hirsutism are noted challenges, as they can function as antiandrogens.

CLINICAL PEARL

Women over the age of 35 who have migraines and use contraceptive methods with systemic estrogen have an increased risk for stroke.

Women of any age who have migraines with aura who use estrogen-containing contraceptives have an increased risk for stroke.

TECHNICAL NOTE

Oral contraceptive progestins are most commonly derived from testosterone.

Progesterone-Only Oral Contraceptives

The mini-pill is an oral tablet taken daily that contains progestin only. It is available in 28-day packs in which all the pills are active. Menstruation (when present) occurs during the fourth week. The mini-pill works by thickening the cervical mucus and may inhibit ovulation and thin the endometrial lining.

CLINICAL PEARL

To maximize the mini-pill's effectiveness, it must be taken at the same time every day, with no more than a 3-hour delay, or it may be rendered ineffective. If the schedule is not adhered to, a backup method is then required for the remainder of the pack.

Advantages
- Minimal maintenance
- Suitable for women who can't use pills containing estrogen
- May be used while breastfeeding

Disadvantages
- Side effects such as nausea, breakthrough bleeding, headaches, sore breasts, acne, and depression
- No protection against STIs
- Less effective than other hormonal methods
- May increase the risk of ectopic pregnancy

Contraindications
- Personal history of liver disease, cardiovascular disease, meningioma, breast cancer, or bariatric surgery

CLINICAL PEARL

Both the mini-pill and the combination pill may be prescribed during lactation; current research evidence suggests that the combination pill does not interfere with lactation.

Fertility Awareness Methods (Natural Family Planning)

Symptothermal

The symptothermal fertility awareness method (FAM) combines the basal body temperature and the characteristics of the cervix, cervical os, and cervical mucus so that the woman can avoid sexual intercourse at the time in the cycle when it could result in pregnancy. At ovulation, cervical mucus is abundant and slippery, the cervical os opens, and the cervix softens and rises.

Billings (Cervical Mucus)

The Billings method is based on the premise that cervical mucus is scant following menses; as ovulation approaches, the mucus becomes more abundant and peaks at ovulation, becoming fluid and slippery. Following ovulation, the mucus becomes thicker, less slippery, and more hostile to sperm.

Basal Body Temperature

The basal body temperature (BBT) rises immediately after ovulation as a result of rising systemic levels of progesterone. The "safe" days begin 3 days after the rise in temperature.

Hormonal Monitoring

Hormonal monitoring involves self-monitoring of the urine for LH. The presence of LH in the urine signals the most fertile days.

Calendar/Rhythm

The formula for calculating safe days assumes that the interval from ovulation to the onset of menses is consistently 14 days. The last safe day is calculated by subtracting 18 from the length of the shortest cycle, and the first safe day is calculated by subtracting 11 from the length of the longest cycle. For example, a woman with cycles ranging from 25 to 29 days is presumed fertile from day 7 ($25 - 18 = 7$) to day 18 ($29 - 11 = 18$).

A female with regular ("like clockwork") 29-day cycles has a last safe day at day 11 (29 − 18) and a first late safe day at day 18 (29 − 11). In the event that intercourse occurs on day 11, by day 14, sperm is nonviable. Ovulation occurs on day 15; within 48 hours, neither egg is viable, and intercourse can resume on day 18.

Standard Days Method

The standard days method (SDM) works for women with cycles ranging from 26 to 32 days. Unprotected vaginal intercourse is prohibited from day 8 to day 18 of each cycle. Color-coded cycle beads alert the user to the days when she is not fertile, meaning vaginal intercourse is safe. Smartphone apps such as iCycleBeads allow for convenient tracking of cycles and fertile days.

The 2-Day Method

The 2-day method is based on the consistency of cervical mucus. Around ovulation, cervical mucus becomes slippery, alkaline, and wet to enable sperm motility toward the cervix. This change in consistency means that around ovulation, vaginal discharge is noticeable in its quantity and consistency. The vaginal opening is assessed for secretions twice each day, beginning immediately after the last day of menstrual bleeding. Evidence of secretions (anything coming from the vagina that is not menstrual blood) indicates fertility. Fertility is assumed until the woman notes 2 consecutive days without vaginal secretions (see Figure 7-1).

Lactational Amenorrhea Method

The lactational amenorrhea method (LAM) works for up to 6 months postpartum and is suited for women who breastfeed exclusively and consistently. Breastfeeding a minimum of every 4 hours during the day and every 6 hours at night creates a hormonal environment that blunts the LH surge, thereby preventing ovulation.

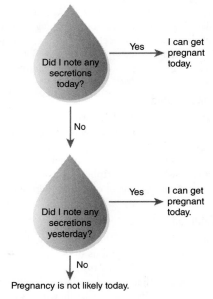

Figure 7-1 TwoDay Method®

Reproduced from Institute for Reproductive Health. (2016). TwoDay® method. Retrieved from http://irh.org/twoday-method/

CLINICAL PEARL

The LAM is not an effective method for women who are breastfeeding but have had a menstrual cycle or who experience bleeding during breastfeeding.

TECHNICAL NOTE

Elevated prolactin levels as observed during regular breastfeeding affect the LH surge and impair ovulation. Neuroendocrine processes occurring postpartum result in dysrhythmia in the pulsed secretions of gonadotropin-releasing hormone (GNRH) and LH, therefore affecting the hypothalamic–pituitary–ovarian axis.

Advantages

- Safe and inexpensive
- Encouragement of mutual responsibility
- No barriers to interrupt lovemaking
- No chemicals or systemic hormones
- Essentially no side effects

Disadvantages

- Not all women have recognizable cervical mucus or BBT patterns.
- Some methods may be perceived as too bothersome.
- Some methods require several months of records and charts.
- Some methods do not work for women with irregular cycles.
- Mutual responsibility is encouraged, but the woman may bear most of the responsibility.
- As a group, these methods do not protect from STIs.

Effectiveness

Effectiveness ranges from 53% to 99%, with an average of 76% to 86% based on compliance.

TECHNICAL NOTE

Typical FAMs assume a sperm life of 3 to 5 days, and ovum life is estimated at 24 to 48 hours.

CLINICAL PEARL

Users of FAMs should be counseled to always have a backup plan. The backup plan may involve abstinence, withdrawal, barrier methods, or emergency contraception.

Fertility Awareness Method Mobile Applications

Many FAM apps are currently available and easily downloaded to iPads, iPhones, and other electronic devices. Several are available at no cost and come with symptom and temperature trackers. Examples include the Ovulation Calendar, Ladytimer Ovulation Calendar, Kindara, Groove, iPeriod, OvuView, Fertility Calendar, My Days, Glow, iCycleBeads, Clue, and Fertility Friend.

These apps differ in focus, with some geared toward enhancing fertility, others designed for contraception, and still others that allow for personalization of information. Some, including Kindara and OvuView, function both as contraception- and fertility-enhancing aids.

Apps documenting evidence-based information include NaturalCycles and iCycleBeads.

The Patch

The patch is a 2-inch-square adhesive that contains ethinyl estradiol and norelgestromin. It is replaced once a week for 3 consecutive weeks, followed by a week of menses. Placement sites include the buttocks, stomach, upper torso, and upper outer arm. Each patch remains effective for up to 9 days but ideally should be replaced once a week on the same day. The patch is less effective for women who weigh more than 198 pounds. The effectiveness of the patch may be impaired by some antibiotics, antifungals, antiseizure drugs, and some herbs, including St. John's wort.

Advantages

- Pregnancy protection for a month without the need to take a daily pill
- Does not interfere with sexual spontaneity
- Lighter and, in some cases, fewer periods
- Reduced incidence of endometrial cancer
- Reduced incidence of ovarian cysts and ovarian cancer
- Reduced incidence of acne in some women

Disadvantages

- Skin irritation at the site
- Decreased libido
- Side effects such as nausea, vomiting, spotting, acne, headaches, weight changes, headaches, depression, and sore breasts
- No protection against STIs

Contraindications

- Smokers over the age of 35
- Personal history of cardiovascular events, liver disease, and diabetes

---

CLINICAL PEARL

The Ortho Evra patch is no longer available. The patch is currently available under the generic name xulane.

Nuva Ring

The Nuva Ring is a flexible circular device that is inserted into the vagina once every month. It releases hormones (ethinyl estradiol and etonogestrel) for 3 weeks and is removed in the fourth week, prompting withdrawal bleeding.

Advantages

- Pregnancy protection for a month without the need to take a daily pill
- Lower systemic hormonal load than other hormonal methods
- Does not interfere with sexual spontaneity
- Lighter and, in some cases, fewer periods
- Reduced incidence of ovarian cysts, ovarian cancer, and endometrial cancer
- Reduced incidence of acne in some women

Disadvantages

- Decreased libido
- Increased vaginal irritation and discharge
- Side effects such as nausea, vomiting, spotting, and sore breasts
- No protection against STIs

Contraindications

- Smokers over the age of 35
- Personal history of cardiovascular events, liver disease, and diabetes

TECHNICAL NOTE

The effectiveness of the ring is impaired if the ring is kept in the vagina for more than 3 weeks, is not kept in the vagina for 3 consecutive weeks, or is not immediately reinserted following expulsion.

CLINICAL PEARL

The effectiveness of the ring is impaired if unopened packages are exposed to very high temperatures or direct sunlight. Use effectiveness is enhanced if the ring is stored in the refrigerator.

Depo-Provera

Depo-Provera is an injection given through the deltoid or gluteus muscles once every 3 months. It is composed of the progestin medroxyprogesterone acetate. To ensure absence of pregnancy, the first administration occurs during the first few days of a normal menses. Depo works by inhibiting ovulation and thickening the cervical mucus, making it more hostile to sperm.

Advantages

- Minimal maintenance
- Convenient
- Pregnancy protection for 3 months
- Useful for women who should not use estrogen

Disadvantages

- Side effects may include depression, acne, weight gain, hirsutism, and headaches
- Ectopic pregnancy
- Loss of bone mineral density
- Bleeding irregularities
- Reproductive cancers
- Thrombosis

Contraindications

There is a significant loss of bone mineral density in women who use Depo-Provera. Women already at risk for loss of bone mineral density should not use Depo-Provera.

CLINICAL PEARL

Depo-Provera negatively affects serum estrogen levels, which results in loss of bone mineral density. Users should be cautioned to avoid using Depo for more than 2 consecutive years.

CLINICAL PEARL

Cycles may not be restored fully for up to 9 months following the last Depo-Provera shot.

Nexplanon (Formerly Implanon)

Nexplanon is a slow-release capsule implanted into the upper arm. Once inserted, it provides protection for up to 3 years. It is composed of the progestin etonogestrel and works by thickening the cervical mucus, inhibiting ovulation, and modifying the uterine lining

Advantages

- Minimal maintenance—once inserted, provides protection for up to 3 years
- Useful for women who should not use estrogen
- Fewer and lighter menstrual cycles
- Can be used while breastfeeding
- In some women, helps alleviate symptoms of premenstrual syndrome (PMS)

Disadvantages

- Does not protect against sexually transmitted diseases
- Menstrual/bleeding irregularities
- Side effects such as depression, acne, headaches, weight gain, mood swings, hair loss, sore breasts, light-headedness, loss of libido, ovarian cysts, and viral infections
- Possible problems at the insertion site

Complications

Some medications and herbs may impair the effectiveness of Nexplanon. These include select oral antifungals, tuberculosis medicines, HIV medications, antiseizure medications, mental disorder medications, and St. John's wort.

CLINICAL PEARL

Cycles (and fertility) are typically restored once the capsule is removed.

Intrauterine Device

The intrauterine device (IUD) is a T-shaped plastic device that may be coiled with copper or coated with progestin derivatives. It is the most popular reversible method worldwide and is experiencing a resurgence in use in the United States; it is currently used by about 6% of women, up from 1% a decade ago (see Figure 7-2).

The IUD irritates the uterine lining, impairs sperm motility, interferes with fertilization, and inhibits implantation. Some brands release low levels of the progestin levonorgestrel, which thickens the cervical mucus, further inhibiting sperm motility and fertilization.

Currently available IUD options include the following:

- The **Paragard Copper T IUD** can provide protection for 10 to 12 years.
- The **Mirena IUD** releases progestin and can provide protection for 5 to 6 years.
- The **Skyla IUD** is a smaller unit that releases progestin and is specifically marketed to younger and nonparous females. It can provide protection for up to 3 years.

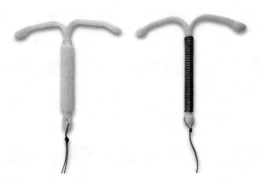

Figure 7-2 Intrauterine device
© Lalocracio/iStock/Getty Images Plus/Getty

- The **Liletta IUD** releases progestin and can provide protection for up to 3 years. Liletta is being marketed as accessible to all females, regardless of income levels.

The **Progestasert IUD** has been discontinued.

Advantages

- Provides long-term birth control with minimal maintenance
- Does not interfere with sexual spontaneity
- Minimal or no systemic hormones

Disadvantages

- Side effects can include abdominal pain, low back pain, pelvic pain, acne, headaches, nausea, sore breasts, dysmenorrhea, menorrhagia, and intermenstrual spotting.
- IUDs do not provide protection against STIs, HIV, or hepatitis B.
- In rare cases, the IUD may perforate or become expelled.

Contraindications

The IUD may be contraindicated in women with multiple sexual partners, a history of pelvic infections, a history of previous IUD expulsion, or a history of fibroids.

Rarely, pregnancy may occur with an IUD in place. Pregnancy with an IUD in place may cause sepsis, septic abortion, premature delivery, and maternal death.

CLINICAL PEARL

IUDs were historically marketed to parous women. With the introduction of smaller versions of the IUD, younger, nonparous women may consider the IUD an appropriate method of contraception.

CLINICAL PEARL

In controlled studies, being under the age of 20 and having heavy menstrual cycles were factors associated with increased risk of IUD expulsion.

Emergency Contraception

Contraceptive Pills

Oral contraceptives containing levonorgestrel or combinations of levonorgestrel and estrogen may be taken within 5 days of unprotected intercourse to prevent pregnancy. Efficacy is improved if the emergency contraception is taken as soon as possible following unprotected intercourse. Some emergency contraceptive pills are available as a single dose; others are available as two dosages taken 12 hours apart. Brand names include Plan B One-Step, Next Choice, and My Way. Emergency contraceptive pills work by preventing ovulation and thickening the cervical mucus.

Advantages
- Available over the counter without prescription
- Approximately 89% effective

Disadvantages
  Side effects include nausea and vomiting.

Copper-Containing IUD

The copper IUD or Paragard IUD, if inserted within 5 days of unprotected intercourse, is the most effective emergency contraception available. It works by preventing implantation.

Advantages
- Approximately 99% effective
- May be inserted up to 5 days following unprotected intercourse
- Once inserted, can continue to provide pregnancy protection for up to 12 years

Disadvantages
- Requires an appointment with a health-care provider
- Can be challenging to locate a qualified health-care practitioner who is available on short notice
- Side effects such as menorrhagia and cramps

The Yuzpe Regimen

The Yuzpe regimen is a method whereby regular birth control pills are used as a form of emergency contraception. Administration is in two dosages, 12 hours apart. Utility is brand specific.

Advantages

- The ability to use pills already on hand to manage an emergency situation

Disadvantages

- Only works with certain brands of birth control pills
- Side effects include nausea, vomiting, intermenstrual spotting, headaches, and breast tenderness
- Requires a prescription

CLINICAL PEARL

Most emergency contraception options work best when used within 24 hours and no more than 72 hours following unprotected intercourse.

ella

Ulipristal acetate, the active ingredient in ella, is a selective progesterone receptor modulator (SPRM) that works as an emergency contraceptive pill by delaying ovulation for up to 5 days.

Advantages

- It provides one-pill protection.
- Unlike most other emergency contraceptive methods, it is as effective at 5 days as it is on day 1.
- There is no minimum age requirement for purchase.

Disadvantages

- Available by prescription only
- Not recommended for women who are breastfeeding
- Side effects such as nausea and cramps

CLINICAL PEARL

According to the Food and Drug Administration (FDA) (2015) ulipristal acetate was found in the breastmilk of lactating women who used ella for 5 consecutive days following use. The effect of ulipristal acetate on the nursing child is currently unknown. The FDA recommends that breastfeeding women should not use ella.

CLINICAL PEARL

Weight considerations in the choice of emergency contraception are as follows:
- The copper IUD is the most effective choice for all women, regardless of weight.
- For women who weigh over 165 lb (75 kilos), ella is more effective than levonorgestrel.
- For women with a body mass index (BMI) greater than 26 or who weigh more than 176 lb (80 kilos), levonorgestrel offers no pregnancy protection.
- For women with a BMI greater than 35 or who weigh more than 195 lb (88 kilos), ella offers no pregnancy protection.

Data from Bedsider.org (2016)

CLINICAL PEARL

Emergency contraceptive pills are not effective for women who have already ovulated.

Sterilization

For women who are absolutely certain that they do not desire to conceive, surgical and nonsurgical sterilization procedures are options.

Sterilization—Nonsurgical

The nonsurgical "Essure" procedure involves inserting metal springs (micro-inserts) into each fallopian tube. The fallopian tubes are accessed through the cervix. The procedure is done in about 30 minutes on an outpatient basis. Over time, the particles create scar tissue, which seals off (blocks) the fallopian tubes.

Advantages
- Nonsurgical procedure
- Permanent birth control
- Safe and effective

Disadvantages
- Other methods of contraception are required for a minimum of 3 months following insertion to allow scar tissue to build up.
- Efficacy in women under 21 or over 45 has not been established.
- Side effects immediately following the procedure include cramping, vaginal bleeding, low back and pelvic pain, and vomiting.
- The inserts may be expelled in some women.
- It does not protect against STIs.
- Carries a slightly higher risk of ectopic pregnancy.

Contraindications
- Ambivalence about terminating fertility
- Pregnancy within 6 weeks of anticipated insertion date
- Recent or current pelvic infection
- Allergy to contrast dye or nickel

Sterilization—Surgical

Surgical options involve reaching the fallopian tubes through incisions made in the lower abdomen, navel, or suprapubic regions.

Laparoscopy

Laparoscopy is a minor surgical procedure whereby the abdominal cavity is distended with carbon dioxide gas. The incision is made in the navel, and a long scope is inserted through the incision into the abdominal cavity. Recovery time is a few days.

Mini-Lap

The mini-laparotomy ("mini-lap") involves incisions made in the suprapubic region. The fallopian tubes are pulled out through the incisions and closed off (tied, cut, or sealed); they are placed back into the abdominal cavity, and the incisions are closed. Recovery time is a few days.

Laparotomy

The laparotomy procedure is less commonly used for sterilization because it involves a larger abdominal incision, requires 2 to 3 days of in-hospital observation, and has a recovery period of several weeks.

Advantages
- Highly effective
- Permanent birth control

Disadvantages
- Requires general or local anesthesia
- Extended recovery time
- Does not protect against STIs

Contraindications
- Ambivalence about fertility
- Known complications from anesthesia

Contraceptive Methods—Summary of Cost, Frequency, and Effectiveness

Cost

Approximate costs for the various methods are as follows:
- Abstinence: $0
- Cervical cap: $0 to $250, including the cost of the cap and fitting
- Cervical sponge: $0 to $5 per sponge
- Condom: $0 to $1 per condom

- Depo Provera shot: $50 to $120 every 3 months
- Diaphragm: $0 to $90 every year
- Fertility Awareness: $0 to $100, including costs for supplies (beads, calendars, thermometers, etc.) and information classes
- IUD
  - Mirena $500 to $1,000 every 6 years
  - Paragard $500 to $1,000 every 12 years
  - Skyla $600 to $800 every 3 years
- Nexplanon (formerly Implanon): $450 to $800 every 3 years
- Nuva Ring: $0 to $75 every month
- Oral contraceptives: $0 to $90 every month
- Patch: $0 to $80 every month
- Sterilization (surgical and nonsurgical): $0 to $5,000

Note: Most insurance plans cover some form of contraceptive services.

Frequency

In Table 7-1, frequency of administration of the various methods is summarized by how often the patient wants to think about contraception.

Table 7-1 Birth Control Methods Compared by Frequency

Frequency	Birth Control Method
With every act of intercourse	Barrier methods
Daily	Oral contraceptives Fertility awareness/natural family planning methods
Weekly	The patch
Monthly	Nuva Ring
Quarterly	Depo-Provera
Annually/every several years	Intrauterine device (IUD) Nexplanon
Never again	Sterilization

Table 7-2 Effectiveness Estimates for Contraceptive Methods

Method	Theoretical Effectiveness, %	Use Effectiveness, %
Cervical cap	n/a	71–86
Cervical sponge	80–91	76–88
Condom—male	98	82
Condom—female	95	79
Depo-Provera	99	94
Diaphragm	94	88
Fertility awareness	95–99	76
IUD	99	99
Nexplanon	>99	>99
Nuva Ring	99	91
Oral contraceptive	99	91
Patch	99	91
Sterilization	>99	>99
Withdrawal	96	78

Data from Bedsider. (n.d.). Birth control methods. Retrieved from https://www.bedsider.org/methods

Effectiveness

For estimates of theoretical and actual use effectiveness of the various contraceptive methods, see Table 7-2.

TECHNICAL NOTE

Mifepristone (the "abortion pill"), also known as RU-486, is not legal or available after the 7th week of pregnancy

INFERTILITY

Infertility is the inability to get pregnant after 1 year of regular sexual activity. Primary infertility implies there is no history of a successful pregnancy. Secondary infertility implies that there has been a previous successful pregnancy. For fertility to occur, the man must produce sperm of sufficient quality and motility, otherwise known as the seminal factor; the sperm must be deposited in the cervix; and the female must produce a healthy ovum, have a healthy uterus, and have patent fallopian tubes. Sterility is the absolute inability to ovulate or produce sperm.

Epidemiology

Statistics show that male infertility accounts for approximately 30% to 40% of all infertility, female infertility accounts for approximately 30% to 40% of all infertility, and shared infertility accounts for approximately 20% to 30% of all infertility.

Etiology

- Anovulation: The eggs are not released.
- Tubal factor: The fallopian tubes are not patent because of scarring from infection, scar tissue from previous medical procedures, or blockage from conditions such as endometriosis. This accounts for approximately 30% of female infertility.
- Inadequate ovulation: Conditions that cause inadequate ovulation include Turner syndrome, premature menopause, premature ovarian failure, and polycystic ovarian syndrome. Inadequate ovulation accounts for approximately 30% of female infertility.
- Cervical patency: Factors that cause problems with the cervix include a pinhole-size cervical os; thickened cervical mucus, which hinders the transport of sperm; and cervical polyps. Problems with cervical patency account for approximately 20% of female infertility.
- Compromised uterine patency (resulting from scarring, a retroverted uterus, endometriosis, or fibroids) accounts for approximately 20% of female infertility.
- Other factors that influence infertility include emotional stress, prolonged contraception, increased age, environmental pollutants, inadequate hormonal function, and misalignment of the spinal vertebrae.

Diagnosis

Signs/Symptoms

- Inability to conceive

Diagnostic Tests

Diagnosis of infertility involves one or more of the procedures listed in the following subsections.

Hormonal Assessment

- Day 3 follicle-stimulating hormone (FSH): A high level of FSH is a signal that estrogen levels are lower than anticipated, which implies that development of the ovarian follicles is inadequate. Healthy follicular development would result in sufficient quantities of estrogen.
- Day 3 LH to determine the FSH-to-LH ratio: A ratio of over 2.5 is an indication of poor ovarian reserve, even in the presence of normal FSH levels. Ovarian reserve is an indication of the quality of the eggs remaining in the woman's ovaries.
- Day 3 Estradiol: This is an adjunct to day 3 FSH that is used to determine ovarian reserve and provide information on the accuracy of the FSH assessment. Normal day 3 assessment findings are low FSH and low estradiol. Elevated estradiol could indicate that estradiol is artificially suppressing FSH levels.
- Clomiphene citrate challenge test (CCCT): The CCCT is used to more accurately assess ovarian reserve. The patient takes a dose of Clomid on days 5–9, and FSH is measured again on day 10. An elevated day 10 FSH is an indication that there will be a decreased response to injectable FSH in assisted reproductive cycles, which is a cause of low pregnancy success rates and high miscarriage rates.
- Thyroid function tests—thyroid-stimulating hormone (TSH), T3, and T4: Hypothyroid and hyperthyroid function can cause anovulatory cycles and miscarriage; hyperthyroidism can also be a cause of fetal malformation and premature labor.

- Human chorionic gonadotrophin (HCG): HCG, which is produced by the blastocyst and placenta, is an indication of pregnancy. HCG sustains the pregnancy in part by signaling the corpus luteum to continue to release progesterone.
- The androgens testosterone and androsterone: Elevated levels can cause anovulatory cycles.
- Hysterosalpingogram (HSG): The HSG allows the uterine cavity and the fallopian tubes to be visualized. It is an x-ray of the uterus following injection of a contrast medium. Patent fallopian tubes permit the contrast material to spill out and be visualized in the abdominal cavity; blocked fallopian tubes will not.
- Rubin test: Carbon dioxide gas is injected into the uterus and fallopian tubes. Shoulder pain as a result of escaping gas is an indication of patent fallopian tubes. This is a low-cost, low-specificity screening procedure. This procedure is rarely used in the United States.
- Laparoscopy: A minor surgical procedure whereby the abdominal cavity is distended with carbon dioxide gas. The incision is made in the navel, and a long scope is inserted through the incision into the abdominal cavity. The patency of the fallopian tubes and uterus is clearly visualized.
- Postcoital test (Sims-Huhner test): This test involves microscopic evaluation of the cervical mucus 2 to 6 hours following intercourse and around ovulation. Cervical mucus should be clear, and sperm should still be active. The presence of inactive sperm indicates cervical mucus with sperm antibodies.
- Endometrial biopsy: A small sample of the lining of the uterus is excised and viewed under a microscope. Cancerous and other abnormal cells are identified, and the endometrium is evaluated for normal stages of change during the menstrual cycle.

CLINICAL PEARL

Recent findings suggest that HCG may be released prior to implantation to support implantation.

HCG injections are frequently administered in fertility treatment for the following reasons:
- To improve implantation rates in in vitro fertilization (IVF)
- To trigger ovulation in women with polycystic ovarian syndrome (PCOS)
- To trigger ovulation in controlled ovarian hyperstimulation situations

Male Infertility

Assessment of infertility should include an evaluation of the male partner's health to ascertain if factors that affect sperm quality, quantity, or viability are present. This evaluation should be undertaken by the male partner's practitioner before or concurrent with evaluation of the female patient because identifying impaired fertility in the male could reduce the need for invasive testing of the female partner.

Management

The management of infertility is based on the outcomes of the previously described diagnostic procedures.

Conventional Therapies

Self-Care and Wellness

- Institute dietary modifications to include intake of whole grains, organic fruits and vegetables, seeds and nuts, and sufficient amounts of water.
- Limit or eliminate tobacco, alcohol, and caffeine.
- Limit refined sugars and processed foods.
- Maintain healthy weight.
- Engage in spiritual practices
  - Studies indicate that prayer, belief in a higher power, and other spiritual practices may enhance fertility through stress-modulating effects.
- Practice other stress-reduction techniques.

- Exercise for general health, and perform specific exercises that facilitate brain impulses crossing the corpus callosum; such as cross-crawl exercises.

Medications

Medications targeted to the identified cause of infertility may include the following:

- Estrogen therapy to induce cervical secretions and to manage thickened cervical mucus
- Clomiphene (Clomid, Serophene) and menotropin (Pergonal), which mature the ovarian follicles and stimulate ovulation
- Bromocriptine (Parlodel), which is used to treat anovulation caused by elevated prolactin levels
- Low-dose corticosteroids to modulate overproduction of androgens and to retard sperm antibody production
- HCG or Ovidrel to time ovulation during IVF
- Progesterone to support the development of the endometrium and to prevent miscarriage, especially during IVF cycles

CLINICAL PEARL

According to research, progesterone is currently the best method of providing luteal-phase support in assisted reproductive technologies. It is associated with higher rates of live birth or ongoing pregnancy than placebos and lower rates of ovarian hyperstimulation syndrome than HCG.

Procedures

- Laparoscopic tubal surgery may be indicated if one or both of the fallopian tubes are plugged.
- Intrauterine insemination (IUI): This procedure involves placing sperm directly inside the uterus to increase the chances of fertilization. IUI is useful for couples when the concerns are low sperm count, altered sperm mobility, thick or scant cervical mucus, and a generally hostile vaginal environment or when a male donor is needed. IUI can be performed with or

without ovulation-enhancing medications. HCG is prescribed to ensure ovulation within 34 to 40 hours.

- Gamete intrafallopian tube transfer (GIFT): This increasingly infrequent procedure involves removing the eggs, combining them with sperm, and immediately placing them in the fallopian tubes, where the egg is fertilized. The female is given follicular-stimulating drugs to increase her chances of producing multiple eggs; the eggs are collected via aspiration and mixed with sperm. The egg-and-sperm mixture is placed in the fallopian tubes by laparoscopy. GIFT is only an option if the female has a healthy uterus and fallopian tubes.

- IVF: This procedure involves removing the eggs via aspiration, combining them with sperm in the lab, and creating a laboratory environment that enables fertilization and early development of the embryo. If fertilization occurs successfully, the embryo is transferred to the uterus. A 2-hour rest period following the procedure is recommended.

- Intracytoplasmic sperm injection (ICSI): This procedure involves obtaining the eggs via aspiration and inserting a single sperm through the zona pellucida (the external covering of the egg) into the cytoplasm of the egg. ICSI is used with couples with male infertility problems, including inability to penetrate the egg, obstructive azoospermia caused by previous vasectomy, scarring from prior infections, or congenital absence of the vas deferens. Sperm for ICSI is retrieved through normal ejaculation, vasectomy reversal, or needle aspiration.

- Zygote intrafallopian transfer (ZIFT): This procedure, also known as tubal embryo transfer (TET), is similar to IVF except the fertilized egg is transferred into the fallopian tubes by laparoscopy. This is an option for couples who have failed prior efforts with ovarian stimulation and intrauterine insemination.

- Preimplantation genetic diagnosis (PGD): In this procedure, the embryos created through IVF are tested for genetic defects. The purpose is to allow the parents to make the decision about whether to continue with implantation or discard the embryos. This procedure is usually performed when either the male or female is a known carrier of specific disease conditions, when the female is over 35 years of age, or where there is a history of repeated miscarriage.

Complementary Therapies

Nutraceuticals

The following nutraceuticals are used to ensure sufficient levels of antioxidants and decrease systemic inflammation:

- Eicosapentaenoic acid (EPA) and docosahexaenoic acid (DHA): EPA and DHA are involved in the synthesis of the anti-inflammatory prostaglandins.
- Vitamin B_6: Food sources include, brewer's yeast, brown rice, whole grains, chicken, eggs, and fish.
- Selenium: Food source includes brewer's yeast, meats, seafood, brown rice, whole grains, and nuts.
- Vitamin E: Food sources include nuts, vegetable oils, and wheat germ.
- Beta-carotene: Food sources include brightly colored fruits and vegetables.
- Zinc: Food sources include most meats, some fish, wheat germ, cashew nuts, cocoa, beans, and spinach.
- Vitamin C: Food sources include citrus fruits.
- Iron: Increased iron is recommended if anemia is found to be a probable cause of the infertility. Food sources include red meats, green leafy vegetables, whole grains, liver, fish, and eggs.
- Chasteberry (Vitex): Chasteberry is recommended if hyperprolactinemia is a cause of infertility.
- Black cohosh (Remifemin) and ginseng: These herbs are purported to influence the hypothalamic–pituitary–ovarian axis.

Acupuncture

- Multiple studies have demonstrated the positive effects of acupuncture alone, electroacupuncture, and acupuncture and herb combinations in infertility management. The results of studies on the efficacy of acupuncture as an adjuvant in IVF are mixed.

Massage

- Massage is used for general relaxation and to decrease hypertonicity and trigger points in the pelvic muscles. Specific muscle-stripping and muscle-release techniques applied to the adductors and psoas are anecdotally reported to restore menstrual bleeding and ovulatory cycles.

Manual Therapies

- Manual therapy, including spinal manipulation and whole-body mobilization of structures affecting reproductive function, are used with women diagnosed as infertile as a result of mechanical causes.

CLINICAL PEARL

Clinics success rates for most of the assisted reproductive techniques are available at the Centers for Disease Control and Prevention (CDC) website. See http://nccd.cdc.gov/DRH_ART/Apps/FertilityClinicReport.aspx or http://www.cdc.gov/art/reports/index.html.

Premature Ovarian Failure

Premature ovarian failure (POF) is the appearance of menopausal symptoms in women younger than age 40. In POF, there is amenorrhea, hypoestrogenism, and elevated serum gonadotrophin.

TECHNICAL NOTE

The hypothalamic–pituitary–ovarian axis is regulated by several hormones, including estradiol, androgens, and inhibins that are secreted by the ovarian follicles. One dominant follicle typically matures with each cycle; however, its maturation is dependent on the development of thousands of nondominant follicles. Conditions that are caused by a reduction in the numbers of these nondominant follicles often manifest with a decline of the ovarian hormones, subsequent elevation of the pituitary hormones, and an overall disruption in the hypothalamic–pituitary–ovarian axis.

Epidemiology

POF can only occur in women under the age of 40. Ovarian failure after the age of 40 is considered to be a normal menopausal state. Approximately 1% of women will experience menopause before the age of 40.

Etiology

POF can be spontaneous or iatrogenically induced. Spontaneous ovarian failure is presumed to fall into two broad categories:

- Follicular depletion as a result of a depleted follicle reserve, a low initial number of follicles, or an accelerated rate of follicle atresia
- Follicle dysfunction as a result of failure to grow and ovulate while under the influence of otherwise normally functioning endocrine systems. (e.g., a follicle that, instead of progressing to normal ovulation, is inappropriately luteinized and persists as a cyst)

Proposed causes for spontaneous POF include the following:

- Genetic defects: X chromosome genes are involved in regulating female fertility. Evidence suggests that half of patients with partial deletions of the short arm of the X chromosome have amenorrhea. Other chromosomal aberrations that have been implicated in POF include the following:
  - Turner syndrome
  - Trisomy 13 and 18, which are associated with ovarian dysgenesis and failure
  - 46 XX, which is affiliated with gonadal dysgenesis
  - Abnormalities of the forkhead transcription factor gene located on chromosome 3q22–23, which are known to result in resistant ovaries (ovaries containing many follicles that do not develop) and subsequent ovarian depletion
- Enzyme deficiencies: Enzyme deficiencies that have been affiliated with ovarian failure include the following:
  - Cholesterol desmolase deficiency, which results in lipid-filled adrenals and a lack of ovarian function

- Deficiency of 17 alpha-hydroxylase, which results in ovarian failure as a result of impaired ovarian and adrenal hormone synthesis
- POF deficiency of the 17–20 desmolase enzyme, a part of the 17 alpha-hydroxylase cytochrome P450 complex, which results in low serum estrogens, high gonadotropins, enlarged ovaries with multiple cysts, and amenorrhea
- Deficiency of the aromatase enzyme needed for synthesis of estrogen and found in adipose tissues, which has been demonstrated to result in a lack of pubertal development, high serum gonadotropin levels, and multiple ovarian cysts
- Autoimmune disorders, including the following:
  - Adrenal autoimmunity
  - Addison's disease
  - Antiovarian antibodies
  - Type 1 diabetes
  - Hashimoto's thyroiditis, with or without hypothyroidism
  - Lupus
  - Rheumatoid arthritis
  - Sjogren's syndrome
- Infection with mumps, malaria, or varicella: These infections have been noted in women with POF; however, a direct cause-and-effect relationship has not been established.
- Cleaning solvents: There is evidence that some women have developed POF following exposure to cleaning solvents containing the agent 2-bromopropane. In some cases, the ovaries recover spontaneously, and regular menstrual cycles may ensue, although reduced fertility and increased serum FSH levels may persist.

Iatrogenic ovarian failure is caused by follicular developmental arrest and follicular depletion resulting from damage to the granulosa cells and the oocytes. In addition, interstitial fibrosis and hyalinization of blood vessels may occur.

Iatrogenic causes include the following:

- Bilateral oophorectomy
- Chemotherapy
- Radiation therapy
- Bone-marrow transplant
- Treatment with Busulfan, a chemotherapy drug used in the treatment of conditions such as leukemia
  - The ovarian cells are sensitive tissues that respond adversely to systemic treatments such as chemotherapy, radiation therapy, gonadal irritation, and various forms of cancer therapy. Following bone-marrow transplant and therapy with busulfan, the majority of women develop ovarian failure.

Signs and Symptoms

- Amenorrhea before the age of 40
- Early onset of menopausal-like symptoms as a result of a prolonged hypoestrogenic state, including the following:
  - Hot flashes
  - Mood swings/irritability
  - Decreased libido
  - Dyspareunia
  - Night sweats
  - Cognitive changes
  - Sleep disturbances
  - Vaginal dryness
  - Atrophic vaginitis
  - Symptoms of hypothyroidism

Diagnosis

Detailed History

- Menstrual history, including last spontaneous menstrual cycle, time of menarche, and previous menstrual patterns
- History of pelvic surgeries, radiation, or chemotherapy
- Prior exposure to toxic environmental agents

- History of infection
- Symptoms of adrenal insufficiency, including the following:
  - Orthostatic hypotension
  - Skin hyperpigmentation
  - Unexplained weakness
  - Salt craving
  - Abdominal pain
  - Anorexia
- Symptoms of hypothyroidism
- Family history of POF
- Family history of male intellectual disability
- Family history of autoimmune disorders

CLINICAL PEARL

The history of a patient with POF can be variable, depending on the pathogenesis. In cases of spontaneous ovarian failure, the typical scenario is a sudden onset of amenorrhea, usually after discontinuation of oral contraceptives or after a pregnancy. In as many as 50% of cases, a long history of oligomenorrhea and polymenorrhea, with or without menopausal symptoms, is present. In 10% of the affected women, POF presents as primary amenorrhea. Occasionally, menopausal symptoms appear before the menses have stopped.

Physical Examination

- Signs of hypoestrogenism
- Presence/absence of palpable ovaries
- Physical signs of Turner syndrome or other genetic syndromes, including the following:
  - Short stature
  - Webbed neck
  - Low position of the ears
  - Low posterior hairline
  - Cubitus valgus

- Shield chest (widely spaced nipples)
- Short fourth and fifth metacarpals
- Signs of autoimmune diseases, Addison disease, and hypothyroidism

Laboratory Testing

- Pregnancy test
- FSH, LH, estradiol
  - Two FSH levels in the menopausal range of over 40 mIU/mL measured at least 1 month apart are diagnostic of POF.
  - LH is typically elevated.
  - Estradiol levels are low.

TECHNICAL NOTE

In some cases, women with POF have spontaneous follicular activity, which may result in erroneous lab results. If the index of suspicion for POF is high, the tests are repeated within 2 months.

Additional Testing

- Standard blood chemistry—fasting glucose, electrolytes, and creatinine
- Karyotyping
- Test for fragile X chromosome (*FMR1* premutation)
- TSH
- Antithyroid peroxidase antibody
- Serum adrenal antibodies
- Screening for other autoimmune disorders
- Bone density by dual-energy x-ray absorptiometry (DEXA) scan
- Screening and testing for exposure to environmental and other toxins

Ovarian biopsy and ultrasound are not recommended in this diagnostic evaluation.

Differential Diagnosis

Differential diagnosis should include the following:

- Pregnancy
- Secondary ovarian failure as a result of factors such as eating disorders and intense exercise
- Systemic diseases, such as Addison's disease
- Medications
- PCOS
- Outflow-tract abnormalities

Other symptoms caused by prolonged hypoestrogenism include osteoporosis and a higher risk for cardiovascular disease.

Management

There is no proven cure for infertile patients with POF. Assisted conception with donated oocytes and hormonal therapy are most commonly used. Embryo ovarian tissue and oocyte cryopreservation is recommended in cases where ovarian failure may be anticipated, such as when chemotherapy, radiation, and other cancer treatments are necessary.

Treatments are designed to manage the accelerated menopausal state and hypoandrogenism.

Conventional

- Medications
  - Hormonal replacement therapy, age-related dose
  - Oral contraceptives
  - TSH and adrenal antibodies
  - Short-term androgen replacement for women with persistent fatigue and low libido
  - DEXA bone-density scan
  - Supplementation with calcium, magnesium, vitamin D, vitamin K, and trace minerals
  - Specific medications for osteoporosis prevention and management

- Weight-bearing exercises to prevent osteoporosis
- Psychological evaluation and counseling for the grief and loss associated with a diagnosis of POF

CLINICAL PEARL

Anecdotal reports have suggested that high-dose, long-term prednisone therapy may be useful in treating autoimmune ovarian failure. However, prednisone, when used in high doses for long periods of time, has substantial side effects, including aseptic necrosis of bone.

Complementary

Complementary and integrative medicine strategies in POF focus on palliative care.

Nutraceuticals

- *Rhodiola rosea*
- Flaxseed
- Milk thistle, dandelion root, beet root, and burdock root for liver support
- Black cohosh, 40 mg of the standardized extract twice daily
- Maca root
- Chasteberry (Vitex)
- Partridge berry
- Yarrow
- Calcium
- Vitamin D
- Trace minerals

Acupuncture

There is preliminary evidence that acupuncture may decrease serum FSH and LH levels and raise serum estradiol levels in women with POF.

> **TECHNICAL NOTE**
>
> The risk of osteoporosis is high in patients with premature ovarian failure. Estrogen therapy is currently the choice method for preventing osteoporosis in women with POF.

> **TECHNICAL NOTE**
>
> Ovarian failure as a result of inappropriate regulatory signals (hypothalamic or pituitary pathology) is secondary ovarian failure. Ovarian failure as a result of a pathological process directly affecting the ovaries (e.g., chemotherapy, irradiation, autoimmunity, chromosomal abnormalities) is primary ovarian failure.
>
> A means of distinguishing between the two conditions is to measure serum FSH and LH levels, which will be elevated in primary ovarian failure and low or normal in secondary ovarian failure.
>
> Many women with POF retain intermittent ovarian function for many years, and unlike in women who are menopausal, pregnancies may spontaneously occur.

> **CLINICAL PEARL**
>
> The human papillomavirus (HPV) vaccine may be a risk factor for POF in adolescence.

Self-Care and Wellness

- Follow a whole-foods diet. A whole-foods diet involves eating a less-processed, predominantly plant-based diet and is increasingly evidenced in the research to be associated with health promotion and disease prevention.
- Facilitate endocrine system detoxification, which involves harnessing the inner strengths of the endocrine organs by maximizing liver function. Endocrine system detoxification begins with a healthy, plant-based diet and may include nutraceutical support, such as maca and silymarin, which are purported to balance hormones and detoxify the liver. Endocrine system

cleansing may involve detailed cleanses for the adrenal glands and liver (see the Appendix for examples of liver and adrenal detox plans).

- Manage stress.

PERIMENOPAUSE AND MENOPAUSE

Perimenopause

Perimenopause is the phase prior to menopause. For many women, this can begin as early as age 35. Perimenopause for some women is an easy transition with minimal symptoms. For other women, perimenopause is rife with adolescence-like symptoms that manifest as the adrenal glands, ovaries, and pituitary gland undergo transition.

Epidemiology

Women experience perimenopausal symptoms primarily in their 30s and 40s.

Etiology

- Perimenopause is a normal phase of transition. It is marked by some of the same symptoms that occur during adolescence, another period of major hormonal transition. The hormonal environment in perimenopause (unlike in menopause) is tumultuous.
- Perimenopausal symptoms may be compounded by factors such as adrenal dysfunction, anovulatory cycles, and poor dietary habits.

Adrenal Dysfunction

The demands of work, family, children, aging parents, and society at large place undue stresses on many women. The result is a perpetual flight-or-fight cycle. The adrenal glands, which are designed to function only in times of danger, function constantly, releasing norepinephrine and epinephrine from the adrenal medulla and corticoids, mineral corticoids, and androgens from the adrenal cortex.

The mineral corticoids (primarily aldosterone) regulate the balance of minerals (sodium, potassium, and magnesium) in the cells. Stress triggers the release of aldosterone, which raises blood pressure by influencing cells to hold on to sodium and lose potassium. Long-term release of stress-level mineral corticoids can cause potassium deficiency, magnesium imbalance, chronic water retention, and high blood pressure. The resultant magnesium insufficiency, as noted by serum red blood cell magnesium levels, can affect many of the enzyme-driven metabolic pathways in the body.

In addition, the adrenal cortex makes all the sex hormones in small amounts and dehydroepiandrosterone (DHEA) in large amounts. DHEA is important in the growth and repair of protein tissues and is a precursor to androstenediol, testosterone, and estrogens. It is not a precursor to progesterone, aldosterone, pregnenolone, or cortisols. Alterations in the normal production of the hormones of the adrenal cortex can predispose women to multiple symptoms of perimenopause, including aggression and anger from too much testosterone; passivity, oversensitivity, mental confusion, and agitation from too much or too little estrogen; and depression from too little estrogen or progesterone.

Anovulatory Cycles

Ovulation becomes increasingly infrequent, the follicular phase is extended, and estrogen levels remain sustained for longer periods. In the absence of ovulation, progesterone is not released in adequate quantities, and progesterone deficiency, estrogen dominance, or both may result.

Poor Dietary Habits

Inadequate intake or absorption of many vitamins and minerals (e.g., vitamins C, E, and A; beta-carotene; and iron) impairs the functioning of many organ systems. The results of these dietary, hormonal, and lifestyle aberrations may manifest as fatigue, high blood pressure, uterine fibroids, mood swings, and several other identified symptoms of perimenopause.

Signs and Symptoms

- Increasing vaginal dryness
- Decreased libido
- Acne
- Generalized fatigue
- Increasing blood pressure
- Endometriosis
- Uterine fibroids
- Symptoms of increased cortisol, which include papery (thin) skin, weight gain around the midsection, memory loss, blood sugar imbalances, and muscle wasting
- Mood swings
- Chronic fatigue
- Diabetes
- Menorrhagia and other menstrual irregularities
- Hot flashes
- Sleep disturbances
- Bladder problems
- Loss of bone mineral density

Diagnosis

- Blood hormonal assays and salivary tests can be performed to guide symptomatic management. These include serum FSH, estrogen, and thyroid function. In addition, saliva may be used to assess DHEA, cortisol, estrogen, progesterone, and testosterone.
- There are no known tests to determine how long a woman will be in perimenopause.

Management

Conventional

Medications

Symptom-specific medications include antidepressants, blood sugar modulators, and hormones.

Complementary

Nutraceuticals

Recommendations include the following:

- Resveratrol
- Tryptophanum
- Glycine
- Vitamin E
- Coenzyme Q10
- EPA/DHA
- DHEA
- Progesterone

Bioidentical Hormones

Bioidentical hormones are hormones manufactured to have similar molecular structures as those naturally produced in the body. An individualized approach is taken in using the information from the hormonal assay to compound specific dosages of estrogen, testosterone, DHEA, and other anabolic steroids. Patients are monitored carefully via symptom evaluation and subsequent hormonal panels.

TECHNICAL NOTE

Prolonged use of high-dose progesterone creams is not recommended. The potential risk of increasing the hormonal load, facilitating an estrogen-dominant state, and predisposing to estrogen-sensitive conditions such as breast cancer, endometriosis, and fibroids warrants caution.

CLINICAL PEARL

- Supplementing with DHEA improves sexual function in perimenopausal and menopausal women.
- DHEA supplementation may cause or worsen acne.

Self-Care and Wellness

- Exercise—a low- to medium-intensity exercise program
- Coping mechanisms such as biofeedback, yoga, and meditation

- Dietary management, including consumption of legumes, phytoestrogens, and filtered water and avoidance of sources of xenoestrogens
- Management for insulin resistance
- A good multivitamin with adequate dosages of calcium, magnesium, and the essential fatty acids
- Psychosocial and psychological factors, such as decreasing stress, developing and nurturing support systems, and recognizing that perimenopause is a phase of transition that can be managed

Menopause

Meno is the root word for *menses*, and *pausis* means "cessation." Menopause is the permanent cessation of menstrual activity. Every woman will go through menopause, which is a natural process of aging. The entire period covering the transition from perimenopause to menopause and beyond is called the climacteric.

CLINICAL PEARL

The principal circulating hormone during menopause is estrone; prior to menopause, it is estradiol. Estrone converts to estradiol and vice versa, with approximately 15% of estradiol converting to estrone and 5% of estrone converting to estradiol. Primary estrogen production shifts from the ovaries to the adrenal glands and peripheral tissues. The adrenal glands increase production of androstenedione. Androstenedione is converted to estrone by aromatase, an enzyme found in considerable quantities in fat cells. Aromatase also converts testosterone to estrone.

Epidemiology

For most women, menopause occurs around age 51.

Etiology

The number of ovarian follicles declines from approximately 6 million at birth to 10,000 at menopause. The ovarian follicles are responsible for the production of estrogen and progesterone. With the decline in the number of follicles, a corresponding decline in the levels of estrogen and progesterone occurs.

Signs and Symptoms

Some women transition through the menopause with minimal or no symptoms; for others, the symptoms are debilitating. Estrogen receptor sites have been found on the surface of virtually every tested cell, including cells of the retina, the skin, and various organs and organ systems. This might explain the broad range of symptoms experienced by women during the transition.

Primary menopausal symptoms include the following:

- Vasomotor—hot flashes, night sweats
- Genitourinary—atrophy, bladder infections, prolapse (including feelings of fullness or lump in the vagina), dragging sensation in the abdomen and lower back, changes in vaginal discharge, difficulty with coitus, and cystitis
- Psychosocial/psychological—depression, mood swings, sleep disturbances
- Cardiovascular—arrhythmia, atherosclerosis
- Skeletal—bone mineral density/osteoporosis

CLINICAL PEARL

Symptoms that have been associated with menopause but that may occur primarily as effects of aging include the following:
- Changes in appearance—weight gain, thinning hair, wrinkles
- Cognitive changes—diminished concentration

Diagnosis

- History and exam elicit amenorrhea for a period of 12 months.
- Blood analysis of FSH: As ovarian production of estrogen declines, the anterior pituitary produces more FSH in an attempt to increase estrogen production

- Levels of FSH that exceed 40 mIU/mL are an indication of menopause.
- Confirmation via hormonal levels requires more than one FSH analysis.

Symptom-Specific Management

Vasomotor

The cause of hot flashes remains unknown. Proposed causes include increased hypothalamic and pituitary activity in an effort to enhance FSH production and heat loss at the level of the arterioles instead of the capillaries and venules.

Conventional

Medications

- Estrogen or estrogen plus progesterone
- Progesterone in the form of megestrol acetate, formerly used for breast cancer treatment, which has been shown to reduce hot flashes
- Synthetic steroids such as tibolone (Livial, Tibofem)
- Antidepressants
  - Low doses of certain antidepressants, including venlafaxine (Effexor XR), and selective serotonin reuptake inhibitors (SSRIs), including paroxetine (Paxil), fluoxetine (Prozac), and citalopram (Celexa), have been found to reduce the depressive symptoms that may be associated with feelings of loss (loss of fertility, loss of youth, loss of family structure, loss of previously defined identity, etc.).
- Clonidine, a medication typically used for high blood pressure, which has been shown to decrease hot flashes in breast cancer survivors and to inhibit norepinephrine, thereby diminishing sympathetic nervous system activity

CLINICAL PEARL

According to Grant et al. (2015) estrogens are the most effective treatment for relieving vasomotor symptoms and are accompanied by the greatest improvement in quality-of-life measures.

TECHNICAL NOTE

The psychological and psychosocial changes in menopause are also partly a result of the changes in the levels of estrogen and progesterone and the concentration of neurotransmitters.

CLINICAL PEARL

Estrogen therapy at doses equivalent to 0.625 mg of conjugated equine estrogen increase the risk for stroke, deep venous thrombosis, and pulmonary embolism, and when combined with progestin medroxyprogesterone acetate, such doses result in increased risk for coronary events and breast cancer.

CLINICAL PEARL

Combined estrogen and testosterone use increases breast cancer risk.

Complementary

Nutraceuticals

- Black cohosh (Remifemin) as a dry herb or extract
- Vitamin E
- Fish oil

CLINICAL PEARL

Significant reduction in total cholesterol and low-density lipoprotein cholesterol (LDL-C) has been observed in perimenopausal and menopausal non-White and White women who received supplements with both vitamin E and fish oil.

CLINICAL PEARL

A significant body of research exists on the value of Remifemin in menopausal management. Earlier studies on the efficacy of black cohosh in the treatment of hot flashes were promising, but current research results are mixed.

Acupuncture

- Research evidence supports acupuncture for reducing the severity of hot flashes in some women. It remains unclear whether acupuncture treatment affects the frequency of hot flashes.

Bioidentical Hormones

- Bioidentical hormones are manufactured hormones that have a similar molecular structure as those naturally produced in the body. An individualized approach is taken in using the information from the hormonal assay to compound specific dosages of the steroid hormones. Careful monitoring via evaluation of symptoms and subsequent hormonal panels is required.

> **TECHNICAL NOTE**
>
> Bioflavonoids have been identified as hot-flash triggers in some women.

Self-Care and Wellness

- Keeping a diary of diet and lifestyle factors that occur with hot flashes might elicit a pattern.
- Dress in layers to facilitate temperature management.
- Engage in regular exercise, such as walking and yoga.
- Identify and avoid hot-flash triggers. Known triggers include stress, heat, caffeine, tomatoes, and berries.
- Taking supplements of the bioflavonoids naturally found in citrus fruit may help to relieve hot flashes.
- Ensure adequate levels of fiber intake.
- Eat a well-balanced diet.

Genitourinary Atrophy/Prolapse

Estrogen's functions include maintaining collagen levels in the skin and epithelial tissues, increasing vascular supply and fluid content of tissues, and enhancing tissue integrity.

Some of the changes resulting from menopausal decline of estrogen include the following:

- Atrophy of the vaginal, cervical, and uterine tissues
- Changes in the consistency and quantity of vaginal lubrication
- Thinning and drying out of the vulvar and vaginal tissues
- Prolapse
- Increased susceptibility to infection

Management

Conventional

- Local vaginal therapies
  - Vaginal estrogen creams
  - Vaginal estrogen ring
    - These may be contraindicated in women with a history of estrogen-dependent conditions such as fibroids and breast and uterine cancers.
  - Pessaries are used to mechanically support the descending tissues (see Figure 7-3)
- Physical therapy
  - Pelvic-floor (Kegel) exercises
  - Electrical therapies to increase the tone of the pelvic floor
- Surgery in severe cases

Complementary

Nutraceuticals

- Chasteberry (Vitex) to restore epithelial integrity
- Black cohosh, dry herb or extract
- Zinc and high-zinc foods, such as seafood (especially oysters), red meat and poultry, wheat germ, oats and other whole grains, beans, nuts, and fortified cereals
- Vitamins and minerals required for collagen synthesis and support of epithelial tissue, including manganese and vitamin C
- Flaxseed oil, which has phytoestrogenic qualities when used as a lubricant

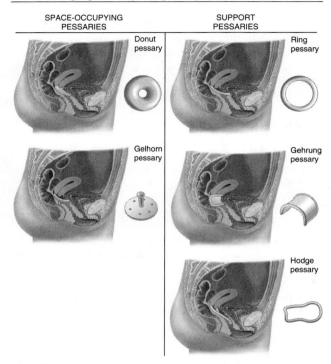

SPACE-OCCUPYING PESSARIES

Donut pessary

Gelhorn pessary

SUPPORT PESSARIES

Ring pessary

Gehrung pessary

Hodge pessary

Figure 7-3 Pessaries, which mechanically supports descending tissues

Manual Therapy/Spinal Manipulation

- Assessment for and correction of leg-length deficiency and other biomechanical factors that affect the patency of the pelvic floor may be recommended.
- Low-force full spine manipulation is anecdotally reported to improve overall sense of well-being during the climacteric.

Massage

- Massage therapy is anecdotally reported to improve overall sense of well-being during the climacteric.

Self-Care and Wellness

- Avoidance medications that cause mucosal dryness, including antihistamines and decongestants
- Kegel exercises (see the Appendix)
- Increased sexual activity (increased foreplay)

Prevention

Uterine and urinary bladder prolapse are best managed prophylactically. Strategies include prenatal and postnatal exercises such as Kegel exercises, knee–chest pulls on a slant board, gluteal contractions, pelvic rocking while squeezing a pillow between the knees, correcting for leg-length discrepancies, appropriate management of birth to prevent excessive tearing of the perineum, and ensuring that the pelvis is in proper alignment. Predisposing factors such as obesity and a chronic cough should be controlled. Heavy lifting and repeated stair climbing should be avoided.

Genitourinary Syndrome of Menopause/Atrophic Vaginitis

Atrophic vaginitis is inflammation of the vaginal epithelium, usually caused by a decrease in estrogen. It is a common manifestation of genitourinary atrophy.

Epidemiology

Atrophic vaginitis occurs primarily in postmenopausal women but can occur in women who have had a hysterectomy, are breast-feeding, are on progesterone-only birth control medications, or have premature ovarian failure. Although very rare, it may occur in premenarcheal children.

Etiology

Estrogens are responsible for keeping the vaginal tissue hydrated, filled with collagen, and elastic. The diminished levels of estrogen that occur in menopause cause the vaginal tissue to become atrophic, thin, and easily traumatized.

Signs and Symptoms

- Vaginal burning
- Pruritus
- Bleeding or spotting
- Pinkish discharge
- Dyspareunia

Diagnosis

- Pelvic exam reveals atrophic changes in the lower genital tract. The vaginal epithelium appears thin and transparent, with decreased rugal folds. It may also appear reddened. The vaginal discharge may be thin, watery, and blood-stained.
- Microscopic evaluation of the vaginal discharge may reveal inflammatory cells and epithelial cells.
- It is atypical to find *Trichomonas vaginalis*, *Gardnerella vaginalis*, or other pathogenic agents.

CLINICAL PEARL

Some of the symptoms of atrophic vaginitis may occur with other, more serious conditions, such as endometrial cancer and vaginal cancer. Women with these symptoms should first be evaluated for these conditions.

Management

Conventional

Medications
- Topical application of intravaginal estrogen cream
- Estrogen replacement therapy

Self-Care and Wellness

- Regular sexual activity, to improve blood circulation to the vagina
- Topical application of flaxseed oil or other lubricants

TECHNICAL NOTE

In 2014, the International Society for the Study of Women's Health and the North American Menopause Society jointly endorsed the term *genitourinary syndrome of menopause* (GSM) in lieu of *vulvovaginal atrophy*. GSM is defined as a collection of symptoms and signs associated with a decrease in estrogen and other sex steroids involving changes to the labia majora and labia minora, clitoris, vestibule/introitus, vagina, urethra, and bladder. The syndrome may include but is not limited to genital symptoms of dryness, burning, and irritation; sexual symptoms of lack of lubrication, discomfort or pain, and impaired function; and urinary symptoms of urgency, dysuria, and recurrent urinary tract infections.

CLINICAL PEARL

Estrogen therapy may be contraindicated in women with a history of liver disease, deep venous thrombosis, thrombophlebitis, or fibroids.

Psychosocial/Psychological

Menopause is a time of transition that is liberating for some but frightening and even depressing for others. Societal views on aging often affect this transition. In societies in which aging is viewed positively, menopausal symptoms do not appear to occur as frequently or with the same severity. It should be noted, however, that these frequently are societies where individuals are generally more physically active, and the diet is rich in cruciferous vegetables, fiber, soy-based products, and lignans. The added benefits of these products in modulating the hormonal transition have been documented.

The psychological and psychosocial changes in menopause are in part a result of the changes in hormonal levels of estrogen and progesterone and the concentrations of neurotransmitters.

Estrogens facilitate the release of the neurotransmitter norepinephrine in the brain and may decrease the action of monoamine oxidase. Estrogen also may aid in the functioning of serotonin, dopamine, and gamma-aminobutyric acid type A (GABAA), all of which have effects on the individual's mental state.

Management

Conventional

Medications

- Antidepressants: SSRIs such as fluoxetine (Prozac), sertraline (Zoloft), and paroxetine (Paxil) are frequently used. Referral to a mental health professional may be necessary.

Complementary

Nutraceuticals

- Hormonal system modulators such as chasteberry (Vitex)
- S-adenosyl-L-methionine (SAMe) to enhance serotonin function
- St. John's wort, which is known to inhibit serotonin uptake in the brain and to inhibit the enzyme catechol-o-methyltransferase, which degrades the neurotransmitter dopamine
  - As with any herb, caution is necessary because St. John's wort may decrease the efficacy of medications such as the protease inhibitors used in the treatment of HIV, the theophylline used in the treatment of asthma, blood thinners such as warfarin (Coumadin), and some chemotherapeutic agents. Patients who have been taking St. John's wort should not discontinue the herb abruptly because this may increase systemic levels of other medications.
- Management of adrenal insufficiency, symptoms of which include depression, loss of libido, and total exhaustion
  - Supplementation with DHEA is anecdotally reported to improve mood. DHEA converts to testosterone, which converts to estrogen, resulting in an increased estrogen load. This is of benefit to women whose symptoms are associated

with estrogen insufficiency; however, the potential negative impact of the increased estrogen load on estrogen-related cancers should not be minimized. Recommendations are for the lowest dosage possible. Levels should be monitored with blood analysis.

- Licorice root as a tea or tincture is used to support adrenal function.
- Ashwagandha root as a capsule or dry herb is used to support adrenal function.

TECHNICAL NOTE

Licorice root can increase blood pressure and cause water retention. To mitigate for this, it is advisable to use deglycyrrhizinated licorice.

Self-Care and Wellness

- Lifestyle factors such as sleeping in the dark and avoiding the use of nightlights can aid the function of the pineal gland, which is responsible for melatonin synthesis. Melatonin is needed for sleep.
- Ensure a well-rounded, whole-foods diet.
- Engage in mild- to moderate-intensity exercise on most days of the week.

CLINICAL PEARL

The major source of estradiol in postmenopausal women is the conversion of estrone to estradiol by the enzyme aromatase, which is present in adipose cells.

For More Information

- Adrenal dysfunction: See the section Adrenal Dysfunction in Chapter 10.
- Bladder Infections in menopause: See Chapter 13.

- Cardiovascular involvement: See Chapter 4.
- Osteoporosis: See the section Osteoporosis in Chapter 10.

TECHNICAL NOTE

Blood levels of estradiol before menopause are 40 to 350 pg/mL; in menopause, blood levels drop to less than 15 pg/mL. The ovaries are the predominant producer of estradiol, with the adrenal glands contributing approximately 4% to total circulating estradiol and the placenta also contributing during pregnancy.

PREGNANCY

Pregnancy is the period marking the development of a fertilized egg. *Pregnancy* is the term used to describe the state in which a person carries and nurtures the fertilized egg within the body. It is the period from conception to birth.

The fertilized egg migrates through the fallopian tube to the uterine cavity and implants in the endometrium. The process from fertilization in the tubes to implantation in the uterine cavity is approximately 6 days (see Figure 7-4). Following implantation and over a period of several weeks, the lining of the uterus will morphologically change to become the decidua, which further differentiates to become the placenta. The placenta provides nourishment for the developing embryo for approximately 9 months.

TECHNICAL NOTE

Terminology for women in relation to pregnancy is as follows:
- Nulliparous: No viable offspring
- Primiparous: First pregnancy completed with viable offspring
- Multiparous: Two to five completed pregnancies with viable offspring
- Grand multiparous: Six or more completed pregnancies with viable offspring

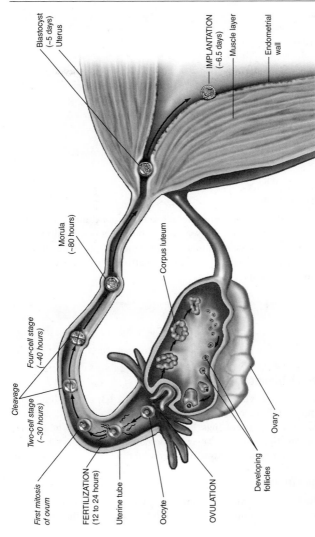

Figure 7-4 The first week

TECHNICAL NOTE

When an app is not available, the estimated due date (EDD) can be calculated as follows:

First day of last menstrual period + 7 days – 3 months + 1 year

For example, if the first day of last menstrual period is May 2, 2015 (5-2-2015):

5-2-2015 + 7 days = 5-9-2015
5-9-2015 – 3 days = 2-9-2015
2-9-2015 + 1 year = 2-9-2016

The EDD is February 9, 2016.

Signs and Symptoms

First Trimester

Maternal symptoms may include but are not limited to fatigue, increased urination, nausea and vomiting, generalized malaise, breast tenderness and enlargement, amenorrhea or oligomenorrhea, increased abdominal girth, heartburn, constipation, food cravings, and dizziness.

CLINICAL PEARL

Sore breasts are one of the first indications that a woman has that she is pregnant.

Second Trimester

Maternal signs and symptoms may include but are not limited to a noticeable increase in weight, greater fatigue, fluid retention, indigestion, food cravings, light-headedness, dizziness, heartburn, gas, constipation, varicose veins, hemorrhoids, and stretch marks. False labor pains (Braxton Hicks contractions) may begin to occur.

Third Trimester

Maternal signs and symptoms may include but are not limited to Braxton Hicks contractions, stretching and pain in the lower ribs, indigestion as the abdominal cavity becomes increasingly cramped, sleeping difficulties, breathing difficulties, frequent urination, low back pain, medial thigh pain, symphysis pubis pain, groin pain, constipation, tingling and numbness in the hands and extremities, swelling in the feet, and anxiety.

Women may also experience lightening, the slight descent of the uterus when the head of the fetus drops into the birth canal in preparation for delivery. This is marked by increased bladder frequency and increased ability to breathe.

Diagnosis

- HCG: The presence of HCG in maternal serum or urine is an indication of pregnancy. Beta HCG is detected in maternal serum and urine 8 to 10 days after conception; at this point, implantation has occurred, and vascular connections have been established between the syncytiotrophoblast and the decidua. HCG is detectable in 98% of patients by day 7 in urine and within 24 to 48 hours in serum.
- By presenting signs and symptoms: See the previous section on first-trimester symptoms.

TECHNICAL NOTE

HCG is a glycoprotein that is similar in structure to FSH and LH. The free beta subunit of HCG is degraded by enzymes in the kidney to a beta subunit core fragment, which is primarily detected in urine samples.

TECHNICAL NOTE

To estimate gestational age in the second trimester and through week 38, measure from the pubic symphysis to the superior aspect of the uterus with a measuring tape. The measurements can be correlated as follows:
- At 16 weeks, the fundus is midway between the pubic symphysis and the umbilicus.
- At 20 weeks, the fundus is at the umbilicus.
- At 14 to 38 weeks, the measurement in centimeters is equal to the number of weeks of gestation.

Diagnostic Tests During Pregnancy

- Fundal height
- Blood pressure
- Pap smears to rule out cervical cancer and sexually transmitted diseases and a vaginal culture to rule out group B streptococcus
- Urinalysis to rule out infections and elevated sugars and proteins
- Ultrasound to evaluate the fetus at various stages of development

Blood Tests—First Trimester

- Blood type and antibody screen, including rhesus factor
- Hematocrit and hemoglobin to rule out anemia
- Hepatitis B virus
- HIV
- Rubella
- Syphilis

Blood Tests—Second and Third Trimesters

- Hematocrit and hemoglobin to rule out anemia
- One-hour screen (oral glucose tolerance test) for gestational diabetes

Specialized Tests

- Maternal alpha-fetoprotein (AFP) or expanded AFP testing, which includes estriol and HCG to screen for neural tube defects, Down syndrome, and other chromosome abnormalities (Note: False-positive results are not uncommon.)
- Amniocentesis
- Evaluation for birth defects
  - This testing is performed at 16 to 18 weeks and may be recommended if either parent has an inheritable disease, if the parents have a child who has an inherited disease, or if the mother is over age 35.

- Evaluation of fetal maturity when repeat cesarean section is planned
  - This testing is performed at 38 to 39 weeks.
- Evaluation of fetal maturity in high-risk pregnancies
  - Pregnancies may be considered high risk when the mother has high blood pressure, diabetes, or rhesus disease; when there is evidence of inadequate fetal growth; and when the mother is overdue by over 2 weeks. The risk of the procedure causing miscarriage is approximately 0.5% to 2%.

Nutrition and Pregnancy

At no other time of life are the nutritional needs of the female more important than during pregnancy. Adequate intake of fresh fruits, whole grains, vegetables, proteins, calcium, vitamin A, vitamin D, iron, and folic acid is critical. A prenatal multivitamin is necessary for most women.

An increased amount of folic acid is recommended preconceptually to prevent open neural tube defects.

CLINICAL PEARLS

- Vegetarian diets may result in deficiencies in protein, iodine, iron, and folate.
- Iodized salt is recommended over sea salt to ensure proper functioning of the thyroid gland.
- Tofu is an excellent source of protein for vegetarians, but it may contain bacteria. Unpackaged tofu should not be eaten during pregnancy, and packaged tofu should be cooked to an internal temperature of 160°F.

Weight Gain in Pregnancy

Emphasis should be placed on the quality of the diet rather than the amount of weight gained; however, during the second half of the pregnancy, caloric intake should increase by about 10%.

Table 7-3 Approximate Weight-Gain Distribution in Pregnancy

Baby: 7–8 lb
Placenta: 2–3 lb
Amniotic fluid: 2–3 lb
Uterus: 2–4 lb
Breasts: 2–3 lb
Blood: 3–4 lb
Fluid retained in body tissues: 2–3 lb
Maternal fat storage required for delivery and breastfeeding: 5–7 lb
Total: 25–35 lb

A total weight gain of 25 to 35 lb is generally recommended. Actual weight gain is patient specific; some women can gain more and still maintain a healthy pregnancy.

See Table 7-3 for approximate weight-gain distribution in pregnancy.

Exercise and Pregnancy

Exercise helps prepare a women's body for labor and delivery, and when done in moderation, it poses no danger to the mother or baby. Exercise may help with constipation, backache, edema, and poor posture.

Continuing an exercise routine or starting a new routine of 30 minutes of moderate exercise daily is advised. (Moderate exercise implies that the patient can carry on a conversation but is slightly out of breath.)

Specific exercises recommended during pregnancy include the following:

- 200 Kegel exercises/day
- 40 squats/day
- 60 pelvic tucks/day
- 20 minutes of walking/day

Pregnancy is not the time to begin a strenuous exercise program, and the following cautions and restrictions should also be considered:

- Activities that may result in decreased oxygen to the fetus should be avoided. These include strenuous activity, scuba diving, sprinting, competitive exercise, high-altitude training, and contact sports. In addition, activities where water can be forced into the vagina should be avoided, including water skiing and surfing.
- Exercise should be avoided or minimized in hot, humid weather because elevated body temperatures have been linked to birth defects.
- Any exercise that causes spotting or bleeding should be discontinued.
- To avoid the risk of dehydration, drinking plenty of fluids while exercising is recommended.

CLINICAL PEARL

Hot yoga should be avoided in pregnancy because there is an increased risk of neural tube defects among fetuses exposed to excessive heat.

According to the American College of Obstetricians and Gynecologists (2015), the following are contraindications to exercise during pregnancy:

- Preeclampsia or pregnancy induced hypertension
- Severe anemia
- Restrictive lung disease
- Hemodynamically significant heart disease
- Premature rupture of membranes
- Premature labor during the prior or current pregnancy
- Incompetent cervix or cerclage
- Persistent second or third trimester bleeding
- Placenta previa after 26 weeks of gestation
- Intrauterine growth retardation

TECHNICAL NOTE

The heart rate should remain in a specific range according to age. The range can be determined with the following equations:

$$\text{lower limit: } (220 - \text{Age}) \times .60$$
$$\text{upper limit: } (220 - \text{Age}) \times .70$$

For example, a 32-year-old female's target heart rate can be determined as follows:

$$220 - 32 = 188$$
$$188 \times .60 = 112$$
$$188 \times .70 = 131$$

$$\text{range} = 112–131 \text{ beats/min}$$

Heart-rate recovery following exercise should be less than 110 at 5 minutes and less than 100 at 10 minutes.

Management

The following section briefly summarizes etiology and protocols for managing select conditions in pregnancy.

Conditions

1. Bleeding gums
2. Breathing difficulties
3. Dehydration
4. Diabetes
5. Diastasis rectus abdominus
6. Dizziness
7. Fluid retention
8. Groin pain
9. Headaches
10. Heartburn
11. Increased vaginal discharge
12. In utero constraint
13. Low back pain

14. Morning sickness
15. Preeclampsia
16. Premature contractions
17. Pubic diastasis
18. Rhesus factor
19. Snoring
20. Spontaneous abortion (miscarriage)
21. Thoracic outlet syndrome
22. Tipped uterus
23. Urinary frequency
24. Urinary urgency

CLINICAL PEARL

Adequate maternal intake of fruits and vegetables decreases the risk of conditions such as diabetes, neural tube defects, and orofacial clefts; however, plant-based diets warrant vigilance to ensure sufficient intake of such nutrients as vitamin B_12, iron, zinc, omega-3 fatty acids, and iodine.

CLINICAL PEARL

Increased maternal consumption of linoleic acid may decrease the risk of autism spectrum disorder.

Bleeding Gums

Etiology
- Inadequate nutrition
- Poor dental hygiene
- Increased vascularity

Management
- Prenatal vitamin with vitamin C
- Vitamin C
- Meticulous dental hygiene
- Dental consult if warranted

Breathing Difficulties

Etiology

The enlarging uterus restricts diaphragm excursion and can lead to anterior rotation of the pectoral girdle.

Management

- Trigger-point therapy and deep-tissue massage for the following muscles: pectoralis major and minor; anterior, middle, and posterior scalenes; levator scapula; sternocleidomastoid (SCM); rhomboids; serratus anterior; trapezius
- Lateral and posterior ribcage expansion techniques to foster deeper diaphragmatic breathing patterns
- Diaphragm release techniques

Dehydration

Management

Dehydration in pregnancy is best managed prophylactically. The patient should be regularly reminded to monitor fluid intake and to drink 8 to 12 glasses of water daily.

Diabetes (Gestational Diabetes)

Gestational diabetes, the more common form of diabetes in pregnancy, occurs in approximately 4% of pregnant women and is more common in women who are overweight, are over age 35, or have a history of larger babies.

Etiology

The actual cause of gestational diabetes is unknown; however, it is thought that the placental hormones may block the action of the mother's insulin, thereby causing insulin resistance and, ultimately, diabetes.

CLINICAL PEARL

Gestational diabetes may increase the risk of developing diabetes mellitus later in life.

Risk Factors

- Female over the age of 35
- A previous baby weighing over 9 lb
- Obesity
- African ancestry
- Hispanic ancestry
- Gestational diabetes in a previous pregnancy
- Recurrent infections

Diagnosis

- Glucose tolerance test
- One-hour postprandial
- Rate of weight gain

Management

- Intense monitoring of nutritional practices, including the following:
  - Carbohydrate content
  - Caloric intake
  - Fat content
- Ketone testing for patients on hypocaloric or carbohydrate-restricted diets
- Regular mild to moderate exercise
- Insulin or other medications

Note: Oral medications can cross the placenta and affect the baby's development. Because of the limited number of studies analyzing the effects of oral diabetic medications on the baby, the American Diabetes Association (2016) does not recommend their use during pregnancy.

CLINICAL PEARL

Diagnosis of gestational diabetes frequently occurs during the second or third trimester, when the rate of weight gain is typically 3/4 to 1 lb/week. Many women are gaining weight at a rate of nearly 2 lb/week when they are diagnosed. Placing less emphasis on the total weight gain and greater emphasis on the rate of weight gain (i.e., approximately 1 lb/week) is an effective strategy.

TECHNICAL NOTE

According to the American Diabetes Association (2016), normal values for blood glucose levels in pregnancy are as follows:

	Whole Blood, mg/dL	Plasma, mg/dL
Fasting	60–90	69–104
Before meals	60–105	69–121
1 hour after meals	100–120	115–138
2 a.m.–6 a.m.	60–120	69–138

Data from American Diabetes Association. (2016). Management of diabetes in pregnancy. *Diabetes Care, 39*(Suppl 1), S94–8.

Diastasis Rectus Abdominus

Diastasis rectus abdominus is a separation of the fascial connection between the bellies of the right and left rectus abdominus muscles.

Etiology

- Unknown
- Familial
- Weakened core abdominal muscles

Signs and Symptoms

- None
- Bulging in the midline of the abdomen
- Separation at the midline of the abdomen
- Low back pain

Diagnosis

- Physical examination
- Observed separation of 1 in. or greater in the sit-up position
- Observed visible bulge

Management

- Core-strengthening exercises
- Assisted abdominal crunches and abdominal exercises on the slant board
- Abdominal surgery if severe

Dizziness or Light-Headedness

Etiology

- Low blood pressure as a result of the decreased blood volume secondary to the rapid dilation of the blood vessels during the first half of the pregnancy
- More common in the second trimester of pregnancy when the blood vessels have dilated in response to the hormones of pregnancy, but the blood volume is not yet enough to fill the blood vessels

Management

- Prenatal multivitamins
- Adequate hydration
- Avoidance of prolonged standing
- Rising slowly from both supine and seated positions
- Avoidance of long, hot showers; saunas; and hot tubs
- Foods rich in iron, such as beans, spinach, red meats, and chicken

Fluid Retention Symptoms

Etiology

- Carpal tunnel syndrome if edema compromises the carpal tunnel
- Tarsal tunnel syndrome if edema results in compression of the tibial nerve in the tarsal tunnel
- Swollen feet and ankles

TECHNICAL NOTE

Rapid fluid retention may be an indication of preeclampsia in pregnancy.

Management

- Ensure adequate protein intake because inadequate protein is a primary cause of fluid retention.

- Complementary and integrative medicine approaches for carpel and tarsal tunnel symptoms include the following:
  - Spinal manipulation and joint mobilization along with rehabilitative exercise, ultrasound, and interferential therapies to the carpel and tarsal tunnels
  - Trigger-point therapy to the supporting muscles
  - Neutral wrist splints
- Complementary and integrative medicine approaches for swollen feet and ankles may necessitate craniosacral release techniques to the pelvic diaphragm if the pelvic fascia is restricted.

Groin Pain

Etiology

- Misalignment of the symphysis pubis bone
- Symphysis pubis diastasis, which produces sharp and sometimes incapacitating pain
- Round ligament pain as the uterus enlarges during pregnancy

Management

- Realignment of the pubic ramus
- Massage and trigger-point therapy to the pelvic muscles and round ligament

Headaches

Etiology

Headaches in pregnancy can be caused by many factors, including the following:

- Hormonal effects on blood vessel dilation
- Suboccipital muscle strain
- Strain and trigger points in the posterior cervical and upper back muscles
- Subluxation of the cervical and cervicothoracic vertebrae
- Elevated blood pressure or preeclampsia
- Overall stress and strain

Management
- Carefully identify and manage the contributing cause or causes
- Teach coping strategies

> **CLINICAL PEARL**
>
> Coping strategies might include the following: cold compresses, deep-breathing techniques, massage, tracking and avoiding headache triggers, biofeedback, adequate sleep/regular sleep schedule, mild to moderate physical activity, and delegation of tasks.

Heartburn

Etiology

Heartburn is caused by the backward flow of stomach acids into the esophagus as a result of factors such as restrictions in the respiratory diaphragm, sluggish digestion, poor dietary choices, and an enlarging uterus.

Management

Lifestyle
- Smaller meals eaten several times during the day
- Avoidance of known heartburn triggers
- Avoidance of lying down within 30 minutes of eating a meal
- Complementary and integrative methods: craniosacral therapy release techniques for the respiratory diaphragm; use of the hiatal hernia maneuver (see the Appendix)

Increased Vaginal Discharge

Etiology

Increased vaginal discharge is an almost universal occurrence during pregnancy that is a result of turnover of the cells lining the vaginal vault. The hormonally induced thickening of the vaginal vault can cause leukorrhea, a thin, white, odorless discharge that is normal but should still be reported to the health-care provider.

Management

This condition usually does not require treatment.

In Utero Constraint

In utero constraint is the term used to describe some of the external forces that obstruct the normal movements of the fetus. This constraint may prevent the developing fetus from achieving the head-down vertex position in preparation for vaginal birth. Breech presentation is a primary reason for many cesarean sections.

Etiology

The causes of in utero constraint are multiple and include sacrum subluxation, hypertonic muscles, and stress and fatigue in the mother.

Management

Complementary and integrative methods include the Webster technique, a technique used specifically with pregnant mothers in the third trimester to relieve the musculoskeletal causes of in utero constraint. The technique involves adjusting the sacrum for misalignment and gentle massage to the round ligament. See the Appendix for a detailed description.

Low Back Pain

Almost half of all pregnant women experience some back pain, especially during the fifth through ninth months. The pain may be localized to the low back and sacroiliac and lumbosacral joints, may refer to the buttocks and legs, and may involve the upper back. Unresolved back and pelvic joint pain in pregnancy can lead to chronic back and pelvic pain years after delivery.

Etiology

- Misalignments of the lumbosacral spine
- Pelvic and lumbosacral instability resulting from ligamentous laxity caused by the hormones of pregnancy

- Sacroiliac joint dysfunction
- Pubic symphysis separation
- Coccydynia
- Diastasis rectus abdominus
- Posturally induced strain to localized segments of the lumbar spine, posterior musculature, and ligaments
- Lumbar and lumbosacral facet imbrication and inflammation as a result of the posterior shift in weight bearing necessitated by the increased abdominal girth
- Referred pain from trigger points in the posterior and anterior musculature
- Referred pain from strained uterine ligaments (see Table 7-4)
- Fetal positioning
- Prolonged standing or sitting

Table 7-4 Common Pain Referral Patterns in Pregnancy

Location	Consider
Low back pain	Lumbopelvic misalignment Broad ligament Postural changes
Sciatica	Lumbopelvic misalignment Broad ligament Postural changes Piriformis hypertonicity or imbalance
Pain in the buttocks	Broad ligament Sacrouterine ligament Lumbar spine misalignment Sacrum misalignment
Diagonal pain from uterus to groin	Pubic misalignment Round ligament
Pain at or below the SI joints	SI joint dysfunction Sacrouterine ligament
Pain directly over the pubic bone or into the medial thigh	Pubic misalignment

- High-heeled shoes
- Insufficient back support while seated or lying down

Management

- Avoid contributing factors.
- Assess and correct for sacroiliac, sacrococcygeal, symphysis pubis, and lumbosacral misalignments.
- Use a sacroiliac belt.
- Assess and treat hypertonicity, strain, and trigger points in the muscles and ligaments of the pelvis.
- Modify posture.
- Engage in individualized progam of home exercises, including corrective exercises for pelvic misalignments, posture training, and body mechanics training.

Morning Sickness

Morning sickness, which causes a sensation of queasiness, nausea, and vomiting, is experienced by as many as 70% of women during the first trimester of pregnancy.

Etiology

The actual cause of morning sickness is unknown. Proposed causes include the following:

- Rising progesterone levels that cause systemic muscle relaxation and slowing down of the peristaltic motions of the digestive tract, resulting in slow elimination and an excess of stomach acids
- Rising levels of HCG
- Enhanced sense of smell

TECHNICAL NOTE

Severe morning sickness, referred to as hyperemesis gravidarium, is a serious medical condition that can result in dehydration, weight loss, and nutritional deficiencies.

Management

There is no known "cure" for morning sickness. A trial-and-error approach is used by many women until they find the strategy that works best for them. Some options are described in the following subsections.

Conventional

- Medications, typically involving a combination of doxylamine and pyridoxine (Diclegis)
- IV fluids

TECHNICAL NOTE

The combination of doxylamine and pyridoxine (Diclegis) causes sleepiness and lethargy and should be taken with caution.

TECHNICAL NOTE

Hyperemesis gravidarium is treated with IV fluids and antinausea medications.

Complementary

- Nutraceuticals
  - Ginger root tea
  - Vitamin B_6 supplementation up to 100 mg daily
- Acupressure
  - Acupressure points for morning sickness include the PC-6 point located between the most lateral two tendons on the anterior surface of the forearm (i.e., the flexor carpi radialis and the palmaris longus tendons, 2 in. proximal to the wrist crease). The point can be stimulated with deep, rhythmic thumb or fingertip pressure four times a day for 10 minutes each time.

- Spinal manipulation
  - This includes a full spine assessment and manipulation, with emphasis on C1 to influence the vagus nerve and potentially enhance production of the food-absorption hormones.
- Massage
  - Generalized relaxation massage is recommended as tolerated.

Self-Care and Wellness
- Eat several small meals during the day.
- Keep hydrated.
- Avoid strong food smells.
- Eat crackers prior to getting out of bed in the morning.
- Eat foods rich in vitamin B_6, such as nuts and legumes.
- Add fresh ginger to foods.
- Try hypnosis.
- Use essential oils containing ginger or mint.

Preeclampsia or Toxemia of Pregnancy

Preeclampsia is a condition marked by edema, elevated blood pressure, and abnormal protein in the urine during pregnancy. True preeclampsia occurs after the 20th week.

Preeclampsia occurs in approximately 7% of births. The rate of preeclampsia in the United States has increased 25% over the last two decades. Preeclampsia is a leading cause of maternal and infant illness and death.

Etiology

The etiology is unknown.

Signs and Symptoms

- Rapid weight gain from fluid retention—5 to 10 pounds within a week

- Prominent swelling of the hands, face, and legs
- Severe headaches
- Blurred vision
- Edema
- Abdominal pain
- Fetal complications as a result of preeclampsia: inadequate fetal growth, premature labor, and fetal distress during labor

Management

There is no known treatment for preeclampsia. Standard interventions include the following:

- Close monitoring
- Early delivery (preeclampsia resolves following the birth)
- Hospitalization to control the blood pressure
- Bedrest—lying on the left side

Prevention

Some studies implicate insufficient riboflavin (vitamin B_2) as a risk factor for preeclampsia.

CLINICAL PEARL

According to the American College of Obstetricians and Gynecologists (ACOG, 2013), treatment is delayed for many patients with preeclampsia because their proteinuria levels do not meet prior established guidelines.

CLINICAL PEARL

According to ACOG, women who had hypertension or preeclampsia in a prior pregnancy have a higher-than-normal risk (as much as 50% higher) of developing it again in a subsequent pregnancy.

Current ACOG Guidelines

Not recommended:

- Screening to predict preeclampsia beyond taking an appropriate medical history to evaluate for risk factors
- Vitamin C or vitamin E to prevent preeclampsia

Recommended:

- Daily low-dose aspirin is recommended to prevent preeclampsia in very high-risk women with a history of preeclampsia and preterm delivery.
- Antihypertensive medication is recommended for severe hypertension during pregnancy.
- A decision to deliver should not be based on the amount of proteinuria or a change in the amount of proteinuria.
- The use of magnesium sulfate is recommended for severe preeclampsia or eclampsia (ACOG, n.d.).

CLINICAL PEARL

Preeclampsia is a serious condition that should be managed by a trained medical professional.

Data from American College of Obstetricians and Gynecologists. (2013). *Hypertension in pregnancy*. Washington, DC: Author.

Premature Contractions

Premature contractions are caused by many factors, some of which are life-threatening and require crisis management, whereas others are amenable to more conservative management protocols. Patients with premature contractions should first consult with their midwives or obstetricians. Premature contractions that occur in rapid succession warrant immediate medical attention.

Dehydration, structural imbalance, and tipped uterus are common causes of premature contractions and are amenable to conservative management.

TECHNICAL NOTE

Risk factors for preterm labor include the following:
- Previous preterm birth
- Multiple pregnancy
- Incompetent cervix
- Uterine abnormalities
- Urinary tract infections
- Vaginal infections, commonly bacterial vaginosis
- Uterine exposure to diethylstilbestrol (DES)
- Diabetes mellitus
- Hypertension
- Thrombophilia and other clotting disorders
- Young maternal age
- Low prepregnancy weight
- Low weekly weight gain
- Nulliparity
- History of three or more abortions
- Late or no prenatal care
- Lifestyle factors such as smoking, drinking alcohol, and using illegal drugs
- Psychosocial factors such as stress, poverty, and lack of social support
- Domestic violence, including physical, sexual, or emotional abuse
- Short time period between pregnancies (less than 6 to 9 months between birth and the beginning of the next pregnancy)

Pubic Diastases (Symphysis Pubis Pain)

Symphysis pubis pain is pain in the pelvic girdle, deep groin, or medial thigh caused by a shift in the pubic and pelvic bones and most commonly occurs during pregnancy.

Epidemiology

Females who are pregnant or in the postpartum period are affected. Estimates of incidence range vastly from 1 in 300 to 1 in 30,000 and demonstrate significant geographic variations.

Etiology

As pregnancy progresses and systemic levels of oxytocin and relaxin increase, the fibro-cartilaginous ligaments at the symphysis pubis become increasingly lax. This increase in laxity predisposes to misalignment of the bony structures of the pelvis.

Signs and Symptoms

- Gradually increasing pelvic and low back pain as pregnancy progresses
- Sciatica
- Moderate to severe pain directly over the symphysis pubis
- Pain deep in the groin or lower abdomen
- Pain with fundal height assessment
- Lower abdominal, pelvic, or pubic pain that occurs in the following activities:
  - Climbing stairs
  - Getting in and out of an automobile
  - Engaging in sexual activity
  - Putting on underwear
  - Walking
- Moderate to severe pain over the pubic bone when turning over in bed or sleeping on the side
- Pain in the lower abdomen over the round ligament
- Clicking or popping in the area of the symphysis pubis with locomotion

Diagnoses

- Biomechanical assessment of the pelvic girdle and surrounding musculature
- Measurement of width of the symphysis by x-ray or real-time ultrasound

Management

Conventional

- Medications include the following:
  - Anti-inflammatory medication, such as naproxen (Aleve, Naprelan)
  - Painkillers, such as ibuprofen (Advil)

Table 7-5 Drug Classifications and Fetal Risk

Category	Risk
A	Generally acceptable. Controlled studies in pregnant women show no evidence of fetal risk.
B	May be acceptable. Either animal studies show no risk but human studies are not available or animal studies showed minor risks and human studies have been done and showed no risk.
C	Use with caution if benefits outweigh risks. Either animal studies show risk and human studies are not available or neither animal nor human studies have been done.
D	Use in life-threatening emergencies when no safer drug is available. Positive evidence of human fetal risk.
X	Do not use in pregnancy. Risks involved outweigh potential benefits. Safer alternatives exist.
NA	Information not available.

- Steroid injection, such as betamethasone (Celestone, Celestone Soluspan)
  - Note: Betamethasone is a Category C medication and should be used with caution and only if benefits outweigh the risks.

The impact of drugs on the developing fetus cannot be overlooked. For drug classifications and fetal risk, see Table 7-5.

Complementary

Manual Therapies

- Manipulation: Pelvic manipulation to include direct adjustments to realign the symphysis pubis
  - Instruction in self-realignment of pelvic joints
  - Activation of pelvic-floor muscle during transitional movements
  - Instruction in compensatory movement strategies
  - Core muscle strengthening
  - Sacroiliac belt

- Massage: Massage to the low back and adductor muscles and over the round ligament

Self-Care and Wellness

- Place an ice pack over the site of pain.
- Sleep with a pillow between the knees to provide some stability to the pelvis.
- Enlist a partner to support the hips by holding them on either side when turning in bed.
- Avoid standing for prolonged periods, and make an effort to ensure the even distribution of weight to both feet when standing.
- Dress while in a seated position, especially when it is necessary to wear clothing that requires inserting one leg at a time.
- Skirts and dresses should be worn instead of pants and pulled down from the top rather than up from the bottom.
- Maternity support belts may be useful.
- Swinging the legs as a unit may be helpful when entering or exiting cars.
- Remain well hydrated.

Prevention

Biomechanical assessment and realignment of the pelvis during pregnancy is recommended and may be especially critical in individuals who have a prior history of pelvic misalignments or low back pain.

Rhesus Factor

The rhesus (Rh) factor is found in the blood of 85% of Whites and 95% of Blacks. People who have Rh factor are known as Rh positive. Those who don't are Rh negative. Rh-negative status has no impact on the general health; however, when the mother is Rh negative, and the father and the baby are both Rh positive, Rh disease, also known as hemolytic disease of the newborn, may occur.

The Rh-positive blood inherited from the father may leak into the mother's circulation during pregnancy, but this more commonly occurs during delivery. The mother who is Rh negative makes Rh-positive antibodies, which can compromise subsequent pregnancies because the antibodies can cross the placenta and destroy some of the fetal red blood cells, producing anemia, which can lead to serious, even fatal, brain damage.

Management

Rh disease is increasingly rare because Rh-negative mothers are given $Rh_o(D)$ immune globulin (RhoGAM) at 28 weeks of gestation and immediately postpartum, which prevents the formation of antibodies in an Rh-negative mother. Rh-positive mothers do not have to worry even if the father is Rh negative. Rh blood typing and testing are currently routinely performed at the first visit. If the mother is Rh positive, there is no cause for concern. If, however, the mother is Rh negative, then the father should be checked. If he is also Rh negative, there is no concern because the baby will be Rh negative, and there is no risk of antibody production. If the father is Rh positive, there is susceptibility for disease, and the test will be repeated to check for antibodies in the sixth and eighth months of pregnancy and at delivery. Amniocentesis may be performed to check for bilirubin, which is released into the amniotic fluid if and when the fetal blood cells are broken down by maternal Rh antibodies.

Snoring

Etiology

The increased blood flow into the mucous membranes causes swelling, which restricts airflow and causes snoring.

Management

- Sleeping on the side instead of on the back prevents the tongue and soft palate from resting against the back of the throat and further blocking the airways.
- Anecdotal reports suggest that wearing a nasal strip might be helpful.

Spontaneous Abortion (Miscarriage)

Spontaneous abortion, also known as miscarriage, is the loss of a pregnancy within the first 20 weeks.

Etiology

Etiology is unknown, but postulated causes for miscarriage include the following:

- Chromosome abnormalities in the sperm or egg
- Maternal factors such as diabetes, smoking, alcohol use, woman over 35 years of age, and anatomical defects of the uterus
- Luteal-phase defects

Signs and Symptoms

- Vaginal bleeding or spotting
- Severe, persistent headaches
- Prolonged vomiting, severe enough to prevent adequate intake of liquids
- Blurred vision or spots before the eyes
- Fever and chills, not accompanied by a cold
- Sudden intense or continual abdominal pains and cramping
- Sudden gush of fluid from the vagina
- Sudden swelling of hands, feet, and ankles
- Frequent burning urination
- Pronounced decrease in fetal movement

Management

- Assessments and interventions for the contributing factors should be undertaken.
- Luteal-phase defect (also known as inadequate progesterone) is diagnosed by endometrial biopsy and treated in subsequent pregnancies with progesterone vaginal suppositories or progesterone creams.

Thoracic Outlet Syndrome

Thoracic outlet syndrome involves pain, numbness, and tingling either in a glove-like distribution or following a specific dermatomal pattern in the hand and along the arm.

Etiology
- Postural compromise as the abdominal girth and breasts enlarge
- Edema

Management

Conventional
- Rehabilitative exercises
- Physiotherapy modalities

Complementary
- Trigger-point therapy for the pectoralis and scalene muscles
- Assessment and manipulation of the cervicothoracic spine as necessary
- Stretching and strengthening of the anterior, middle, and posterior scalene muscles
- Assessment and modification of postural inadequacies
- Rehabilitative exercises
- Physiotherapy modalities

Tipped Uterus

A tipped uterus is a uterus that tips forward in a pelvic cavity that has typically endured prior undiagnosed or untreated trauma. The added pressure and weight of the amniotic fluid and the growing baby apply stress to the unstable sacral segments, causing them to buckle.

TECHNICAL NOTE

The uterus is anchored by several ligaments, which must evenly distribute the tension for maximum balance (see Figure 7-5). If the ligaments on the anterior surface of the uterus contract more than those in the back, the uterus is pulled forward. Pressure on the nerves and arteries that supply the muscles of the groin and upper thigh may result, and movement, especially walking, is compromised. Extreme cervical pressure occurs, and premature labor may result.

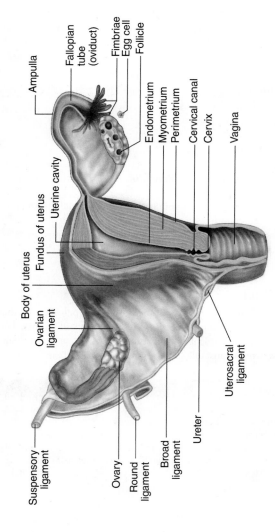

Figure 7-5 Uterine ligaments

Management

Complementary

- Manual therapy: Buckled sacrum maneuver (see the Appendix)

> **CLINICAL PEARL**
>
> "My feet flew out from underneath me before I fell on my bottom" is a typical scenario elicited in the prior history from a woman with premature labor that may be caused by a buckled sacrum.

Urinary Frequency/Urgency

Etiology

- Increased pressure on the bladder as the size of the uterus increases
- Urinary tract infection (UTI) or bladder infection

Management

- Identify and treat any pathogens. The most common are those causing bacterial vaginosis and candidiasis.
- Assess for contributing factors, such as diet.
- Perform pelvic-floor muscle (Kegel) exercises (see the Appendix)

Urinary Stress Incontinence

Etiology

The muscles of the pelvic floor may become overstretched and weakened in pregnancy. One-third of pregnant women report urinary incontinence.

> **CLINICAL PEARL**
>
> Women with incontinence during pregnancy are more likely to suffer long-term symptoms of urinary incontinence.

Management
- Pelvic-floor muscle training in pregnancy

> **CLINICAL PEARL**
>
> Pelvic-floor muscle training in pregnancy is known to reduce the risk for urinary incontinence postpartum.

Fetal Development

- First trimester (months 1 through 3): Fetal development includes the formation of the head, brain, spine, heart, body, and limbs and development of the sex organs. Caution about drugs and chemicals is warranted in this trimester because drugs and chemicals may cross the placenta and influence the development of the fetus.
- Second trimester (months 4 through 6): Fetal development includes the maturation of the circulatory system and skeletal movements. Assessing the mother's daily activities to ensure frequent rest is recommended.
- Third trimester (months 7 through 9): This is a period of rapid fetal growth. The fetus multiplies its weight three to four times. It is important to ensure that the mother remains well hydrated and that protein intake is adequate.

> **CLINICAL PEARL**
>
> Seafood intake in pregnancy is positively associated with birthweight; however, mercury exposure is negatively associated with birthweight. Types of seafood known to have higher levels of mercury include shark, albacore tuna, swordfish, king mackerel, and tilefish.

LABOR AND DELIVERY

There are three stages of labor and delivery:
- The first stage is the time of dilation of the cervix and includes the early, active, and transition phases. The early phase manifests

as 3 to 4 cm of dilation and is the most comfortable of the three stages. The active phase manifests as approximately 4 to 7 cm of dilation, and the contractions become more intense. Breathing techniques may be useful. The phase of transition manifests as approximately 8 to 10 cm of dilation, and the pain and pressure are most intense.

- The second stage begins when the cervix is completely dilated and ends when the baby is born. It typically averages 20 minutes to an hour but can last for several hours. It is marked by a tremendous urge to bear down and push the baby out.
- The third stage is delivery of the afterbirth, or placenta, and usually occurs within 30 minutes after the birth.

Labor Induction

Procedures to induce labor in women who are considerably past the due date are described in the following subsections.

Conventional

Medications

- Oxytocin (Pitocin, Syntocinon), typically given through an IV
- Prostaglandin gels or vaginal inserts, which soften and dilate the cervix

CLINICAL PEARL

Pitocin use is associated with Apgar scores of less than 7 at 5 minutes and unexpected admission to the newborn intensive care unit (NICU) lasting more 24 hours for full-term infants.

Procedures

- Amniotomy, in which the amniotic sac is ruptured.
- "Stripping the membrane," in which the membrane that connects the amniotic sac to the uterine wall is stripped, causing the release of prostaglandins that help prepare the cervix for delivery and may induce contractions

Complementary

Massage

- Muscle-stripping techniques for the adductors

Acupressure

- Bone-to-bone pressure to the uterus and ovary zones at the midpoint of the medial and lateral calcaneus, respectively

Acupuncture

Acupuncture points that are commonly needled to promote uterine contractions include the following:

- Spleen 6—four client finger widths proximal to the malleolus along the medial tibial border
- Kidney 3—on the superior border and just posterior to the medial malleolus
- Liver 3—at the proximal border of the first and second metatarsal bones
- Hoku hand point at the junction of the thumb and index finger

Spinal Manipulation

- Emphasis on the sympathetic nervous system

Self-Care and Wellness

- Exercise: Walking, especially up and down a hill
- Nipple stimulation with a rough face towel

Back Labor

Etiology

One of the causes of back labor is the baby exiting in the occiput posterior position. The front of the baby's head is turned toward the pubic bone, and the back of the head is turned toward the sacrum. The converse is the ideal. The back of the head against the sacrum puts pressure on the parasympathetic nerves exiting the sacral foramen, which can be very painful for the mother.

Management

Conventional

- Medications, such as the opiates Stadol, fentanyl, and Demerol
- Epidural
- Spinal tap

For a complete list of commonly used medications in labor and delivery and their side effects, see the Appendix.

CLINICAL PEARL

Morphine is no longer routinely used during labor because it depresses the baby's ability to breathe.

Complementary

- Craniosacral therapy
  Respiratory and pelvic diaphragm release techniques
  The side lying maneuver (see the Appendix)

Self-Care and Wellness

- Pressure applied to the sacrum, usually with the fists of the partner
- Warm poultices applied to the low back
- Use of a birth ball
- Pelvic tilt exercises
- Hydrotherapy/water therapy immersion
- Heated rice sock
- Frequent position changes
- Soliciting the attendance of a doula (trained birth support personnel)
- Meditation/guided meditation to address concerns and fears about the delivery
- Assesment of the environment
  - A peaceful, quiet, and dimly lit environment allows for relaxation and may promote the progression of labor.
- Development of a birth plan (see the Appendix for a sample)

> **CLINICAL PEARL**
>
> Factors that may interfere with the natural progression of labor include being restricted to the bed, electronic fetal monitoring, lack of support, and emotional concerns.

Episiotomy

An episiotomy is a surgical cut in the perineum, the muscular area between the vagina and the anus. Historically, episiotomies were thought to prevent more extensive tears during childbirth. Current research suggests that is not the case and that episiotomies are sometimes more problematic than a natural tear. Episiotomies are further associated with infection, fecal incontinence, bleeding, and uncomfortable recovery.

There are two types of episiotomy incision: the midline or median incision, which is performed vertically, and the mediolateral incision, which is done at an angle. The midline incision has a higher risk of extending to the anus, but it is easier to repair. The mediolateral incision is more painful and more difficult to repair, but it affords protection from a tear to the anus.

Current thinking is that episiotomies should only be performed if the baby is very large, needs to be delivered quickly, or is in an abnormal position or if the risk of extensive tearing is imminent.

Management

The wound is sutured together, and the typical healing time is 4 to 6 weeks.

Women should be counseled to wait for 6 weeks before using tampons, having sex, or engaging in high-impact exercise.

IMMEDIATE/EARLY POSTPARTUM

In a process called involution, which lasts approximately 6 weeks, the uterus returns to its normal size. The process occurs by a series of uterine contractions, often termed "after pains." The multiparous woman may experience more contractions than the primiparous woman because the uterus of a multiparous woman tends to be a little more lax. Involution is under the control of oxytocin, the same hormone that causes the milk letdown reflex during breastfeeding.

Conditions and concerns of the postpartum period include the following:

- Abdominal laxity
- Breast pain
- Caesarian management
- Constipation
- Engorgement
- Itching from the stitches
- Loss of bladder sensitivity
- Nipple pain
- Sore perineum
- Vaginal drainage
- Weight loss

Abdominal Laxity

Etiology

A certain degree of abdominal laxity is expected in the postpartum period. Abdominal laxity may result in diastasis recti.

Management

To minimize the possibility of diastasis recti and to restore the abdominal girth to its regular tone, it is recommended to follow a progression of abdominal exercises, beginning with abdominal breathing and followed carefully and cautiously with abdominal isometrics, pelvic rocking, and curl-ups. Activation of the transverse abdominus muscle is recommended to initiate abdominal muscle recovery.

Filling of the Breasts (Engorgement)

Etiology

The presence of the infant at the nipple is a stimulus to the anterior pituitary gland to release prolactin. Prolactin is responsible for initiating milk production. When the infant begins to suckle, the suckling effect stimulates the neurohypophysis to release oxytocin. Oxytocin causes contraction of the myoepithelial cells that line the alveoli, propelling the fluid forward into the lactiferous ducts behind the areola. The result is the letdown reflex, often described as the filling of the breasts with milk. The woman may simultaneously experience contraction of the uterus.

> **TECHNICAL NOTE**
>
> The initial fluid that the infant gets from the breast is colostrum, which contains valuable protein, mineral, and vitamin content (vitamins A and E) and nitrogen. The cathartic effects of colostrum enable the infant to eliminate any meconium that is in the gastrointestinal tract as a result of the birth.

Management

- Comfort measures

Breast Pain

Etiology

The "coming in" of the milk occurs on or about the third day following birth and results in marked engorgement of the breasts. This is often accompanied by pain, tenderness, and throbbing of the breasts and sometimes a mild fever.

Management

- Frequent nursing and the use of a supportive bra are recommended.
- Provide reassurance that the discomfort commonly resolves in 7 to 10 days once the mother and baby are on a regular nursing schedule.

- If the mother does not plan to nurse, she should wear a supportive bra and avoid expressing any milk, using ice therapies for relief and pain medications as prescribed.

Cesarean Section
Management
- Wound and scar management
- Rehabilitation
- Bracing body mechanics
- Modifications in activities of daily living (ADLs): no lifting over 15 lb, no heavy household duties, and avoidance of any activities that cause pain

Constipation
Etiology
The first bowel movement may not occur until a few days after delivery, and constipation is common. The mother's fear of exerting pressure as a result of soreness in the perineal region, hemorrhoids, healing episiotomy scars, sluggish intestinal peristaltic action, and lax abdominal muscles all contribute to constipation.

Management
If the mother has not returned to normal bowel functioning by the third day, stool softeners such as Colace or laxatives such as Metamucil may be recommended. She should be encouraged to increase her intake of fiber (fruits, vegetables, whole grains) and water as tolerated and to take short walks to facilitate bowel motion.

> ### CLINICAL PEARL
> The safest laxatives to take while breastfeeding are the bulk-forming laxatives, such as Metamucil. Stimulant laxatives, such as Correctol and Senokot, should be avoided while breastfeeding.

Itching from Episiotomy Stitches

Management

The itching caused by stitches will resolve spontaneously, but the mother can be advised to sit on an inflatable doughnut pillow and to use cold compresses.

Loss of Bladder Sensitivity

The early postpartum is a period of diuresis as the excess fluid accumulated during the pregnancy is eliminated.

Management

The mother should be reminded to be attentive to cues to urinate because there might be a slight loss of bladder sensitivity to fluid pressure as a result of the trauma resulting from the birth process. (See Chapter 13 for further information.)

Nipple Pain

Nipple pain may occur as a result of the infant's suckling and suckling techniques.

Management

- Prepare the nipples by rubbing them with a rough towel in the weeks approaching the due date.
- In the postpartum period, expressing some of the milk immediately prior to nursing may allow the infant to find the nipple more easily.
- Use cold compresses on the breasts and nipples.

Sore Perineum

As a result of the tremendous stretching of the perineum during birth, there is often postpartum soreness in this area even if an episiotomy was not performed.

Management

Self-Care and Wellness

- Reinstitute pelvic-floor muscle (Kegel) exercises as soon as possible.
- If tolerated, sitting meditation style places the pressure evenly on the ischial tuberosities, instead of on the perineum.
- The vaginal area should be washed regularly with warm water. A squeeze bottle can be used.
- Cold packs can be applied to the perineum.
- Sitz baths may help to alleviate the soreness.

Vaginal Drainage

Vaginal drainage, known as lochia, occurs for the first few days after childbirth but may be plentiful for 2 to 3 weeks and may last for up to 6 weeks. This process, which feels to many women like a heavy menstrual period, enables the endometrium to heal by sloughing off the superficial layer of cells and necrotic tissue from the placental site, with concurrent regrowth of healthy new epithelium. The lochia changes in color from red or pink to brown or yellow and eventually becomes whitish.

Management

- Comfort measures are recommended, such as rest and frequent urination (a full bladder may impair uterine contractions).
- The patient should be counseled about warning signs of more serious conditions (see the Clinical Pearl).

CLINICAL PEARL

Women who fear the blood loss that occurs postpartum can be reminded that the body has taken on a greater volume of blood during pregnancy.

CLINICAL PEARL

Excessive bleeding (more than one pad per hour, clots larger than a plum, heavy menstrual flow after 4 days, return of spotting or bleeding following several days without bleeding), foul odor, and fever are indications of more serious conditions that should be evaluated.

Weight Loss

The expulsion of the uterine contents results in a weight loss of approximately 10 to 12 lb. Diuresis and diaphoresis result in the loss of an additional 5 lb. The increased caloric demands that accompany nursing (for milk production) typically result in additional weight loss over the subsequent months.

Management

- Encourage appropriate dietary modifications.

TECHNICAL NOTE

Breastfeeding women need more of most nutrients than they did during pregnancy. The body requires more energy to produce milk, and milk production requires substantial caloric intake. To produce 1 quart of milk per day when breastfeeding, the woman needs to consume approximately 500 extra calories daily. No nourishing foods need to be eliminated from the diet.

TECHNICAL NOTE

Some foods may have undesirable effects on the breastfeeding infant. These include the following:
- Chocolate, which may have a laxative effect
- Broccoli, brussel sprouts, cabbage, dried beans, and cauliflower, which may create gas
- Spicy foods, which may flavor the milk or cause gas pains

> **CLINICAL PEARL**
>
> Brown spots on fairer-skinned women or white spots on darker-skinned women, referred to as the "mask of pregnancy," "pregnancy cap," or melasma, that do not disappear within a few months after delivery might indicate folic acid deficiency. Supplementation with folic acid and a diet that contains foods high in folate, such as green leafy vegetables and whole grains, should facilitate restoration of normal skin tone within 2 to 3 weeks.

LONGER-TERM POSTPARTUM CONCERNS

Diabetes

Appropriate follow-up for all patients diagnosed with gestational diabetes includes the following:

- Diabetes prevention strategies, including physical activity and breastfeeding, should be recommended.
- A postpartum glucose tolerance test should be performed to determine the patient's risk for developing type II diabetes.
- The patient should be screened for type II diabetes yearly or every 3 years depending on the results of the initial postpartum tests.

Postpartum Depression

- As many as 80% of women experience the "postpartum blues," which is a brief period during which women are tearful and sensitive. Postpartum blues should resolve within 1 to 2 weeks.
- Postpartum depression may occur immediately or several months after the birth and can last for days, weeks, months, and even years in some cases. As many as 14% of women develop postpartum depression. Postpartum depression is thought to result from the rapidly fluctuating internal (hormonal) and external (physical) environments.

CLINICAL PEARL

Postpartum depression is a serious condition that warrants intervention from trained psychologists and psychiatrists. Providers should be alert to postpartum depression whenever there are concerns regarding the development of attachment between the mother and child.

TECHNICAL NOTE

Many additional symptoms have been linked to the postpartum period. These include but are not limited to impaired mother–infant interactions, bipolar disorder, posttraumatic stress disorder, back pain, pelvic pain, postpartum anxiety disorders, frequent headaches, various forms of psychosis, dyspareunia, stress incontinence, anemia, and hemorrhoids. Refer to the guidelines on postpartum conditions in the *Diagnostic and Statistical Manual of Mental Disorders* (American Psychiatric Association, 2013) and to the following websites for additional information on these concerns:

http://www.mentalhealth.gov

http://www.nimh.nih.gov.

http://www.mayoclinic.org/diseases-conditions/postpartum-depression
    /basics/definition/con-20029130

Management

Conventional

Medications

- Avoid premature use of hormonal birth control methods.
- Antidepressants such as Prozac may be necessary.

Counseling

- Talk therapy with a trained professional

Self-Care and Wellness

- Management of psychosocial issues, including the following:
  - Obtaining experienced help for baby care

- Getting adequate rest and sleep
- Finding a support system
- Stress management
- Exercise
- Relaxation measures
- Adequate nutritional support

CLINICAL PEARL

Large population studies have indicated that a process for integrated and systematic postpartum depression screening, detection, and referral performed by nurses is overwhelmingly supported by postpartum women.

CLINICAL PEARL

Depression screening tools validated across cultures include the Edinburgh Postnatal Depression Scale (EPDS), Center for Epidemiologic Studies Depression Scale (CES-D), and Beck Depression Inventory II (BDI-II). Cutoff points may need to be adjusted with different demographic populations. (See the Appendix for further information.)

LACTATION

Lactation is associated with an abundance of health benefits for both mother and baby.

Practitioners are therefore encouraged to recommend breast-milk for all infants unless there are significant contraindications. They should also provide assistance/education/instructions on the most effective breastfeeding positions. These include the laid-back position, the cradle hold, the cross-cradle hold, the football/clutch position, and the side-lying position.

Dyad Bonding

- Laid-back breastfeeding: Also referred to as biological nurturing, this is an instinctive approach to breastfeeding. The mother is encouraged to lean back while slightly elevated on a comfortable surface, with the head and shoulder supported. The baby is placed with his or her whole front to the mother's whole front, with the baby's cheeks resting close to the bare breast. The mother is encouraged to provide as much or as little assistance as she wants.

- Cradle hold: This position is most commonly used after the first few weeks. The baby is in a side-lying position, resting on his or her side, with the shoulder, hip, and mouth level with the breast. The baby's head is on the mother's forearm, with the baby facing the mother. The mother supports the breast with a "U" or "C" hold. The baby's mouth should cover at least half of the dark area around the nipple.

- Cross-cradle hold: This is similar to the cradle hold, except the baby is supported on a pillow across mother's lap to aid in raising the nipple. The pillow should support both of the baby's elbows. The mother supports the baby with the fingers of the opposite hand.

- Side-lying position: This is most commonly used for night feeding. The mother and baby lie on their sides facing each other. A pillow is placed behind the baby's back for stability and behind the mother's back for comfort and support. The baby is cradled in the mother's arm, with the baby's back along the mother's forearm; the baby's hips are flexed, and the baby's ear, shoulder, and hip are in a line.

See the Appendix for more detailed explanations and pictures of breastfeeding positions.

Achieving Good Latch

To encourage good latch of the baby to the breast, the mother uses her nipple to tickle the center of the baby's bottom lip. This encourages the baby to open his or her mouth widely, as in a yawn. The mother brings the baby in and aims her nipple toward the roof of the baby's mouth.

CLINICAL PEARL

With the first offering of the breast, the baby will suck without swallowing to position the nipple, alerting the breast to let down the milk.

CLINICAL PEARL

If the latch is uncomfortable, the mother can place her finger in the baby's mouth between the gums to detach and then try again.

Effective Feeding

Checkpoints for effective feeding include the following:

- The baby's nose is almost or essentially touching the breast.
- The baby's lips are flanged.
- At least half of the areola is in the baby's mouth.
- The mother can observe the baby's jaw "working" all the way to the ear.
- The baby's temples wiggle.
- The mother can hear the baby swallow.

CLINICAL PEARL

Positioning the baby can pose additional challenges for large-breasted women. Tips for providers include the following:

- If the mother experiences difficulty lifting the breast, she can place a diaper or rolled cloth under the breast to lift it up.
- She may need to hold the breast with her fingers underneath and thumbs on top during the entire nursing session.
- She should not lean over the baby while nursing because this can cause the infant's jaws to compress the areola, limiting the flow of milk and irritating the mother's breasts.
- She should be encouraged to vary the nursing positions to ensure complete emptying.
- She may find the football hold to be most comfortable.
- Massage of stretch marks can provide relief.
- Nursing bras made of cotton may help with heat rashes.

Tips for assisting the mother who doesn't want to breastfeed or has tried unsuccessfully to breastfeed include the following:

- Support and encourage the patient, and address possible feelings of guilt.
- Reassure the woman that the process of achieving good latch may take several days to weeks.
- Cold compresses/packs over the breasts or cold cabbage leaves placed in the bra can be used to reduce discomfort.
- Wearing a sports bra night and day will keep the breasts supported.
- To prevent mastitis, she should avoid binding the breasts.
- NSAIDs and pain medications can be used to relieve the pain from engorgement.
- Expressing a small amount of milk can relieve the pain from engorgement; however, this must not be done regularly to avoid establishing a milk supply.
- Avoid passing judgment on mothers who choose not to breastfeed.

Mastitis

Mastitis is inflammation or infection of the breasts.

Etiology

- Improper drainage of the milk duct, leading to inflammation
- Entry of bacteria through a crack in the nipple

Signs/Symptoms

- Area of redness (triangular flush) on the underside of the breast
- Swelling of the breast
- Moderate to severe pain and tenderness in the breast
- Sensation of heat on the breast
- Mild to moderate fever
- Flu-like symptoms

Diagnoses

- History and physical exam (history of breastfeeding)

- Needle aspiration/biopsy, especially in females who are not breastfeeding
- Mammography in females who are not breastfeeding

Management

Conventional

Medications

Antibiotics such as cephalexin (Keflex) and dicloxacillin (generic only) may be recommended in the following circumstances:

1. The infection/inflammation has exceeded 72 hours.
2. The nipple is discharging pus or blood.
3. Signs and symptoms are sudden, severe, or bilateral.
4. Worsening fever and flu-like symptoms persist.
5. Nipples are cracked, predisposing to bacteria entering the breast tissue.

CLINICAL PEARL

Mothers may continue to breastfeed while on antibiotics; however, more conservative methods should be the first line of treatment. There is a risk of a candidal infection that includes the nipples following administration of antibiotics.

Complementary

Nutraceuticals

The following supplements have been anecdotally reported to improve symptomatology; however, research evidence is lacking:

- Thymus support
- Sage tea in small quantities for engorgement
- Lecithin
- Green tea

CLINICAL PEARL

The infant's pediatrician should always be informed of herbal supplements taken by the mother while breastfeeding.

> **TECHNICAL NOTE**
>
> Although chasteberry (Vitex) is an effective treatment for cyclic mastalgia, it is not an appropriate treatment for mastitis. Its prolactin-lowering abilities are contraindicated in the nursing mother.

Ancillary Support

Spinal Manipulation

The mothers' thoracic spine and cervicothoracic spine are evaluated for misalignments, particularly if the mother is complaining of tingling and numbness in the fingers.

Soft-Tissue Techniques

Comfort measures include massage therapy for the muscles of the shoulder girdle and cervical and thoracic spines.

Self-Care and Wellness

- The nursing bra should accommodate changes in breast size.
- The infant should be nursed on demand.
- Nursing should be frequent to unplug the duct and to keep the breasts from becoming engorged. The affected side should be nursed first, with the feeding position altered to allow the breast to hang freely.
- Adequate rest is necessary for both mother and infant.
- Hot packs may be placed on the breast, and the breast may be massaged toward the nipple from behind the site of inflammation. Immediately following this application, the baby should be breastfed, or the breast should be pumped. Hot packs increase circulation and accelerate healing. Hot packs may be used with a compress, such as comfrey. Treatment with hot packs can also be followed with cold packs to decrease inflammation.
- Cold cabbage leaves placed in the bra can decrease inflammation.
- The mother should drink plenty of fluids, ensure good nutrition, and supplement as needed with a multivitamin.

Prevention

- Fit of the bra: The pressure on the tissues from a snugly fitting bra may restrict flow and predispose to inflammation.
- Feeding schedule: Missed or shortened feedings predispose to engorged and inflamed breasts.
- Position of the baby: The infant should be positioned in a manner that enables him or her to suckle effectively.
- Relaxed, unhurried, thorough nursing is mandatory, with care taken to ensure cleanliness around the nipple.
- The infant should be encouraged to suckle from both breasts uniformly. Inability to suckle comfortably from both breasts may be a result of factors such as trigger points and hypertonicity in the cervical muscles.
- The infant should be assessed for his or her ability to suckle effectively. Inability to suckle effectively may be a result of the infant's feeding position, trigger points in the muscles of the infant's jaw, or misalignment of the infant's cervical spine.

CLINICAL PEARL

Weaning increases the risk of developing a breast abscess that may require surgical drainage. Cold cabbage leaves placed in the bra can help to decrease the milk supply in women who wish to discontinue breastfeeding.

CLINICAL PEARL

Mastitis is a condition that is directly correlated with the infant's well-being. Strategies to enhance the infant's ability to latch and suckle effectively include the following:

- Assessment for trigger points and hypertonicity around the temporomandibular joint, including the temporalis, masseter, and pterygoids
- Assessment for upper cervical spinal misalignments and/or torticollis when the infant is favoring one breast.

Where these factors exist, mild and gentle trigger-point therapies accompanied by gentle stretching, mobilization, and craniosacral therapy may enable the infant to latch on and suckle appropriately.

PREGNANCY LOSS

Spontaneous Abortion (Miscarriage)

Spontaneous abortion, or miscarriage, is the loss of a pregnancy from natural causes prior to the 20th week of gestation

Epidemiology

- Approximately 15% to 20% of pregnancies end in miscarriage.

Etiology

- Genetic anomalies/chromosomal disorders
- Inadequate endometrial stem cells
- Maternal infections
- Endocrine disorders
- Uterine anomalies
- Incompetent cervix
- Age
  - According to the ACOG, one-third of pregnancies in women over the age of 40 results in early pregnancy loss.

Signs and Symptoms

- Bleeding
- Cramping

CLINICAL PEARL

Heavy bleeding, fever, chills, or severe pain following miscarriage warrants immediate attention.

Diagnosis

- Ultrasound
- Serologic testing of HCG levels

Management

Conventional

- Dilation and curettage
- Medications
- Vacuum aspiration

CLINICAL PEARL

It is medically safe to conceive after 2 or 3 normal menstrual periods following childbirth.

TECHNICAL NOTE

Classification of the types of spontaneous abortion is as follows:

Threatened: Vaginal bleeding and uterine cramping occur that may or may not result in the loss of the fetus. The patient is advised to avoid sexual activity, tampons, douches, and strenuous exercise and to report any bleeding.

Inevitable: Uterine cramping occurs, the amniotic membranes rupture, and the cervix dilates. Dilation and curettage (D&C) may be necessary; however, products of conception are sometimes expelled without intervention.

Incomplete abortion: Symptoms include severe cramping and menorrhagia. The products of conception are not fully expelled. Medications such as oxytocin are required, and D&C is performed.

Complete abortion: All the products of conception, including the fetus and placenta, are expelled. The cervix closes, and cramping and bleeding stop. The patient should contact the provider if any symptoms of infection are observed, including foul-smelling discharge and additional bleeding.

Missed abortion: The fetus expires but is not expelled immediately. Expulsion may not occur for several weeks. A D&C may be needed.

Recurrent/habitual spontaneous abortion: Three or more consecutive spontaneous abortions have occurred. Causes include incompetent cervix, uterine defects, and genetic anomalies.

Induced Abortion

Induced abortion occurs when procedures or medications are used to terminate a pregnancy. In countries where induced abortions are legal, they are provided in either the first trimester (prior to the 14th week) or the second trimester (after 13 weeks of gestation).

First-trimester abortions involve oral or vaginal medications alone or in combination with surgery. When medications only are used, the pregnancy is terminated over time. Bleeding will occur for days to weeks until completion. Surgery involves local anesthesia and suction curettage. The cervix is dilated, a tube is inserted into the uterus, and the contents are removed by suction. In rare cases, general anesthesia may be used.

Second-trimester abortions are most commonly surgical and involve regional or general anesthesia, dilation, and evacuation.

Epidemiology

According to Henshaw (2008), the annual worldwide elective abortion rate is 20 to 30 per 1,000 women. The peak age range for women who undergo induced abortions in the United States is 20 to 24; in this demographic, the rate is approximately 39 per 1,000 women (see the Technical Note).

Etiology

Women elect to have abortions for various reasons, including unwanted pregnancy, unplanned pregnancy, sexual assault, cultural views, concerns about fetal health, concerns about maternal health, lack of information about family planning, socioeconomic factors, personal beliefs and feelings, influence of others, concern about people's opinions, and easy access.

Management

- Complications include cramps, bleeding, spotting, retained tissue, perforation, and injury to the uterine lining

- For many women, the emotional loss is as significant as that experienced in a spontaneous abortion.
- Home care: See the following "Home Care" section.

Stillbirth

Stillbirth is defined by the Centers for Disease Control (2016) as the death of a baby before or during delivery.

Epidemiology

Of all pregnancies, 1 in 100 results in a stillbirth.

Etiology

- Placental abruption
- Preeclampsia
- Chromosomal disorders
- Bacterial infections between 24 and 27 weeks
- Growth restriction/asphyxia

Signs and Symptoms

- Decreased activity of the baby

Diagnosis

- Ultrasound

Prevention

- Avoiding drugs, alcohol, and smoking
  - Blood flow to and through the placenta is impaired by drugs and smoking, and heavy drinking during pregnancy is known to cause birth defects.
- Assessing the baby's daily kick count

CLINICAL PEARL

Smoking, illicit drug use, cannabis use, and secondhand smoke exposure have been associated with an increased risk of stillbirth.

Home Care

The patient must understand the warning signs of further complications, which include the following:

- Foul-smelling discharge
- Pelvic pain
- Ongoing or excessive vaginal bleeding

Other home-care recommendations include the following:

- Sexual activity should be avoided, and the patient should avoid inserting anything into the vagina, such as tampons and douches, for at least 3 weeks and up to 6 weeks.
- Rest is encouraged.
- Diet supplementation with iron and iron-rich foods is warranted.
- The patient should be encouraged to allow for mental, physical, and spiritual healing prior to attempting another pregnancy.
- Assist in managing the patient's feelings of loss.
- Assess and address the patient's stage of grieving.
- Practice active listening; the grieving patient may want to talk about the baby.
- Anticipate and provide recommendations for coping with physical reactions to grief, including the following:
  - Poor appetite
  - Disturbed sleep patterns
  - Lethargy
  - Panic
  - Anxiety
- Encourage communication.
- Connect the patient with other support services, including counseling/therapy, and grief support.

CHAPTER 8

Menstrual and Reproductive Tract Disorders

Amenorrhea

Amenorrhea is the absence of menstrual bleeding. It is a symptom, not a diagnosis.

- Primary amenorrhea is the absence of spontaneous uterine bleeding and secondary sexual characteristics by age 14 or the absence of spontaneous uterine bleeding by age 16 with otherwise normal development.
- Secondary amenorrhea is a 6-month absence of menstrual bleeding in a woman with regular menses or a 12-month absence of menstrual bleeding in a woman with previous oligomenorrhea.
- Oligomenorrhea is a reduction in the frequency of menses, with an interval longer than 35 days but less than 3 months.
- Cryptomenorrhea is hidden menstruation; menstruation occurs but makes no external appearance because of uterine or vaginal obstruction. It is a rare condition more commonly observed in the developing world.

Etiology

Causes of amenorrhea are multiple and include but are not limited to changes in the hypothalamus, pituitary gland, ovaries, uterus, adrenal glands, outlet tract, thyroid gland, and spine; systemic or chronic disease; extremes of weight and exercise; physical or mental stress; medications; and normal physiologic processes, such as pregnancy, breastfeeding, and menopause.

Hypothalamus

Alterations of the rhythmic secretions of gonadotropin-releasing hormone (GNRH) from excessive exercise, stress, or medications can cause a decrease in follicle-stimulating hormone (FSH) and luteinizing hormone (LH). The subsequent decline in estrogen and progesterone results in amenorrhea. In addition, extreme or rapid changes in weight and anorexia nervosa also influence the neuroendocrine function of the hypothalamus.

Pituitary Gland

Adenomas, prolactinomas, and other benign tumors of the pituitary gland can cause excessive production of prolactin (hyperprolactinemia), which results in amenorrhea. Other causes of hyperprolactinemia include stress, frequent or vigorous activity, nipple stimulation, and medications (including some birth control pills, ulcer medications, and psychotropic medications). Hyperprolactinemia causes amenorrhea by a negative feedback mechanism to the anterior pituitary that results in decreased production of FSH and LH.

TECHNICAL NOTE

- Prolactin secretion is under the influence of thyroid-releasing hormone (TRH), which is secreted by the pituitary in response to nipple stimulation. Inhibition of prolactin is controlled by prolactin-inhibiting hormone (PIH) and dopamine.
- Hypopituitary malfunction caused by conditions such as empty sella syndrome, Sheehan's syndrome (postpartum ischemic necrosis of the anterior pituitary), and Simmonds' syndrome (atrophy of the pituitary) results in decreased production of FSH and LH and subsequent amenorrhea.

Ovaries

Turner syndrome (XO) is a genetic disorder whereby ovaries are not present at birth or are devoid of germ cells; the karyotype 45 X instead of 46 XX. The absence of ovaries implies no or minimal production of estrogen and progesterone.

In premature ovarian failure, the ovaries do not respond to pituitary hormones.

Infections, tumors, and radiation therapy all have the potential to affect ovarian hormone secretion and can result in amenorrhea.

Polycystic ovarian syndrome (PCOS) is a condition that frequently manifests with increased levels of estrogen, the absence of ovulation, and minimal or no progesterone, resulting in amenorrhea.

Uterus

Intrauterine adhesions as seen in Asherman's syndrome and endometriosis disrupt the ability of the endometrium to respond appropriately to estrogen and progesterone, possibly resulting in amenorrhea.

Adrenal Glands

Causes of amenorrhea attributable to adrenal gland dysfunction include the following:

- Tumors, which frequently cause hypercortisolemia
- Cushing's syndrome (i.e., hypersecretion of the adrenal cortex)
- Administration of large doses of the adrenocortical hormones, such as prednisone

TECHNICAL NOTE

Benign tumors of the pituitary and adrenals are common, and the presence of a tumor does not imply that this is the cause of Cushing's syndrome.

Outlet Tract

Mechanical problems such as transverse vaginal septum, imperforate hymen, cervical stenosis, and agenesis affect patency from the uterus to the vaginal introitus and interfere with the outflow of menstrual blood.

Thyroid

Hypothyroidism results in increased production from the pituitary. Increased TRH induces an increase in prolactin secretion, which in turn causes amenorrhea. Hyperthyroidism causes amenorrhea by interfering with the production of FSH and LH.

Chronic or Systemic Disease

Chronic or systemic diseases that can cause amenorrhea include chronic kidney disease; chronic liver diseases, such as cirrhosis and nonalcoholic or alcoholic liver disease; and systemic diseases, such as systemic lupus erythematosus.

Pregnancy

Pregnancy is the most common cause of secondary amenorrhea in women of reproductive age. Once implantation occurs, the lining of the uterus, which normally sheds as menstrual blood, changes morphologically to become the decidua. The decidua ultimately becomes the placenta, which nourishes the fertilized egg and subsequently the fetus.

Extremes of Weight

Low body weight, as seen in athletes or in conditions such as anorexia nervosa or bulimia, results in diminished levels of estrogen, a decrease that predisposes to amenorrhea. In addition, estrogen is stored and synthesized in adipose tissue under the influence of the enzyme aromatase. In obesity or excessive weight, there is the potential for excess estrogen, which can also cause amenorrhea.

Excessive Exercise

Activities that require rigorous training, such as ballet, long-distance running, swimming, or gymnastics, may interrupt ovarian function, resulting in amenorrhea. The hormone leptin alerts the brain to the amount of body fat in the body. If the percentage of body fat is too low (less than 15% to 17%), menstrual function is compromised.

Stressors

Physical, emotional, or mental stress can cause amenorrhea by interfering with the delicate neuroendocrine processes.

CLINICAL PEARL

Nerves of the sympathetic trunk innervate the uterus and ovaries via the hypogastric plexus. From this plexus, branches follow paths to the pelvic plexuses that supply the pelvic viscera. Inadequate or aberrant innervation can interfere with normal ovarian and uterine function.

Diagnosis

Diagnosis requires a comprehensive history, physical exam, blood analysis, and special studies, where indicated. Blood analysis may include a pregnancy test, FSH, LH, TSH, prolactin, testosterone, and estrogen. Special studies may include a progesterone challenge, ultrasound of the reproductive organs, computed tomography (CT) scans of the ovaries and kidneys, and hysteroscopy.

History

See Table 8-1 for diagnostic clues in the history.

Physical Exam

See Table 8-2 for diagnostic clues in the physical examination.

Pelvic Examination

- A pelvic exam is performed to rule out conditions such as imperforate hymen or cervical stenosis.

Blood Analysis

See Figure 8-1 for a blood analysis flow chart.

Advanced Diagnostic Procedures

See Table 8-3 for advanced diagnostic procedures.

TECHNICAL NOTE

Cushing's syndrome is hypercortisolism or hyperadrenocorticism caused by high blood levels of cortisol. The most common causes include tumors and glucocorticoid drugs.

Cushing's disease is an adenoma (noncancerous tumor in the pituitary) that produces excessive ACTH. Excessive ACTH results in increased cortisol levels.

Cushing's disease causes Cushing's syndrome; however, not all cases of Cushing's syndrome are caused by Cushing's disease.

CLINICAL PEARL

Prolonged stress causes hypercortisolism.

Table 8-1 Diagnostic Clues: History

Amenorrhea with comorbid symptoms of	Is suggestive of
Depression and mood swings	Cushing's syndrome
Ease of bruising	Cushing's syndrome
Feelings of constipation	Imperforate hymen
Fever or cough	Pulmonary tuberculosis
Galactorrhea	Pituitary tumor, hyperprolactinemia
Generalized fatigue	Cushing's syndrome
Headaches	Pituitary tumor
Hirsutism	Adrenal or ovarian tumor, Cushing's syndrome
Hot flashes or night sweats	Menopause
Increase in skin pigmentation	Adrenal cortex failure
Intolerance to cold	Hypothyroidism
Intolerance to heat	Hyperthyroidism
Loss of axillary or pubic hair	Adrenal cortex or pituitary insufficiency
Loss of vision	Pituitary tumor
Low back pain	Imperforate hymen, lumbopelvic misalignments
Lower abdominal cramping	Imperforate hymen
Monthly or cyclic lower abdominal pain	Imperforate hymen
Nausea and vomiting	Pituitary tumor, pregnancy
Purple striations of the abdomen	Cushing's syndrome
Rectal pressure or cramping	Imperforate hymen
Vaginal pressure	Imperforate hymen
Weight gain	PCOS, pregnancy
Weight loss	Anorexia nervosa, other eating disorders

Table 8-2 Diagnostic Clues: Physical Examination

Amenorrhea with physical examination evidence of	Is suggestive of
Centripetal obesity	Cushing's syndrome
Distended abdomen	Imperforate hymen
Edema of the hands and legs	Turner syndrome
Enlarged thyroid	Thyroid disease
Enlarged uterus	Pregnancy, imperforate hymen
Hirsutism	Cushing's syndrome, androgen excess
Hyperglycemia	Cushing's syndrome
Lactation in the absence of breastfeeding	Hyperprolactinemia, pituitary tumor
Low-set ears, widely spaced eyes	Turner syndrome
Moon facies (rounded and red)	Cushing's syndrome
Muscle wasting	Cushing's syndrome
Osteoporosis	Menopause, Cushing's syndrome
Poor wound healing or thinning skin	Cushing's syndrome
Purple striations of the abdomen	Cushing's syndrome
Short stature	Turner syndrome
Webbing of the neck	Turner syndrome

TECHNICAL NOTE

Skin pigmentation is determined in part by the interplay between melanin and hemoglobin and is a function of the ratio of eumelanin (brown/black) and pheomelanin (yellow/red). ACTH stimulates melanin production, resulting in increased skin pigmentation. ACTH is equipotent with melanocyte-stimulating hormone.

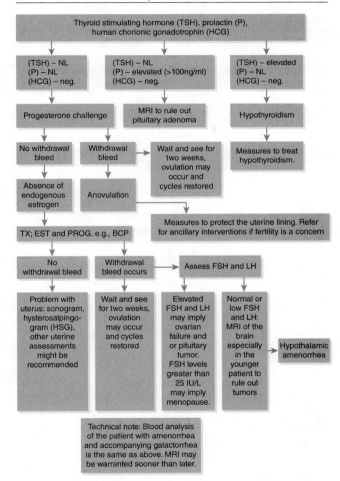

Figure 8-1 Amenorrhea blood analysis flow chart

Data from Zavanelli-Morgan, B.A. (2005). Presentation at Institute of Women's Health and Integrative Medicine, Portland, OR, October 2005; Speroff, L., & Fritz, M.A. (2005). *Clinical gyencologic endocrinology and infertility*. 7th ed. Philadelphia, PA: Lippincott Williams & Wilkins.

Table 8-3 Advanced Diagnostic Procedures

Amenorrhea caused by	May be diagnosed by
Asherman's syndrome (intrauterine adhesions)	Hysteroscopy
Cushing's syndrome	24-hour urinary free cortisol levels ≥ 50–100 mcg/day Dexamethasone suppression test to determine the source of the excess adrenocorticotropic hormone (ACTH) Corticotropin-releasing hormone (CRH) stimulation test to distinguish between pituitary adenomas, ectopic ACTH syndrome, or cortisol-secreting adrenal tumors Note: Dexamethasone and CRH tests also help to differentiate between Cushing's and conditions that may mimic Cushing's, such as PCOS and syndrome X. These conditions do not manifest elevated cortisol levels. CT scan or MRI of the pituitary and adrenals to determine presence of a tumor Petrosal sinus sampling to differentiate between pituitary adenoma and ectopic ACTH syndrome
Pituitary tumors	Magnetic resonance imaging (MRI)
Turner syndrome	Karyotyping

Management

Conventional

Management is predicated on an accurate diagnosis and management of the underlying pathology, including managing for conditions such as PCOS.

Oral contraceptives may be used to induce bleeding and to protect against osteopenia and osteoporosis.

Amenorrhea caused by a pituitary tumor or hyperprolactinemia may require specialized medical management, including the following:

- Estrogen replacement therapy: Careful monitoring of the tumor is necessary.
- Dopamine agonists such as cabergoline, bromocriptine, or pergolide: The goal of these medications is to increase estrogen levels by reducing prolactin levels. An added bonus is that they can help to restore fertility. There is some concern about fetal malformation occurring as a result of dopamine agonists.
- Transsphenoidal surgery for resection of adenoma

Amenorrhea caused by imperforate hymen is uncommon and is surgically corrected by a skilled gynecologist following estrogenization of the hymen and vagina to prevent scarring and potential recurrence.

Complementary

Nutraceuticals

- Herbs, such as chasteberry (Vitex), one capsule of the standardized extract daily, or *Rhodiola*, 200 mg/day, may be employed.
  - Vitex is a choice in the management of amenorrhea caused by hyperprolactinemia. Studies demonstrate that women with hyperprolactinemia who were given Vitex extract noted a reduction in prolactin release, shortened luteal phases, and elimination of defects in luteal progesterone synthesis (Męczekalski and Czyżyk, 2015; Van die et al., 2013).
- Acupuncture with herbs, naturopathy, and chiropractic treatments are employed as warranted to treat the underlying causes of amenorrhea.

> **CLINICAL PEARL**
>
> Hypogonadotropic states (e.g., prepubertal, hypothalamic dysfunction, pituitary dysfunction):
> Serum FSH less than 5 IU/L
> Serum LH less than 5 IU/L
> Hypergonadotropic states (e.g., postmenopausal, castration, ovarian failure):
> Serum FSH greater than 20 IU/L
> Serum LH greater than 40 IU/L

Self-Care and Wellness
- Stress-induced amenorrhea requires modifications to the activities that promote stress.
- Amenorrhea caused by excessive exercise or inadequate diet requires modifications to these activities and may necessitate collaboration with coaches, athletic trainers, dietitians, physicians, and family members.

Cervical Polyps
- Benign growths on the cervix that frequently occur at or close to the cervical os

Epidemiology
- Most commonly occur in parous women in the reproductive phase and menopausal phases

Etiology
Although the etiology is unknown, proposed causes include the following:
- Altered response to normal hormonal fluctuations
- Estrogen dominance
- Chronic inflammation
- Clogged blood vessels in the cervix

Signs and Symptoms

- Frequently asymptomatic
- Menorrhagia
- Spotting
- Intermenstrual bleeding
- Contact bleeding
- Postmenopausal bleeding
- Leukorrhea
- Discolored discharge

Diagnosis

- Pelvic exam
- Cervical biopsy

Management

Conventional

In-office procedures include the following:
- Gently twisting the polyp off at the base
- Ring forceps
- Surgical strings and suturing
- Laser
- Liquid nitrogen
- Electrocautery for larger polyps

Dysmenorrhea

Dysmenorrhea is painful menses; there are two types:

- Primary dysmenorrhea is painful menses that is not related to any definable pelvic lesion. Primary dysmenorrhea begins with the first ovulatory cycles in women under the age of 20, and in most women, it resolves or subsides by age 30, with the onset of sexual activity, or with childbirth.
- Secondary dysmenorrhea is painful menses that is related to the presence of pelvic lesions or pelvic disease (e.g., endometriosis, fibroids, episiotomy, and pelvic inflammatory disease).

Epidemiology

- The prevalence of dysmenorrhea among adolescents and young adults is 60% to 85%.
- It is the most common reason for absences from work or school among women.
- Of all women, 75% will experience some type of dysmenorrhea.

Etiology

Primary

Increased Uterine Activity/Forceful Contractions

- As the uterus contracts to expel menstrual blood, the force of the contractions can temporarily cause ischemia by occluding uterine blood supply.
- Excessive production of vasopressin causes contraction of the smooth muscle of the uterus and the small muscles within the blood vessels. Excess can stimulate very powerful contractions, which increases pain. Vasopressin is formed in the supraoptic and paraventricular nuclei of the hypothalamus and is transported to the posterior lobe through the hypothalamo-hypophyseal tract.
- Prostaglandins are a group of chemicals, some of which are formed locally at the endometrium. Similar to vasopressin, some prostaglandins cause smooth muscle contractions. Overproduction of prostaglandins can cause platelet aggregation, vasoconstriction, intense and irregular contractions, and ischemia.

TECHNICAL NOTE

Prostaglandins are not stored in the tissues; they are produced locally in situ from arachidonic acid and other fatty acids during the luteal phase of the menstrual cycle. Prostaglandins with predominantly inflammatory effects include prostaglandin E2 (PGE2); those with predominantly anti-inflammatory effects include PGE1 and PGE3.

Cervical Stenosis

- The cervical os is narrow in nonparous females. The expulsion of a nonliquefied clot through a narrowed cervical os is a potential cause of pain.
- Parous females can experience pain from the expulsion of a large nonliquefied clot.
- Women have described clots the size of a plum and larger.

Biomechanical and Neuromusculoskeletal Factors

- The uterus is situated in the middle of the pelvis, between the symphysis pubis and the sacrum. Misalignment of the pelvic girdle, including the sacrum and ilia; trigger points within the pelvic muscles; and hypertonicity of the supporting muscles can cause dysmenorrhea.
- The uterus is supported within the pelvic cavity by the two broad ligaments, the two round ligaments and the two uterosacral ligaments, in addition to other ligaments (Figure 8-2). Imbalance of the tension within the ligaments can predispose to dysmenorrhea.
- Nerves of the sympathetic trunk innervate the uterus and the ovaries via the hypogastric plexus. From this plexus, branches follow paths to the pelvic plexuses that supply the pelvic viscera. Inadequate or aberrant innervation can interfere with normal ovarian and uterine function.

Psychosocial and Constitutional Factors

- Factors such as diabetes, anemia, stress, and learned behavior are all possible causes for dysmenorrhea, either because of a lower pain threshold or increased sensitivity to pain.

CLINICAL PEARL

Nongynecological causes of pelvic pain are a component of the presentation in one-third of patients.

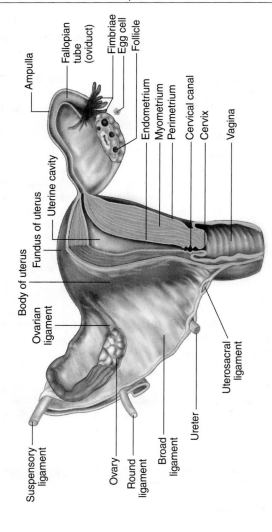

Figure 8-2 Illustration of uterus with ligamentous support

Secondary

- Postsurgical adhesions caused by caesarean section, episiotomy, or tearing with birth
- Cervical stenosis occurring after surgical procedures to the cervix
- Trigger points in the muscles that alter tension and the normal dynamics of the uterus
- Use of an intrauterine device (IUD)
  - Anecdotal reports suggest that IUDs promote dysmenorrhea in some women while relieving dysmenorrhea in others.
- Endometriosis, a condition characterized by the presence of endometrial tissue outside the uterus, which causes local inflammation, scar tissue, and pain
- Fibroids, benign tumors of the uterus, which cause pain by creating inflammation in the uterus and placing pressure on the spine and other pelvic organs
- Pelvic inflammatory disease (PID), which may result in scar tissue in the endometrial and abdominal cavities and result in subsequent predisposition to dysmenorrhea

Signs and Symptoms

Primary

- Dull, midline cramping or spasmodic lower abdominal pain begins shortly before or at the onset of menses and may radiate to the lower back or the inner thighs.
- Ancillary symptoms include nausea, diarrhea, vomiting, headache, anxiety, and fatigue.

Secondary

- Secondary dysmenorrhea is characterized by a dull ache in the lower abdomen, which may begin several hours to several days before the onset of menses and is frequently accompanied by headache, lower back pain, depression, and fatigue.

- Duration depends on the cause and may begin with ovulation and extend for 2 weeks through the next menses.

Management

Conventional

Medications

Primary Dysmenorrhea

- Nonsteroidal anti-inflammatory drugs (NSAIDs), including naproxen (Naprosyn, Aleve, Anaprox) and ibuprofen (Advil, Motrin, NeoProfen)
- Prolonged-cycle oral contraceptives, such as Seasonale and Seasonique, or intravaginal use of oral contraceptive pills
- Continuous progestogens or progestogen-releasing IUD

Secondary Dysmenorrhea

- Symptom-specific medications, including naproxen (Naprosyn, Aleve, Anaprox) and ibuprofen (Advil, Motrin, NeoProfen)

Management of the Underlying Cause

Physical Therapy

- Transcutaneous electrical nerve stimulation (TENS) is a modality that uses electrical impulses to interrupt pain signals. A combination of TENS and biofeedback has merit in managing patients with pudendal nerve distribution pain and vestibulodynia.
- Direct digital compression, stretching, and relaxation of the pelvic-floor muscles is used for relief of pelvic-floor spasm and pain.
- Botulinum toxin type A may be injected into the muscles of the pelvic floor in severe cases.
- Additional physical therapy techniques to relieve pelvic-floor tension myalgia.

Complementary

Nutraceuticals

- Calcium 1,200 to 1,800 mg/day
  - Dietary sources include dairy, green leafy vegetables, broccoli, and sardines.
- Magnesium 500 mg/day
  - Dietary sources include green leafy vegetables, molasses, soybeans, dairy, and some nuts and seeds.
- Eicosapentaenoic acid (EPA) and docosahexaenoic acid (DHA) 400 mg/day to 1,000 mg/day
- Ginger
  - Randomized clinical trials provide suggestive evidence that 750 to 2,000 mg ginger powder taken during the first 3 to 4 days of the menstrual cycle is an effective treatment for primary dysmenorrhea.
- Valerian
  - Valerian, an herb with known antispasmodic effects on smooth muscle, has demonstrated pain-relieving effects on dysmenorrhea in randomized placebo-controlled trials.
- Red raspberry leaf tea (see Technical Note)

TECHNICAL NOTE

Calcium and magnesium together are known to promote overall muscle health and muscle relaxation. EPA and DHA are known to decrease systemic inflammation.

TECHNICAL NOTE

Raspberry leaf tea has been used for centuries as a medicinal herb to treat a host of conditions, including the management of labor pain. The mechanism of action is purported to be through its antioxidant properties. Numerous anecdotal reports support the claim that for some women, red raspberry leaf tea reduces the pain and cramping associated with dysmenorrhea. Red raspberry leaf tea may impair iron absorption.

Spinal and Pelvic Manipulation

The goal of spinal and pelvic manipulation is to ensure proper pelvic alignment of the bony structures that serve as origin and insertion points for the pelvic-floor muscles and all muscles providing support for the pelvic organs.

TECHNICAL NOTE

The levator ani muscle is supplied by a branch from the fourth sacral nerve and by a branch that is sometimes derived from the perineal and sometimes from the inferior hemorrhoidal division of the pudendal nerve. The coccygeus is supplied by a branch from the fourth and fifth sacral nerves. The muscles within the pelvis include the obturator internus and the piriformis, which are muscles of the lower extremity, and the levator ani and coccygeus, which together form the pelvic diaphragm and are associated with the pelvic viscera.

CLINICAL PEARL

Misalignment of the sacrum is anecdotally reported as a common finding in dysmenorrhea.

Massage Therapy

- Assessment and management of the muscles of the pelvic girdle and abdomen for trigger points and hypertonicity
- Generalized relaxation massage techniques and additional massage techniques to address abdominal myofascial pain

CLINICAL PEARL

Of women with chronic pelvic pain, 85% have musculoskeletal dysfunction (Won & Abbott, 2010).

Lymphatic Drainage

- The sacral pump and other lymphatic drainage techniques are anecdotally reported to reduce feelings of congestion and bloating in the lower abdomen and pelvis.

TECHNICAL NOTE

In the sacral pump technique, the sacrum is tractioned caudally and pumped two or three times. This can be repeated for up to five cycles.

Acupuncture

- Acupuncture treatments have been found to significantly reduce the duration of menstrual pain and affect mood in women and can be beneficial for patients who decline NSAIDs and oral contraceptives.

Self-Care and Wellness

- Rest: Tense muscles contract more forcefully. Relaxed muscles contract with less intensity.
- Exercise: Exercise tones the muscles of the pelvic floor and the core abdominal muscles, releasing pressure on the articular facets in the lumbar spine. Beneficial exercises include knee/chest stretches and core abdominal strengthening.
- Correction of poor posture: Swayback is a cause of strain to the pelvic muscles.
- Kegel exercises: The deep pelvic-floor contractions in Kegel exercises tone the levator ani muscle (see the Appendix). The levator ani is composed of the pubococcygeus, puborectalis, and iliococcygeus muscles.
- Heat packs: Heat packs are applied to the abdomen to relax the muscles of the uterus.
- Orgasm: orgasm draws blood to the muscles of the pelvis, which aids in relaxation and decreases pain.

- Childbirth: Childbirth increases uterine vascularity, which enables the uterine muscles to relax.
- Diet: The following should be ingested sparingly:
  - Red meats and dairy—precursors to the inflammatory prostaglandins via arachidonic acid
  - Alcohol—a liver stressor that may impair the functioning of the detoxification pathways
  - Caffeine—a sympathetic nervous system stimulant that can intensify smooth muscle contractions of the uterus

Dyspareunia

Dyspareunia is painful sexual intercourse.

Epidemiology

- Sexually active women of all ages
- Experienced by an estimated 10% to 20% of women in the United States

Etiology

Proposed causes for dyspareunia include the following:

- **Biomechanical factors:** The pelvic floor is composed of nine muscles in three layers that form a sling hinged on the anterior surface by the pubic bones and on the posterior surface by the coccyx. Within this sling of muscles is the opening for the vagina; the anus, the opening to the rectum; and the urethra. Any change to the biomechanics of the pelvic girdle can result in dyspareunia. In addition, the sacral plexus lies on the piriformis and may be affected by injuries or biomechanical factors that cause piriformis strain. The levator ani is comprised of the pubococcygeus, puborectalis, and iliococcygeus muscles and is supplied by the fourth sacral nerve and by a branch that is sometimes derived from the perineal and sometimes from the inferior hemorrhoidal division of the pudendal nerve. The coccygeus is supplied by the fourth and fifth sacral nerves (see Figure 8-3).

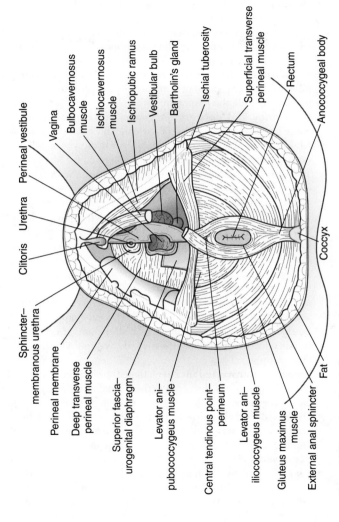

Figure 8-3 Illustration of pelvic floor musculature

- **Postural alterations:** The support of the pelvis is controlled by the larger gluteus maximum, medius, piriformis, psoas, and transversus abdominal muscles. When these are weakened by factors such as poor posture, the smaller muscles are recruited to help stabilize the pelvis. This is not their primary function, and as a result, they rapidly become strained, leading to pain, inflammation, trigger-point formation, and vaginismus. These muscles include the levator ani.
- **Pregnancy and delivery:** Pregnancy and childbirth may cause alterations in the tone of the core abdominal muscles. Maintaining posture necessitates recruiting the smaller muscles of the pelvis, which are not equipped for this task. The result is muscle inflammation, strain, and the development of trigger points. Several of these muscles support the vagina. Episiotomy caused by tearing of the perineum during vaginal birth can also cause scar tissue, which results in soft tissue hypomobility. Nerve supply to the pelvic girdle may be impaired by damage during delivery.
- **Postpartum changes:** As many as 40% of women report problems with sexual activity 3 months after birth, and 20% report such problems 12 months after birth. Almost half of all breastfeeding women report some problems with sexual activity. The elevated prolactin and decreased estrogen state that occur with breastfeeding can lead to vaginal dryness, fragility in the epithelial tissue of the vaginal vault, and dyspareunia.
- **Tipped or retroverted uterus:** A tipped or retroverted uterus alters the position of the cervix in the vaginal vault, which can cause dyspareunia.
- **Drug side effects:** Medications such as those used for allergies, hypertension, and depression may reduce the amount of vaginal lubrication, causing vaginal dryness and dyspareunia.
- **Psychosocial/psychological issues:** Issues such as depression, substance abuse, expectations attitudes and fears about sexuality, partner expectations, previous or current domestic

and or sexual abuse, and gender-role expectations may all cause vaginismus, which causes dyspareunia.

- **Stress and anxiety:** Muscles respond to stress and anxiety by becoming tense, hypertonic, and contracted. Contracted muscles do not stretch, causing pain. Vaginismus involves painful spasms of the vagina as a result of contraction of the muscles surrounding the vagina.
- **Inflammation or infection:** The deep fascia of the perineum is connected to the fascia surrounding the levator ani, the coccygeus muscles, and the pelvic viscera. Inflammation or infection of any of these intertwined structures in the pelvic girdle may predispose to dyspareunia. Conditions that cause inflammation and infection include the following:
  - Ovarian cysts
  - PID
  - Endometriosis
  - Fibroids
  - Fibromyalgia
  - Irritable bowel syndrome (IBS)
- **Pelvic adhesions and trigger points:** These can cause local and referred pain.
- **Vulvodynia:** See the section on vulvodynia.
- **Menopause:** Menopause results in a decline in estrogen and other hormones. Estrogen maintains the integrity of epithelial tissues and facilitates lubrication of the vaginal vault. In menopause, the vagina may not receive adequate lubrication, and the tissues atrophy, resulting in petechial hemorrhaging of the vaginal vault and a condition known as atrophic vaginitis (see the section on atrophic vaginitis/genitourinary syndrome of menopause).
- **Trauma:** Past or present injury, such as trauma to the tailbone or groin from a fall, sports activity such as horseback riding, or gymnastics can result in dyspareunia.
- **Coccydynia:** See the section on coccydynia.
- **Constipation:** Impacted stools create pressure on the rectum and vagina and can lead to dyspareunia.

Signs and Symptoms

- Painful intercourse
- Feeling of pelvic or vaginal heaviness
- Back pain with vaginal penetration
- Rectal pain with vaginal penetration
- Involuntary vaginal spasms

CLINICAL PEARL

- Pain with initial penetration may suggest vaginismus, trigger points in the pelvic diaphragm, or scars from an episiotomy.
- Pain with deep penetration may suggest infections, endometriosis, ovarian cysts, fibroids, trigger points in the abdominal muscles, or pudendal nerve dysfunction.
- Pain with either initial or deep penetration or both may suggest pudendal nerve dysfunction, pelvic misalignments, infection, scars from an episiotomy, trauma, and any irritation of the fascia.

Diagnosis

- By symptoms
- Screening tests for any of the conditions described previously
- Careful, nonjudgmental patient history progressing from the medical history to the sexual history

Management

Conventional

- Lubricants
- Estrogen creams for dyspareunia caused by atrophic vaginitis
- Physical therapy
  - Pelvic floor physical therapy
  - Biofeedback
  - Electrical therapies to the pelvic floor
  - Internal and external myofascial release
- Surgical intervention

Complementary

Massage Therapy

- Muscle therapy
- Trigger-point therapy to any affected muscle groups
- Myofascial and scar-tissue release techniques
- Massage of the perineum, abdominal cavity, and gluteal muscles
- Systemic massage for relaxation
- Postpartum massage of the perineum beginning 2 to 3 weeks postpartum to minimize the risk of adhesions

Laser Therapy

Laser therapy is well tolerated and may increase the thickness of the squamous epithelium and improve the vascularity of the vagina, which may alleviate the symptoms of dyspareunia. The duration of the therapeutic effects and the safety of repeated applications are not yet clear.

Self-Care and Wellness

Foremost, encourage patients to seek help; far too many women live for years with the pain of dyspareunia instead of consulting with a women's health-care provider or psychologist. Beneficial self-care and wellness measures include the following:

- Postpartum exercises to strengthen the core and pelvic outlet, such as Pilates and pelvic tilts
- Kegel exercises to draw blood to the region, increase the tone of flaccid muscles, and relax the muscles experiencing spasms
- Self-massage or partner massage of the perineum
- Gentle stretches of the vaginal orifice
  - If self-performed, the thumb is inserted into the vaginal opening and stretches the lower border from superior to inferior (the thumb is inserted into the vaginal vault, and downward pressure is applied at the 5, 6, and 7 o'clock

positions until a slight burning sensation is felt). Two to three repetitions should be performed daily. If performed by the partner, the index finger is used.

- Dilators, which come in graduated sizes and are utilized in place of the fingers to stretch the vaginal vault and treat trigger points
- Hot and cold packs to the lower abdomen and pelvic diaphragm
- Postural mindfulness
- Exercises to strengthen the core
- Counseling for psychosocial and psychosexual concerns

Endometriosis

Endometriosis is the growth of endometrial tissue in ectopic sites. The endometrium is the inner lining of the uterus. In endometriosis, uterine cells migrate or develop abnormally in ectopic sites, such as the ovaries, bladder, cervix, rectum, neck, upper arm, and axillary area. This endometrial tissue responds to hormones as if it is in the uterus, proliferating and multiplying during the first half of the cycle and imbibing, specializing, and disintegrating after ovulation. This can lead to bleeding, inflammation, adhesions, scars malformation, deformity, infertility, and pain that is often debilitating.

Epidemiology

Endometriosis occurs in menstruating women or females during their reproductive years and is frequently diagnosed in the mid-20s to early 30s. The precise incidence and prevalence remain undetermined. Geographic variations, limitations in the understanding and interpretation of the pathophysiology, and the fact that laparoscopy is required for absolute diagnosis all contribute to the difficulty in accurately assessing incidence and prevalence. What is known is that endometriosis is the third leading cause of gynecologic hospitalization in the United States and one of the most prominent causes of pelvic pain and infertility.

TECHNICAL NOTE

Types of endometriosis and their descriptions are as follows (data from Koninckx et al., 2016):

Subtle endometriosis	Nonpigmented/microscopic endometriosis—small superficial active lesions without sclerosis and without black spots
Typical endometriosis	Black puckered lesions surrounded by a sclerotic area Possess a typical vascular pattern suggesting angiogenesis
Cystic ovarian endometriosis	Strongly associated with adhesions May manifest as chocolate cyst with adhesions Differentiated from a cystic corpus luteum by the presence of adhesions Best diagnosed by ultrasound and CT scanning.
Deep endometriosis	Significantly associated with pain and infertility Tissue infiltrates deeper than 5–6 mm Type 1: covers a large pelvic area Type 2: involves retraction of the bowel Type 3: involves the rectovaginal septum; dark blue cysts in the posterior fornix Type 4: invades the sigmoid

CLINICAL PEARL

Ovarian cysts can develop from ovarian downregulation.

Etiology

The etiology of endometriosis is not fully understood; proposed causes are described in the following subsections.

Retrograde Menstruation

The theory of retrograde menstruation is that a narrow uterine outlet can cause blood to pool in the uterus, resulting in backflow out of the fallopian tubes into the abdominal cavity. Some have suggested that the use of tampons and antifungal creams may contribute to endometriosis by delaying the expulsion of menstrual blood, thereby causing pooling and backflow. The evidence to support this is lacking.

Hereditary Factors

There is significant evidence of a familial or genetic cause for endometriosis. For example, the European Society for Human Reproduction and Embryology (Stefansson et al., 2002) published a study providing further evidence that there is a genetic link to endometriosis. The study was conducted on 750 women in Iceland who had a surgical diagnosis of endometriosis between 1981 and 1993. Researchers found that a woman has more than five times the normal risk of developing endometriosis if her sister has the disease and that even having a cousin with endometriosis raises a woman's risk by over 50%. Many studies have described the contribution of genetic variants to endometriosis, the specific genetic variants as yet remain unclear. Genome-wide association scanning is demonstrating evidence of genetic associations with endometriosis in individuals of European and Japanese origin (Steinthorsdottir et al., 2016).

Lymphatic and Vascular Flow (Halban's Theory)

Endometrial tissue has been identified in distal sites, including the neck, arms, and feet. This has led some to suggest that endometrial tissue may travel via blood and lymph channels.

Coelomic Epithelium

Mucous membranes of the uterus, fallopian tubes, ovaries, vagina, external ovarian lining, and the internal lining of the pelvis are all embryologically derived from coelomic epithelium. This theory suggests that coelomic epithelium may differentiate abnormally in these sites.

Signs and Symptoms

- Pain in any or all of the pelvic organs
- Dysmenorrhea
- Dyspareunia
- Mittelschmerz (pain at ovulation)
- Intermenstrual spotting or bleeding
- Infertility
- Low back pain

CLINICAL PEARL

The severity of the disease does not necessarily correlate with the severity of symptoms. Endometriosis is a multi-faceted and multi-layered disorder that because of its chronicity may necessitate both physical and psychological support.

Diagnosis

History and exam might elicit any one or several of the following:

- History of infertility
- Moderate to severe menstrual cramps
- Pain with intercourse
- Abnormal bleeding patterns
- Constipation
- Pain with bowel movements
- Bloating and abdominal swelling
- Endometriomas (chocolate cysts) observed on examination

The pelvic examination may be painful and reveal a uterus that is retroverted, rigid, or not freely moveable; palpable nodules in the uterosacral ligaments; and cystic ovarian enlargements.

The speculum examination may reveal the presence of blue dome-like bulges in the vagina and cervix.

Definitive diagnosis of endometriosis requires either laparoscopy or MRI of the pelvis. In the laparoscopic evaluation, carbon dioxide gas is infused into the abdomen, causing distention. This enables the structures to be better visualized. A scope is inserted into the abdomen through an incision made in the navel, and the presence of scar tissue, adhesions, chocolate ovarian cysts, or powder-burn lesions provides evidence of endometriosis. In addition, the patency of the fallopian tubes can be determined.

CLINICAL PEARL

When endometriosis is suspected in adolescence, diagnosis by laparoscopy is frequently delayed. This may result in lesions compromising the ovaries and fallopian tubes and fecundability. Consideration should be given to transvaginal ultrasounds and transvaginal access with a less invasive needle endoscopy to facilitate early diagnosis before severe lesions develop.

TECHNICAL NOTE

The incidence and severity of endometriosis in adolescents are comparable to those in adult women; however, there is a mean delay of 5 years (11 years versus 6 years) from the onset of symptoms to the time of final diagnosis between adolescents and adult females.

Management

Conventional

Medications

- Birth control pills: The hormones in either the mini-pill or the combined pill diminish the intensity of endometrial symptoms by inhibiting the growth of endometrial tissue.
- NSAIDs such as Motrin, Anaprox, and Naprosyn inhibit the production of the inflammatory prostaglandin PGE2. This helps to decrease inflammation, scarring and adhesions, and pain.
- Danazol, a testosterone derivative, causes the endometrial implants to shrink by inhibiting gonadotropin release from the hypothalamus and subsequent FSH and LH release from the pituitary.
- Lupron (leuprolide acetate) and Synarel (nafarelin) are GNRH agonists, which create a low-estrogen (menopausal) state, resulting in decreased symptoms.

Procedures

Scenarios that might warrant surgery include infertility and severe pain. If fertility is desired, removal of the ectopic endometrial tissue will occur typically at the time of laparoscopy. The ectopic endometrial tissue is destroyed by either laser or electrocautery. Laser surgery to restore fertility is successful in about 50% of cases. A total hysterectomy occurs in cases where fertility is not a concern and the scars from endometriosis are extensive. It is recommended that the ovaries are preserved whenever possible to prevent premature menopause.

TECHNICAL NOTE

Pre- and postoperative assessment of serum anti-Müllerian hormone (AMH) suggests that the excision of endometriomas has a negative effect on the ovarian reserve. Ovarian endometriomas adversely affect the ovarian reserve, and cystectomy of endometriomas may cause greater damage to the ovarian reserve.

Complementary

Nutraceuticals

- Nutraceuticals that are purported to inhibit the production of the inflammatory prostaglandin PGE2 in favor of the anti-inflammatory prostaglandin PGE1 and/or decrease oxidative stress, including the following:
  - L-carnitine
  - Gamma linolenic acid (GLA)
  - EPA/DHA
  - Vitamin C
  - Pyridoxine
- Nutraceuticals that are purported to enhance liver function, including the following:
  - Methionine
  - Choline
  - Inositol
  - Milk thistle (Silymarin)

TECHNICAL NOTE

Red meats and dairy increase systemic production of arachidonic acid, a precursor to the inflammatory prostaglandins.

- Phytoestrogens, which are found in cruciferous vegetables, including kale, collard greens, cauliflower, cabbage, broccoli, and brussel sprouts, and legumes, such as lentils, chickpeas, and mung beans.
- Calcium, magnesium, and potassium found in fruits such as kiwi, figs, raspberries, and oranges, which help relax the muscles and decrease menstrual pain and cramping.

CLINICAL PEARL

Large population studies suggest that greater predicted plasma 25(OH) D levels and higher intake (more than three servings) of dairy foods (total and low-fat products) are associated with a decreased risk of endometriosis.

Acupuncture
- There is research-based evidence to indicate that acupuncture enhances female reproductive functioning, although the specific mechanism is not clear.
- In traditional Chinese medicine (TCM), specific acupuncture points of the Ren Meridian and Spleen Meridian are treated with needling and Moxibustion, a warm heat source from burning herbs or needling.

Spinal Manipulation
- Comprehensive musculoskeletal examination and treatment to address biomechanical imbalances in the pelvis, hips, and pelvic floor

Massage/Myofascial Release

- Low back and abdominal massage to break up scar tissue, work out trigger points, and "free" the uterus
- Heat pack application over the abdomen either by itself or along with castor oil or vitamin E oil application as a precursor to myofascial release techniques

Vag Packs (Vaginal Depletion Packs)

Vag Packs are small suppositories containing vitamins, minerals, and herbs that are placed deep in the vagina, close to the cervix. They are purported to function by the following mechanisms:

- Improving circulation of the pelvic organs by suspending the uterus higher in the pelvis
- Drawing fluid and infectious exudates out of the uterus
- Inhibiting local bacterial growth
- Stimulating the body to slough off abnormal cervical cells
- Promoting lymphatic drainage

Self-Care and Wellness

Diet

- Decreasing refined sugars and simple carbohydrates
  - Insulin resistance results in elevated levels of estrogen, which worsens the symptoms of endometriosis. Insulin resistance can occur under conditions of prolonged stress and with high-carbohydrate diets.
- Eliminating caffeine
- Increasing dietary fiber
  - Whole grains in the form of oats, rice, buckwheat, and millet are excellent sources of fiber. They enhance the function of the elimination pathways and provide B vitamins, which are useful in the body's synthesis of the anti-inflammatory prostaglandins.
- Minimizing exposure to endocrine system disruptors, such as pesticides

- Modifying exposure to xenoestrogens and exogenous estrogens by drinking pure filtered water; eating meats, poultry, and dairy products from nonhormonally fattened livestock; eating organic vegetables; and minimizing the use of high-estrogen hormone replacement therapy

Psychosocial Factors

- Stress causes a rise in cortisol, which affects other hormones, such as estrogen. Attending to psychosocial stressors is essential to the management of endometriosis.

Fibroids/Uterine Leiomyoma

Fibroids are noncancerous tumors of the uterus and can vary in size from very small like an apple seed to larger than a grapefruit (Figure 8-4).

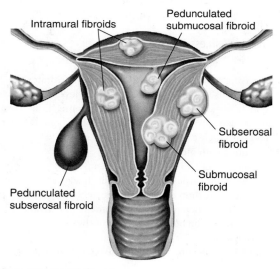

Figure 8-4 Uterus with fibroids

Epidemiology

Fibroids occur in females during their reproductive years. Symptoms of fibroids often onset during the early to mid-30s; however, evidence suggests that fibroids may be present but asymptomatic as early as the mid-20s. Some research studies suggest that as many as 70% of women have fibroids, but only 20% to 50% are symptomatic. Women who are overweight are at higher risk, as are women of African descent. The lifetime risk of fibroids in women over the age of 45 is estimated at 60%.

Etiology

The actual cause of fibroids remains unknown. Risk factors include the following:

- Nulliparity
- Obesity
- PCOS
- Diabetes
- Hypertension
- Black race
- Heredity

CLINICAL PEARL

African American women are estimated to be three times more likely to develop fibroids and experience more severe symptoms than their Caucasian counterparts.

There are racial differences in fibroid growth between Black and White women. In women over the age of 35, the growth rate of fibroids declines in White women but not in Black women.

CLINICAL PEARL

Studies have found that the risk of fibroids in African American women is positively associated with current consumption of alcohol, particularly beer. Cigarette smoking and caffeine consumption were not found to affect overall risk.

Proposed causes include the following:

- Hereditary factors: There is evidence of a genetic component to fibroids. Minimally, there is clustering between first-degree relatives and twins.
- Estrogen/progesterone imbalances: Fibroids increase in size and number when the estrogen load is high, such as during pregnancy; with the use of high-estrogen birth control pills; and in insulin resistance. Fibroids shrink when estrogen levels decline, such as in menopause. Progesterone and progesterone receptor (PR) have been implicated in the cause of fibroids. Progesterone promotes growth by increasing proliferation, cellular hypertrophy, and deposition of extracellular matrix.
- Systemic inflammation: Systemic inflammation has been proposed as a contributor to fibroids.

TECHNICAL NOTE

Estrogen stimulates the growth of fibroids leiomyomas through ovarian steroidogenesis and through local conversion of androgens by aromatase within the fibroid itself.

Progesterone stimulates fibroid growth of leiomyomas through a set of genes that regulate both apoptosis and proliferation.

Signs/Symptoms

When they occur, symptoms are potentially severe and include the following:

- A feeling of hardness in the lower abdomen and/or pelvic area
- Frequent urination
- Menorrhagia
- Anemia as a result of months (sometimes years) of menorrhagia
- Blood clots associated with menses
- Hemorrhage
- Dysmenorrhea
- Dyspareunia
- Mittelschmerz (Pain at ovulation)

- Reproductive problems such as miscarriage and infertility
- Low back pain
- Possible associated symptoms of thinning hair or male-balding hair patterns

Diagnosis

- Enlarged and lumpy appearance of uterus on routine pelvic exam
- Pelvic ultrasound
- MRI
- CT
- Laparoscopy
- Hysteroscopy
- Hysterosalpingogram (HSG), an x-ray of the uterus with contrast, to visualize submucous, interstitial, and subserous fibroids
- Dilation and curettage (D&C)

CLINICAL PEARL

Definitive diagnosis of fibroids is by ultrasound of the uterus.

Management

Management is based on factors such as symptoms, age, desire for pregnancy, and the size and location of fibroids.

Conventional

Medications

- Medications such as the GNRH agonists leuprolide acetate (Lupron) and Synarel (nafarelin), which create a low-estrogen (menopausal) state
- Low-dose emergency contraception pill, such as Ella (Esmya)
- Progesterone-releasing IUD, such as Mirena
- Progesterone injections, such as Depo-Provera
- Ulipristal acetate in 1- to 3-month doses to induce apoptosis, decrease proliferation of uterine fibroid cells, and decrease fibroid size

TECHNICAL NOTE

Ulipristal acetate is not approved by the U.S. Food and Drug Administration (FDA) for the treatment of fibroids. Ulipristal acetate is approved in Europe as a treatment for fibroids and FDA approved in the United States as emergency contraception.

TECHNICAL NOTE

Multiple research studies are under way to evaluate the efficacy of injectable drugs, such as the selective *PR* modulators and new drugs that include *Clostridium histolyticum* collagenase, in fibroid treatment.

Procedures
- Insertion of the levonorgestrel IUD
- Surgical removal of the fibroid (myomectomy)
- Surgical removal of the uterus and ovaries (hysterectomy and oophorectomy)
  - Scenarios that might warrant surgery include excessive bleeding, risk of hemorrhage, an inability to determine that the tumor is benign, and family history of endometrial and other reproductive tract cancers
- Uterine artery embolization, occlusion of the portion of the uterine artery, which supplies the fibroid
- MRI-guided ultrasound

CLINICAL PEARL

Fibroids are the leading cause of hysterectomy in women in the United States.

CLINICAL PEARL

Fibroids in the same woman do not all grow at the same rate and will sometimes spontaneously regress. Fibroid size does not predict growth rate.

CLINICAL PEARL

- Ultrasound studies suggest that 29% of women had fibroids left behind after myomectomy.
- Studies suggest that symptom recurrence rate 30 months following fibroid embolization is 17%. Fibroid size and number are predictive factors for recurrence.
- Pregnancy is possible following uterine artery embolization (UAE), and studies suggest that pregnancy rates following UAE are similar to those of the general population; however, the risk of miscarriage is higher following UAE.

Complementary

Significant evidence suggests that the development of fibroids may be triggered in part by a chronically active inflammatory immune system. A primary goal of treatment is to decrease systemic inflammation.

Nutraceuticals

- Nutraceuticals that are purported to decrease systemic inflammation and/or decrease oxidative stress, include the following:
  - L-carnitine
  - GLA
  - EPA/DHA
  - Vitamin C
  - Pyridoxine
  - Milk thistle (Silymarin)
- Curcumin: Curcumin has demonstrated an antiproliferative effect on leiomyoma cell lines in lab studies.
- Green tea (epigallocatechin gallate): In small population studies, the green tree substrate epigallocatechin gallate was found to enhance quality-of-life indicators in women with fibroids.
- Black cohosh (REMIFEMIN): In small population studies, Remifemin was found to have decreased fibroid size and symptomatology.

Acupuncture

Fibroids are influenced by the functions of the hypothalamus and pituitary. Although the mechanism remains unclear, there is evidence that acupuncture influences pituitary gland function. Based on current research, the effectiveness of acupuncture as a primary treatment for fibroids remains uncertain. Acupuncture has been found to improve the symptoms of menorrhagia, a common finding in patients with fibroids.

Manipulation

Large fibroids may place pressure on the spine, causing diffused low back pain. Spinal manipulation anecdotally provides temporary relief from the discomfort.

Massage

- Myofascial release

Vag Packs (Vaginal Depletion Packs)

Vag Packs are small suppositories containing vitamins, minerals, and herbs that are placed deep in the vagina, close to the cervix. They are purported to function by the following mechanisms:

- Improving circulation of the pelvic organs by suspending the uterus higher in the pelvis
- Drawing fluid and infectious exudates out of the uterus
- Inhibiting local bacterial growth
- Stimulating the body to slough off abnormal cervical cells
- Promoting lymphatic drainage

Self-Care and Wellness

- Follow dietary protocols to manage for insulin resistance, including increasing complex carbohydrates and decreasing refined sugars and simple carbohydrates insulin resistance may result in elevated estrogen levels and may occur under conditions of prolonged stress.

- Encourage overall lifestyle habits that promote regular exercise, eliminate cigarette use, and minimize alcohol and caffeine intake.

CLINICAL PEARL

Stress causes a rise in cortisol, which affects estrogen and other hormones. Attending to psychosocial stressors is essential to the management of fibroids.

- Increase intake of dietary fiber. Whole grains in the form of oats, rice, buckwheat, and millet are excellent sources. They enhance the function of the elimination pathways and provide B vitamins, which are useful in the body's synthesis of the anti-inflammatory prostaglandins.
- Minimize exposure to endocrine system disruptors, such as pesticides.
- Modify exposure to xenoestrogens and exogenous estrogens by drinking filtered water; eating meats, poultry, and dairy products from nonhormonally fattened livestock; eating organic vegetables; and minimizing the use of high-estrogen hormone replacement therapy.
- Ensure adequate intake of phytoestrogens, including cruciferous vegetables, such as kale, collard greens, cauliflower, cabbage, broccoli, and brussel sprouts, and legumes, such as lentils, chickpeas, and mung beans.
- Fruits such as kiwi, figs, raspberries, and oranges are sources of calcium, magnesium, and potassium, which help relax the muscles and decrease menstrual pain and cramping.

TECHNICAL NOTE

Oxidative stress status is elevated, and antioxidant capacity is diminished, in the serum of women with fibroids.

Menorrhagia

Menorrhagia is excessive menstrual bleeding and can imply menses that lasts longer than 7 days, menses that occurs more frequently than every 21 days, menses that is very heavy and requires lifestyle modifications, and excessive clotting and intermenstrual bleeding.

Epidemiology

- Women of childbearing age, although it is more commonly seen in women in their 30s and 40s.
- Affects 30% of women in the reproductive age range

Etiology

- Fibroids
- Endometriosis
- Abortion or threatened miscarriage
- Use of some IUDs for birth control
- PID

- Underlying bleeding disorders, such as von Willebrand's disease
- Platelet disorders
- Uterine polyps
- Congenital uterine anomalies
- Stress
- Insufficient nutrient intake
- Some birth control pills
- Abnormal hormonal fluctuations
- Increased prostaglandin activity
- Medications such as the anticoagulants and some anti-inflammatory agents, which may contribute to prolonged or heavy menstrual bleeding

Signs and Symptoms

- Excessive menstrual bleeding that may or may not be accompanied by pain

Diagnosis

Diagnosis involves one or several of the following:

- Careful comprehensive history
- Assessment for iron deficiency anemia
- Assessment for reproductive tract cancers
- Pelvic exam and Pap smear
- Complete blood count (CBC)
- Endometrial biopsy
- D&C if the biopsy is normal and bleeding persists
- Ultrasound to evaluate for fibroids and ovarian cysts/tumors
- HSG
- Hysteroscopy

Management

- Identify and manage the causative factors.

Conventional

Medications

- Birth control pills: Oral contraceptives help to regulate the timing and intensity of each cycle. Either the combined pill or the progesterone-only pills may be used. These help to maintain a uterine lining that is less vascular resulting in lighter periods.
- Depo-Provera: The progestin-only birth control injection, which is administered every 3 months, reduces the thickness of the endometrial lining, thereby reducing blood loss.
- GNRH agonists: GNRH agonists create a menopausal state by depleting FSH and LH secretion from the pituitary, thereby reducing or eliminating menstrual flow. GNRH agonists are more commonly utilized to minimize blood loss during myomectomy and are rarely used as a long-term strategy for menorrhagia management.
- NSAIDs: NSAIDs and prostaglandin synthetase inhibitors, such as naproxen (Naprosyn, Aleve, Midol) and ibuprofen (Advil, Motrin), reduce bleeding and modulate the pain that is sometimes associated with menorrhagia.
- Antibiotics: Antibiotics may be prescribed for menorrhagia caused by PID.

Procedures

- Endometrial ablation to destroy the entire internal lining of the uterus
- Endometrial resection to remove the lining of the uterus
- D&C
- Insertion of progestin-releasing IUD, which released small amounts of levonorgestrel locally into the uterus, thereby reducing menstrual blood loss.
- Laparoscopy or myomectomy if fibroids or endometriosis are identified as the causative factors
- Hysterectomy or hysterectomy with bilateral salpingo-oophorectomy

CLINICAL PEARL

The most common complication of menorrhagia is iron-deficiency anemia. Iron is needed by the blood to make hemoglobin, the oxygen-carrying component of red blood cells. Menorrhagia is the most common cause of anemia in premenopausal women.

Symptoms of iron-deficiency anemia include weakness, fatigue, shortness of breath, brittle nails, tinnitus, headaches, rapid heart rate, light-headedness, memory loss, general mental confusion, irritability, pale skin, and restless leg syndrome.

Management of iron deficiency anemia may include the following:

- Dietary alterations (foods high in iron include liver and other red meats, green leafy vegetables, fish, beans, fortified cereals and breads, chicken, and turkey)
- Iron supplementation
- Vitamin C to enhance iron absorption

CLINICAL PEARL

Menorrhagia in a postmenopausal woman who is not on combined hormonal replacement therapy warrants evaluation and assessment for reproductive tract cancer.

CLINICAL PEARL

Some studies have found that endometrial thinning with GNRH agonists and danazol before hysteroscopic surgery improves operating conditions and short-term postoperative outcomes.

CLINICAL PEARL

The levonorgestrel IUD has been identified in systemic reviews as the most effective and first choice for management of menorrhagia.

Complementary

Nutraceuticals

Approaches to menorrhagia management focus on control of blood loss and prevention and treatment of anemia. Recommendations based on indigenous practices and anecdotal reports include the following:

- Vitamin A
- The bioflavonoids
- Chasteberry extract (*Vitex agnus*) to normalize the menstrual cycle
- Ginger to modulate prostaglandin synthesis
- Shepherd's purse (contains tannin) to manage hemorrhage
- Ragwort/life root to improve uterine tone (based on the premise that uterine tone determines ease of flow and that a hypotonic uterus may result in heavy bleeding)
- Blue cohosh to regulate menses
- Yarrow to stimulate the uterus
- Chinese formulas specific to the patient's presentation

Self-Care and Wellness

Diet

- Foods high in beta-carotene, including watermelon and other brightly colored fruits and vegetables such as sweet potatoes, red yam, peppers, carrots, beets, and squash
- Foods high in iron, including fish, poultry, red meats, green leafy vegetables, and legumes

Pelvic Inflammatory Disease

Pelvic inflammatory disease (PID), as described by the Centers for Disease Control and Prevention (CDC), (2016) is a general term that refers to a spectrum of inflammatory disorders of the upper female genital tract, including any combination of endometritis, salpingitis, tubo-ovarian abscess, and pelvic peritonitis. All women who have acute PID should be tested for *Neisseria gonorrhea* and *Chlamydia trachomatis* and should be screened for HIV infection. PID is a common and serious complication of some sexually transmitted diseases (STDs), especially chlamydia and gonorrhea. PID can damage the fallopian tubes and tissues in and near the uterus and ovaries. Untreated PID can lead to serious consequences, including infertility, ectopic pregnancy, abscess formation, and chronic pelvic pain.

Epidemiology

- PID affects as many as 1 million women every year in the United States.
- It occurs primarily during the menstruating years, most commonly in women under 25 years of age.
- One in eight sexually active adolescent girls will develop acute PID.

Etiology

- Organisms migrate from the vagina and cervix into the uterus and pelvis. Infection spreads along the mucosal surface of the endometrium to the fallopian tubes, then to the ovaries, and then into the peritoneum.
  - The two most common pathogens implicated in PID are *N. gonorrhea* and *C. trachomatis*.
  - Other pathogens implicated in PID include *Streptococcus agalactiae*, *Escherichia coli*, *Hemophilus influenza*, *Staphylococcus* species, *Mycobacterium tuberculosis*, and *Mycobacterium bovis*.
  - Microorganisms that comprise the vaginal flora, such as the anaerobe *Gardnerella vaginalis* and the gram-negative rods, also have been associated with PID.
- Approximately 10% of PID is iatrogenically induced as a result of an abortion, IUD insertion, or D&C.
- PID also can result from transperitoneal spread of infection from a ruptured appendix or intraabdominal abscess.

Risk Factors

- Sexual activity
- Menstruation
- Prior history of PID
- Use of the IUD as a contraceptive device
- Recent procedures involving instrumentation or genital tract invasive procedures
- Douching
- Procedures or processes that involve dilation of the cervical canal, including menses, childbirth, abortion, miscarriage, D&C, and IUD insertion

Signs and Symptoms

Acute PID

- Symptom onset during or immediately after menstruation
- Presenting complaint of dull lower abdominal pain that is less than 7 days in duration and is exacerbated by movement or sexual intercourse
- Increased vaginal discharge
- Fever or chills
- Nausea and vomiting
- Right upper quadrant abdominal pain referring to the corresponding shoulder and perihepatitis with mild liver function test abnormalities (Fitz–Hugh–Curtis syndrome [FHC])
- Rebound tenderness
- Fatigue or generalized weakness
- Dyspareunia
- Urinary frequency and urgency

Subacute PID

- Symptoms as in acute, but mild to moderate severity and slower onset
- Low back pain

- Symptoms that may persist for a while before the patient seeks treatment

Chronic PID

- Constant or intermittent abdominal pain
- Persistent low-grade infection
- History of acute infection that never completely resolved
- Menstrual irregularities
- Infection of Bartholin's glands
- Constant or intermittent low back pain

Diagnosis

- Differential diagnosis
  - Ectopic pregnancy: pregnancy test, abdominal ultrasound, and serum human chorionic gonadotropin (HCG) that doesn't double in 48 hours
  - Appendicitis: rebound tenderness, fever, nausea vomiting, leukocytosis, fever, location of pain, onset, and intensity of pain
- Careful history
  - Timing, with symptoms often beginning during or immediately after menstruation
  - History of IUD insertion or abortion
- Pelvic exam that reveals pain with movement of the cervix, colored pus discharge from the cervix, and pain or a mass in the adnexa
- Leukocytosis and erythrocyte sedimentation rate (ESR)
- STD screening that reveals yellow or green discharge

TECHNICAL NOTE

Women in high-risk categories (i.e., sexually active young women and women with multiple partners) should be routinely screened for STDs.

Management

Conventional

Medications

- Broad-spectrum antibiotics with activity against gram-negative aerobes and anaerobes, such as metronidazole (Flagyl) and the cephalosporins (see CDC guidelines in the Appendix)
- Pelvic rest (bedrest and sexual abstinence)
- Fluids
- Treatment of partner for STDs
- Hospitalization and imaging if symptoms do not improve within 48 to 72 hours with oral antibiotics
  - Imaging to rule out tubo-ovarian abscess
- Surgery, if warranted—laparoscopy, laparotomy, or needle aspiration of an abscess

Self-Care and Wellness

Prevention

- Extra care should be taken whenever the cervix is dilated. Nothing should be placed into the vaginal vault during menses; for 2 to 3 weeks after miscarriage, abortion, or D&C; and for 6 weeks after childbirth.
- Wipe from front to back after a bowel movement.
- Promptly treat all vaginal infections.
- Practice "safer sex" techniques. These include low-risk sexual activities that don't involve fluid exchange; observing the genitals for discharge, sores, and odors; getting tested and treated for STDs; and sterilizing sex toys.
- Practice abstinence.

Premenstrual Syndrome/Premenstrual Tension/Premenstrual Disorder

Premenstrual syndrome (PMS), premenstrual tension (PMT), and premenstrual disorder (PMD) are "catch-all" terms for a broad range of symptoms that begin after ovulation, peak prior to menstruation, and diminish after menses.

Epidemiology
- PMS affects women in their menstruating years.
- PMS most commonly affects women of ages 25 to 40.
- Some studies suggest that 40% to 80% of women in the United States experience some premenstrual symptoms.

Etiology
Proposed causes include the following:
- Alterations in the normal ratios of estrogen to progesterone, with a preponderance of estrogen during the luteal phase
- Altered serotonin and dopamine levels
- Altered prostaglandin levels, with the inflammatory prostaglandins dominating
- Vitamin and mineral insufficiencies
- Suboptimal liver function
- Suboptimal gastrointestinal function
- Emotional, physical, or sexual abuse in early life

Signs and Symptoms
- Irritability
- Mood swings
- Swelling of the abdomen, breasts, and ankles
- Restlessness
- Tension
- Depression
- Anxiety
- Sore and tender breasts
- Headaches
- Food cravings
- Weight gain
- Memory loss
- Decreased concentration and forgetfulness

There are several classification systems, and currently, no consensus on a universal classification system exists. Select classification systems are summarized here.

The Guy Abrahams classification chart system identifies four subgroups for PMT:

- PMT-A (Anxiety)—marked by nervous tension, mood swings, irritability, anxiety, and insomnia.
- PMT-C (Craving)—marked by cravings for sugars and sweets, occasional episodes of arrhythmia, dizzy spells, fainting, fatigue, and increased appetite
- PMT-H (Hyperhydration)—marked by weight gain (greater than 3 lb [1.4 kg]) swelling of the extremities, breast tenderness, and abdominal bloating
- PMT-D (Depression)—marked by episodes of depression, forgetfulness, crying, and confusion

PMT-A, PMT-C, and PMT-H are thought to be caused in part by estrogen dominance.

PMT-D is thought to be caused in part by fluctuations in mean blood progesterone.

The International Society for Premenstrual Disorders (ISPMD) advocates for the term *premenstrual disorder* (PMD) and classifies PMD in two key categories: core PMD and variant PMD. Core PMD is more typical and more closely correlated with spontaneous ovulatory menstrual cycles. Variant PMD has more complex features.

Core PMD has three categories, as follows:

- Predominantly physical symptoms
- Predominantly psychological symptoms
- Predominantly mixed symptoms

Variant PMD has four different types, as follows:

- Premenstrual exacerbation
- PMD with anovulatory ovarian activity
- PMD with absent menstruation
- Progestogen-induced PMD

TECHNICAL NOTE

Insulin resistance predisposes to estrogen dominance, in part by increasing fat and consequent fat-cell synthesis of estrogen.

Diagnosis

- Assessment of daily record of symptoms for 2 to 3 months, with symptoms ranked from most distressing to least distressing
- Timing of symptoms in relation to the menstrual cycle
- Thyroid hormone assessment, including TSH, T4, T3 uptake, and T3, to ensure that there is no evidence of hypothyroidism
- Nutritional status assessment
- Comprehensive hormonal assay, including estrogen, progesterone (serum and saliva), dehydroepiandrosterone (DHEA), and cortisol

A diagnosis of PMS can be made if there is a clear pattern of symptoms that begin after ovulation and resolve or subside with menses.

Premenstrual dysphoric disorder (PMDD) is a severe form of PMS that is classified in the *Diagnostic and Statistical Manual of Mental Disorders*, 5th edition (*DSM-5*; APA, 2013) as a psychiatric disorder. Some authorities suggest that all levels of PMS are best assessed and managed as psychological or psychiatric disorders.

Management

Conventional

Medications

For affective symptoms:

- Alprazolam (Xanax, Niravam)
- Fluoxetine (Prozac/Sarafem)
- Paroxetine (Paxil)
- Zoloft (Sertraline HCL)
- Citalopram (Celexa)

- Venlafaxine (Effexor)
- Escitalopram (Lexapro)

  For primary symptoms of edema:

- Aldactone (spironolactone) during the luteal phase

  For primary symptoms of mastodynia:

- Daily oral contraceptives
- Bromocriptine (Parlodel, Cycloset)
- Tamoxifen (Nolvadex, Soltamox)

Complementary

Nutraceuticals

- Vitamin B_6 in a B complex up to 500 mg/day for 3 months facilitates the excretion of estrogen and estrogen by-products and aids in the synthesis of anti-inflammatory prostaglandins. Doses less than 200 mg do not appear to offer benefit for PMS symptoms.
  - The B vitamins are necessary for neurotransmitter synthesis, a factor that may affect PMS symptomatology.
- Iron (nonheme), potassium, and zinc have demonstrated utility in decreasing PMS symptomatology.
- Vitamin D: Studies have indicated that women with a vitamin D intake of an average of 706 IU per day were at significantly lower risk for PMS than those with an intake of 112 IU/day (Tartagni, et al., 2016; Johnson et al., 2005).
- Vitamin E: Studies have indicated that women with an intake of up to 100mg/ day of Vitamin E experienced some relief from PMS symptoms (Dadkhah et al., 2016).
- Calcium: Women with an average intake of 1,280 mg/day calcium from food were found to have lower PMS risk than those with an intake of 529 mg/day (Hollins-Martin, et al., 2014).
- L-tryptophan: Some women with PMDD when given 6 g of L-tryptophan during the luteal phase noted improvements in dysphoria, mood swings, tension, and irritability (Shaw et al., 2002).

- Progesterone creams are anecdotally reported to improve PMS symptoms of estrogen dominance. Progesterone creams in non-menopausal females are introduced during the luteal phase beginning on or around day 12 and extending through day 26. A low-dose of approximately 15 to 20 mg/day of the cream is applied to the cheeks, chin, neck, upper chest, and inner thighs.

TECHNICAL NOTE

Research on oral micronized progesterone in doses of 100 to 400 mg daily shows no improvement for symptoms of PMS.

CLINICAL PEARL

Case-controlled studies reveal significantly lower risk of PMS in women with high dietary intakes of thiamine and riboflavin from food sources. Similar results were not observed when the B vitamins were taken as supplements.

Primary Symptoms of Mastodynia

- Gingko biloba (80 mg twice a day taken during the luteal phase)
- Evening primrose oil (EPO) (320 mg/day for 3 to 6 months)
  - EPO is fat soluble and best taken with meals.
- Chasteberry in the form of *V. agnus* extract (20 mg three times a day during the luteal phase)

CLINICAL PEARL

Chasteberry (*V. angus*) regulates the hypothalamus–pituitary axis by acting directly on the pituitary to stimulate LH secretion and inhibit FSH secretion. This can result in an increase of progesterone, which decreases the ratios of estrogen to progesterone in the premenstruum, thereby providing relief for symptoms of headache, breast tenderness, mood swings, and bloating.

Primary Symptoms of Depression

- St. John's wort (*Hypericum perforatum*) inhibits serotonin uptake and is useful for primary symptoms of depression (900 to 1,800 mg/day for 2 months).

CLINICAL PEARL

St. John's wort is an inducer of the cytochrome P450 metabolic pathway. Many prescription drugs are metabolized through this pathway. Use of St. John's wort may impair the function of many drugs, including oral contraceptives, antiretrovirals used for HIV, antihypertensives, and antiseizure medications.

TECHNICAL NOTE

Systematic reviews affirm the efficacy of gingko biloba and *V. agnus* for improving PMS symptoms. Results from studies on the efficacy of evening primrose oil and St. John's Wort are mixed.

CLINICAL PEARL

PMS is a complex condition, and there is no one treatment that is efficacious for all patients.

Manual Techniques

- Manipulative techniques to the upper cervical spine and sacrum and techniques such as spinal touch and Logan basic (see the Appendix) have been anecdotally reported to improve sympathetic-dominant PMS symptoms.

Talk Therapy

- Talk therapy (therapeutic communication) and reassurance are integral parts of PMS management.

CLINICAL PEARL

Research has identified alterations in serotonin activity resulting from falling levels of estrogen in the luteal phase.

Self-Care and Wellness

- Ensure regular moderate aerobic exercise.
- Drink filtered drinking water.
  - Water from municipal drinking systems may contain estrogen, estrogen by-products, and other endocrine disrupters.
- Increase dietary intake of flaxseed and other lignans, which have the following effects:
  - Modulate estrogen levels by upregulating the production of the sex-hormone-binding globulins (SHBGs)
  - Activate selective receptor sites with less potent net estrogenic activity
  - Facilitate the elimination of more potent estrogens
- Avoid/minimize red meat and dairy, which are sources of arachidonic acid, a precursor to the inflammatory prostaglandins.
- Minimize exposure to exogenous estrogens (xenoestrogens) and other known endocrine disruptors, including fuels and pesticides.
- Minimize intake of refined sugars.
- Minimize alcohol and other substances that may interfere with the utility of some of the B vitamins, magnesium, and chromium.
- Limit caffeine and other substances that can intensify anxiety.

TECHNICAL NOTE

Estrogen is transported through the blood system bound to SHBGs. While bound, estrogen is unavailable to tissue.

REPRODUCTIVE TRACT MALIGNANCIES

Preinvasive Vulvar Cancer

Malignancy of the vulva is a rare form of cancer that primarily affects the labia.

Epidemiology

The most common form of vulvar cancer, which is squamous cell carcinoma, occurs in postmenopausal women in their 60s and 70s. The average age at diagnosis is 65; however, diagnosis can occur in women in their 80s and 90s. Melanoma, which is a rare form of invasive vulvar carcinoma, has been reported in females in their 40s.

Other forms of vulvar cancers include basal cell carcinoma (1.4%), adenocarcinoma (1.2%), and sarcoma (2%). Basal cell carcinoma and adenocarcinoma affect the elderly age group; melanomas and sarcomas more commonly manifest in premenopausal women.

Etiology

- The cause of vulvar carcinoma is unknown; however, the herpes simplex virus (HSV) and the human papillomavirus (HPV) have been implicated.

Signs and Symptoms

- Pruritus around the vulva
- Vulvar pain
- Bleeding, discharge, or the presence of a lump
- Possible dysuria and dyspareunia
- Affected areas that may be thicker and lighter
- Red, pink, or white bumps
- Darkly pigmented growth
- Mass on either side of the opening of the vagina
- Soreness of the vulva
- Growths on the vulva

Diagnosis

- Pelvic exam and Pap smear, followed by incision biopsy
- Pelvic exam that may reveal a lesion or lump close to the Bartholin's gland; palpable lymph nodes in the inguinal and femoral areas
- CBC, liver, and renal function tests, including serum creatinine, glomerular filtration rate, and blood urea nitrogen
- Staging to determine treatment, including chest radiograph, MRI, CT scan, cystoscopy, proctoscopy, and intravenous pyelogram

Management

Conventional

- Management is determined by the stage of the disease; stages include 0, 1, II, III, IVA, and IVB.
- Simple vulvectomy may be indicated.
- Radical vulvectomy with inguinal and femoral lymphadenectomy may be indicated.
- Modified radical vulvectomy, which involves radical excision of unilateral disease while leaving the contralateral vulva intact, is considered if the squamous cell invasion is less than 5 mm and the lesion is less than 2 cm in diameter.
- Sexual rehabilitation of the patient may be augmented by plastic surgery procedures, such as vulvar reconstruction with gracilis flaps or coverage of the inguinal region with tensor fascia lata flaps or skin grafts.
- Emotional support should be provided as needed.
- Survival rate is 75% at 5 years unless metastasis involves more than three inguinal lymph nodes, in which case 5-year survival is approximately 20%.

Vaginal Cancer

Vaginal cancer is a rare form of cancer that affects the vagina. Of all gynecological malignancies, only 1% to 2% arise in the vagina, of which 95% are squamous cell cancers occurring in women ages 55 to 65; approximately 2% are adenocarcinomas occurring in younger females, with an average age of 19 years.

Epidemiology

Squamous cell carcinoma occurs primarily in postmenopausal females aged 55 to 70.

Adenocarcinoma occurs primarily in younger females with previous exposure to diethylstilbestrol (DES). Incidence rates vary significantly by race, ethnicity, and age group, with higher incidence and a high proportion of late-stage disease in Black, Asian Pacific Islander, and Hispanic women. The rate for in situ squamous cell carcinoma appears to peak at age 70 and subsequently decline, whereas the rates for invasive squamous cell carcinoma appear to increase with advancing age.

Etiology

- The cause of squamous cell carcinoma is unknown.
- Risk factors are similar to those for cervical cancer and include persistent HPV infection.
- Adenocarcinoma and clear cell carcinoma have been linked to in utero exposure to DES prior to the 18th week of gestation.

Signs/Symptoms

- Vaginal bleeding in approximately 60% of cases
- Increased vaginal discharge
- Color and consistency changes in vaginal discharge in approximately 20% of cases
  - Discharge becomes more watery and brown in color and may cause itching.
- Pain on urination
- Pressure in the rectum
- Pain with bowel movements
- Vaginal and bladder pain as the disease progresses

CLINICAL PEARL

Reproductive tract malignancy should be suspected when there is a resumption of bleeding in a postmenopausal female who has ceased menses for a year in the absence of hormonal replacement therapy.

Diagnosis

- Four-quadrant Pap smear
- Colposcopy
- Biopsy (lymph node and tissue)
- Chest x-rays, CT scan, and MRI for metastasis and staging

Management

Conventional

- Lesions in the lower vagina may be treated with pelvic exenteration (surgical removal of all organs from the pelvic cavity) and radical vulvectomy.
- Radiation therapy is recommended for smaller lesions less than 2 cm to conserve bladder and rectal function.
- Larger lesions are treated with a combination of external beam radiation therapy and interstitial or intracavitary brachytherapy.
- Younger women with adenocarcinoma typically have a lesion in the upper half of the vagina and may be treated by radical hysterectomy with upper vaginectomy combined with pelvic lymphadenectomy.

Cervical Cancer

Cervical cancer is a malignancy of the cervix. Most cervical cancers arise from the squamous cells on the outer surface of the cervix and the transitional zone. A small proportion of cervical cancer is adenocarcinoma, which arises from the glandular mucus-secreting cells of the endocervix.

Epidemiology

Cervical cancer is typically diagnosed in women in their 40s and 50s, with an average age of 48. It is the third most common gynecologic cancer diagnosis and cause of death among gynecological cancers in the United States. This represents a decline, in that cervical cancer used to be the leading cause of cancer death for women in the United States. It accounts for half a million new cancer cases worldwide. In the United States, approximately 12,000 women are diagnosed annually, and 4,000 deaths are reported from cervical cancer each year.

Etiology

Cervical cancer arises from unmanaged cervical dysplasia. Cervical dysplasia is a precancerous condition that is treatable.

Risk factors for cervical dysplasia and cervical cancer are as follows:

- History of infection with the HSV
- History of infection with the HPV
- Early age of sexual activity
- Multiple sexual partners without the use of barrier methods of birth control
- Oral contraceptive use
  - Women utilizing oral contraceptives may have a higher incidence of cervical dysplasia. Whether this is a result of the fact that women in this group are more likely to schedule Pap smear consistently or that they are less likely to use a barrier method of birth control remains undetermined.
- Smoking
- DES exposure
- Decreased immunity, such as that observed in chronic systemic diseases (diabetes, HIV, kidney failure, etc.)
- STDs such as chlamydia, which may also increase the risk of cervical dysplasia

CLINICAL PEARL

HPV has been detected in the sperm of men who had no visible symptoms of HPV. Women with recurrent episodes of cervical dysplasia should have their partners evaluated for HPV.

Signs and Symptoms

- Approximately 70% of women with early-stage cancer have no unusual bleeding, and in 60%, the cervix appears normal.
- Vaginal bleeding or spotting between menses or as a result of activity such as exercise, with straining, or with bowel movements may occur.
- Postcoital bleeding may occur.
- Vaginal discharge that is watery, blood-tinged, or yellow-brown in color may occur.
- Invasive cervical cancer often appears as an irregular, fleshy growth.
- As the condition progresses, the patient experiences pain and pelvic or rectal pressure.

Diagnosis

- Pap smear (also known as cervical smear): A sampling of cells is taken from the cervix to aid in the diagnosis of precancerous cells.
- Thin prep Pap: The thin prep pap is similar to the conventional Pap smear in that a sampling of the cells from the cervix is obtained. However, the sample is deposited into a fluid medium instead of onto a slide, which allows for subsequent evaluation for HPV, DNA testing, and simultaneous screening for chlamydia and gonorrhea.
- Colposcopy: Colposcopy involves bathing the cervix in an acidic (vinegar water) solution, followed by subsequent evaluation under magnification with the use of a colposcope. Colposcopy with biopsy is done to confirm the diagnosis of cervical cancer.

Management

- Management is determined by the stage of the disease (see the Appendix for staging recommendations from the American Cancer Society).
- Screening includes regular Pap smears (see Table 8-4).

Conventional

Conventional therapies differ depending on the severity of cervical cancer.

- Treatments for noninvasive cancers include the following:
  - Cone biopsy: A cone-shaped tissue sample is removed from the cervix and examined under a scope.
  - Cryotherapy: Liquid nitrogen or another cold substance is used to freeze and remove the lesion.
  - Loop electrosurgical excision procedure (LEEP): Also known as large loop excision of the cervix (LLEC) and loop cone biopsy, this is a procedure whereby a special wire loop connected to an electrical source is used to evaluate and remove predetermined areas of abnormality on the cervix. The procedure requires local anesthesia.
- Treatments for invasive cancers include the following:
  - Microinvasive carcinoma: The lesion is typically less than 3 mm, and the probability of lymphatic metastasis is less than 1%. Treatment is by extrafascial vaginal or abdominal hysterectomy.
  - Invasive carcinoma: Procedures utilized are dependent on the severity of the condition, the age of the patient, and the ability of the patient to tolerate radical surgery. Additional considerations include the desire to preserve ovarian function, vaginal function, and sexual satisfaction.
  - Radiation therapy: High doses of radiation are directed to the pelvis in the form of external beam irradiation and intracavitary irradiation (brachytherapy). Generally, the pelvic viscera can tolerate relatively high doses of radiation before complications arise. Brachytherapy means "short therapy" and involves implanting radioactive sources in or near the malignancy. Brachytherapy is available in two forms: high dose rate (HDR) and low dose rate (LDR).
  - Radical hysterectomy (Wertheim hysterectomy): This procedure involves complete resection of the uterus, cervix, and parametrial tissues.

- Pelvic lymphadenectomy: This procedure is performed for both staging and treatment purposes and involves extensive dissection of the base of the bladder and terminal ureter, in addition to deep pelvic dissection. Hemorrhage and injury to the bladder, ureter, or rectum are potential complications.

Self-Care and Wellness

Prevention

- Early diagnosis of cervical dysplasia
- Regular Pap smears
- Use of barrier methods of birth control, such as condoms, diaphragms, and cervical caps.

Table 8-4 American Cancer Society Guidelines for Pap Smear

- **Cervical cancer screening (testing) should begin at age 21.** Women under age 21 should not be tested.
- **Women between ages 21 and 29** should have a Pap test every 3 years. HPV testing should not be used in this age group unless it is needed after an abnormal Pap test result.
- **Women between the ages of 30 and 65** should have a Pap test plus an HPV test (called "co-testing") every 5 years. This is the preferred approach, but it is also OK to have a Pap test alone every 3 years.
- **Women over age 65** who have had regular cervical cancer testing with normal results should not be of tested for cervical cancer. Once testing is stopped, it should not be started again. Women with a history of a serious form cervical pre-cancer should continue to be tested for at least 20 years after that diagnosis, even if testing continues past age 65.
- **A woman who has had her uterus removed (and also her cervix)** for reasons not related to cervical cancer and who has no history of cervical cancer or serious pre-cancer should not be tested.
- **A woman who has been vaccinated against HPV** should still follow the screening recommendations for her age group.
- Because of their health history (HIV infection, organ transplant, or DES exposure, etc.), some women may need to have a different screening schedule for cervical cancer.

- Avoidance of intercourse if visible warts are apparent on the partner's genitals
- Stress management
  - Mild cervical dysplasia may be an indication of excessive stress.
- Diet and nutritional supplementation to enhance overall immune health
  - Folate supplementation: In a clinical trial, folic acid supplementation of 10 mg per day resulted in improvement or normalization of Pap smears in women with cervical dysplasia. Folate supplementation for mild dysplasia in the absence of clear evidence of HPV might be useful. The recommended dose is 10 mg of folic acid daily.

Ovarian Cancer

Ovarian cancer is a catchall term for several different malignancies of the ovaries. Each of these cancers has different characteristics, treatments, and survival rates. Epithelial ovarian cancer arises from the germinal epithelium of the ovary, comprises 80% of ovarian cancers, and occurs primarily in postmenopausal women but can occur as early as the mid-30s.

The other forms of ovarian cancer are germ cell cancers, which occur primarily during childhood and adolescence, and gonadal, mesenchymal, stromal, and sex cord tumors, which are much less common and can arise anytime throughout a woman's life, although they are more common in women over the age of 35.

Epidemiology

- One-quarter of all ovarian cancer deaths occur in women aged 35 to 54.
- Half of all ovarian cancer deaths occur in women aged 55 to 75.

Etiology

The cause of ovarian cancer is unknown; however, it appears that women with the breast cancer gene mutations BRCA1 and BRCA2 and women with a history of breast cancer are at higher risk.

Reported risk factors include the use of talcum powder, living in industrialized nations, and the use of some fertility drugs.

Epithelial ovarian cancer is thought to be linked to ovulation. This hypothesis appears to be supported by the increased risk of developing epithelial ovarian cancer that is observed in nulliparous women and diminished risk in women who have had two or more pregnancies.

CLINICAL PEARL

Pregnancy, lactation, use of oral contraceptives, and other scenarios where the ovaries gain physiological rest appear to decrease the risk for ovarian cancer.

Signs and Symptoms

Signs and symptoms, when they occur, include the following:

- Abdominal pain
- Abdominal swelling
- Irregularities in bladder and bowel function
- Varicose veins
- Hemorrhoids
- Swelling of the legs or vulva
- Feelings of fullness or heaviness in the pelvic region
- Changes in weight
- Low back pain
- Vaginal bleeding
- Serosanguineous vaginal discharge
- Gastrointestinal symptoms such as flatulence, indigestion, loss of appetite, nausea, and vomiting
  - Many of the symptoms of ovarian cancer appear to be related to the gastrointestinal tract. This is in part because ovarian cancers shed malignant cells that then implant on organs of the reproductive and gastrointestinal systems, including the uterus, bladder, bowels, and omentum. These cells become sites for the growth of additional tumors.

Diagnosis

- Regular pelvic exams
- Pelvic ultrasound
- Blood tests for the ovarian-cancer-associated antigen, CA 125
  - A palpable adnexal mass on pelvic exam and an elevated CA 125 is positive for ovarian cancer in 80% of the patients.

TECHNICAL NOTE

Definitive diagnosis of ovarian cancer is based on surgical pelvic exploration by laparotomy and pathologic review.

- Additional diagnostic protocols: CBC, HCG, alpha-fetoprotein, urinalysis, a complete gastrointestinal series, abdominal and pelvic CT or MRI scan, and ultrasound

CLINICAL PEARL

Diagnosis of ovarian cancer by symptomatology is difficult because symptoms are vague and often mimic those of gastrointestinal disorders. As a result, by the time the female presents for treatment, the disease has often progressed to other areas of the reproductive tract and abdominal cavity.

Management

Conventional

Treatment is dependent on a number of factors, such as the stage and grade of the disease and the patient's age and overall health, but may include the following:

- Surgical removal of the ovaries
- Chemotherapy and or radiation

> **CLINICAL PEARL**
>
> Complications from chemotherapy include pancytopenia, sepsis, alopecia, hepatic toxicity, pulmonary toxicity, neurotoxicity, and nephrotoxicity; long-term complications can include pulmonary fibrosis and leukemia.

The survival rate for ovarian cancer is approximately 15% at 5 years because of the spread via epithelium and lymphatic channels into the peritoneal/abdominal cavity as a result of delayed diagnosis. If the diagnosis is made while the malignancy remains confined to the ovaries, the survival rate is approximately 90%.

Self-Care and Wellness

Prevention strategies might include the following:

- Dietary folate: Studies indicate that high levels of folate obtained from food sources may protect against ovarian cancer.
- Acetaminophen: There is some evidence that acetaminophen may lower the risk for ovarian cancer. In a small-scale study, women who regularly used acetaminophen were found to have a 50% to 60% decrease in the rate of ovarian cancer when compared with those who did not.
- Aspirin: According to the National Institutes of Health (NIH), women who take aspirin daily may reduce their risk of ovarian cancer by as much as 20%.

Fallopian Tube Cancer

Malignancy of the fallopian tube is the rarest of all the gynecological malignancies, accounting for 0.1% to 0.5% of the gynecological cancers. Fallopian tube cancer sometimes occurs concurrently with ovarian cancer.

Epidemiology

- Women of low parity with an average age of 55 years at the time of diagnosis.
- Estimated incidence rate of 0.41 per 100,000

Etiology

- Although etiology is unknown, women with breast cancer gene mutations BRCA1 and BRCA2 and women with a history of breast cancer may be at higher risk.

Signs and Symptoms

- Vague
- History of mild but chronic lower abdominal and pelvic pain
- Vaginal bleeding
- Vaginal discharge

Diagnosis

- The physical exam may reveal an adnexal mass.
- Because fallopian tube cancer is so rare, it may be suspected in a patient with Pap smear evidence of adenocarcinoma and negative fractional D&C.

Management

Treatment for fallopian tube cancer is similar to that outlined for epithelial ovarian cancer and may involve a total abdominal hysterectomy, bilateral salpingo-oophorectomy, omentectomy, peritoneal cytology, and selective lymphadenectomy followed by chemotherapeutic agents.

Overall survival is approximately 18% for stage III disease and between 40% and 75% for stage 1 and stage 2 diseases.

Uterine Cancer

Also known as endometrial cancer, uterine cancers are malignancies primarily of the endometrial lining of the uterus.

Epidemiology

- Uterine cancer is the leading invasive gynecologic malignancy encountered in the United States, with approximately 38,000 cases diagnosed yearly.

- Most uterine cancers (~75%) occur in postmenopausal women; less than 3% occur in women 40 years of age and younger.

Etiology

- Unopposed or excess estrogen

Risk Factors

- Obesity
- Late menopause (after age 53)
- Nulliparity
- Hypertension
- Diabetes
- Ovarian disorders such as PCOS and granulosa tumors of the ovary
- Estrogen replacement therapy (ERT)
  - Case-controlled studies demonstrate that the risk of developing endometrial carcinoma in patients taking ERT was increased from 3-fold to 12-fold. This risk is closely tied to the dosage and duration of ERT.
- Previous history of reproductive and other cancers
- Hereditary factors
- Tamoxifen given to treat breast cancer, may increase the risk of uterine cancer
- Early menarche and/or late menopause
- History of benign polyps or other growths of the endometrial lining
- High-fat diet

Signs and Symptoms

- Painless vaginal bleeding, which is a hallmark of uterine cancer and occurs in 90% of cases
  - Uterine cancer should be considered in any case of a postmenopausal woman who has stopped bleeding for over one year and resumes bleeding in the absence of hormonal replacement therapy.
- Bleeding between periods in premenopausal women

- Pain—pelvic pain, lower abdominal pain, low-grade and diffuse low back pain
- Pelvic mass
- Discharge—serosanguineous vaginal discharge and vaginal discharge that may be profuse and malodorous and may occur in bursts, particularly after heavy exertion or straining

Diagnosis

- History that reveals symptoms of vaginal bleeding
- Pap smear
- Endometrial and endocervical biopsy
- Fractional D&C performed under general or spinal anesthesia

Management

Conventional

Treatment is based on disease progression and staging, as follows:

> **TECHNICAL NOTE**
>
> The American Joint Commission on Cancer stages uterine cancer as follows:
>
> Stage 0: Carcinoma in situ. Cancer cells are only found in the surface layer of the endometrium.
>
> Stage 1: The cancer is only growing into the body of the uterus and perhaps into the glands of the cervix.
>
> Stage 2: The cancer has spread from the body of the uterus into the connective tissue (stroma) of the cervix.
>
> Stage 3: The cancer has spread outside of the uterus into the nearby tissues of the pelvis.
>
> Stage 4: The cancer has spread to the inner surface of the urinary bladder, the rectum, the lymph nodes in the groin, and/or distant organs such as the bones, omentum, or lungs.
>
> Data from American Diabetes Association. (2016). Management of diabetes in pregnancy. *Diabetes Care, 39*(Suppl 1), S94–8.

- Stage 1: abdominal hysterectomy to include bilateral salpingo-oophorectomy
- Stage 2: surgery and combination radiation therapy

Table 8-5 Five-Year Survival Rates for Uterine Cancer

Stage	5-Year Survival
Stage 0	90%
Stage IA	88%
Stage IB	75%
Stage II	69%
Stage IIIA	58%
Stage IIIB	50%
Stage IIIC	47%
Stage IVA	17%
Stage IVB	15%

Data from American Cancer Society. (2016). Endometrial cancer survival rates, by stage. Retrieved from https://www.cancer.org/cancer/endometrial-cancer/detection-diagnosis-staging/survival-rates.html

- Stage 3: surgery, radiation therapy, and the possibility of chemotherapy or hormonal therapy such as progestins or antiestrogens
- Stage 4: extensive surgery, radiation therapy, chemotherapy, or hormonal therapy such as progestins or antiestrogens

Table 8-5 lists 5-year survival rates for uterine cancer from the American Cancer Society.

VULVODYNIA

Vulvodynia is an all-encompassing term to describe several conditions, including cyclic vulvovaginitis, vulvar vestibulitis syndrome, and essential vulvodynia, all of which manifest with acute or chronic vulvar pain.

Epidemiology

- Vulvodynia appears to afflict primarily Caucasian women.
- The prevalence among sexually active women of any age is estimated at 8%.

Etiology

The etiology for vulvodynia is unknown. Proposed causes include the following:

- Allergic reactions to food, female hygiene products, soaps, toilet paper, other sanitary products, and clothing fibers
- Previous vaginal infections
- Irritation or injury to the nerves around the vulva
- Autoimmune disorders
- Chronic tension
- Muscle spasms
- Sexual abuse
- History of cryotherapy to the vulva
- History of laser therapy to the vulva
- Lichen sclerosis

TECHNICAL NOTE

Lichen sclerosis is a condition that presents with inflammation and white plaques on the vulva and progressive pruritus, dyspareunia, dysuria, or genital bleeding. The inflammation can be so intense that is causes blisters, which may mimic the trauma of sexual abuse or other genital ulcerative disease. Autoimmune disorders are suspected to be the primary cause of lichen sclerosis.

Signs and Symptoms

- Raw feeling around the vulva
- Vulvar burning, soreness, itching, or stinging
- Dyspareunia
- Pain in the vulva that is frequently aggravated by activities of daily living

Diagnosis

- Detailed history
- Physical examination, including pelvic exam
- Screening for bacterial, viral, and fungal infections

Management

Conventional

Medications

- Local anesthetics for pain relief, such as a 4% liquid solution of xylocaine administered 5 to 10 minutes before intercourse
  - Lidocaine and benzocaine are also reported to provide short-term relief.
- Cortisone and other topical creams
- Antihistamines to reduce itching
- Antidepressants for chronic pain
  - Studies suggest that antidepressants such as amitriptyline, desipramine, and nortriptyline in doses ranging from 10 mg/day to 225 mg/day for 4 weeks to 30 months in duration provided some relief for some women. Lower doses of 50 mg to 100 mg of amitriptyline and desipramine are reported to have an analgesic effect.
- Anticonvulsants
  - Studies suggest that gabapentin and pregabalin in dosages of 300 mg per day to 300 mg per week provided some relief for some women.
- Estrogen creams
- Treatment for identified infections or fungi, which may include oral metronidazole, intravaginal clindamycin cream, or metronidazole gel (for candidiasis, oral fluconazole or intravaginal clotrimazole)

Therapy

- Physical therapy, including biofeedback and other relaxation training procedures to release pelvic muscles experiencing spasms and decrease the pain response
- Psychologic therapy, including cognitive-behavioral therapy
- Sexual therapy

Surgery

- Nerve stimulation via implanted electrodes and regional nerve blocks, which is anecdotally reported to offer some relief
- Modified vestibulectomy, which involves excising the hymen ring and the superficial vestibular mucosa
- Vestibuloplasty, which involves a hymenectomy and removal of the painful mucosa and other painful sites in the anterior vestibule and removal of the minor vestibular glands

Complementary

- Pelvic-strengthening exercises and therapies
- Spinal manipulation as needed to release irritation to the spinal nerves supplying the vulva
- Acupuncture, which has been purported to help turn off overactive or malfunctioning pain fibers

Self-Care and Wellness

- Kegel exercises to assess awareness and control of the pelvic-floor muscles (10 sets of contractions three times a day)
- Reverse Kegel maneuver (Valsalva) to push out the pelvic floor; can increase the capacity of the introitus
- Superficial perineal massage to desensitize the area through touch and increase the pliability of the superficial pelvic-floor muscles
  - The patient inserts the lubricated thumb into the vagina and presses down toward the anus until the stretch is uncomfortable but not painful. The position is held for 1 minute, with the focus being to relax the pelvic floor. The vagina is slowly massaged using a U-shaped movement from 3 o'clock to 9 o'clock for up to 3 minutes daily. The partner may also be trained in this technique but will use the index finger.
- Avoidance potential allergens, such as soaps, vaginal creams, and feminine deodorant sprays

- Wearing of cotton underwear and loose clothing
- Frequent washing of the genital area with water alone
- Avoidance of deodorized sanitary products
- Avoidance of tight-fitting clothing, including underwear, pantyhose, and tight jeans
- Cold compresses applied directly to the genital area
- Baking soda douche
- Sitz baths
- Avoidance of exercises that put direct pressure on the vulva, such as bicycling
- Low-oxalate diet
- Calcium citrate to reduce vulvar burning sensation
- Vulvar pain support groups

CLINICAL PEARL

Some research suggests that the burning sensation associated with vulvodynia is a result of oxalic acid in the urine irritating the vulvar tissues.

CHAPTER 9

Mental Health and Eating Disorders

MENTAL DISORDERS

The mental disorders most common in women are as follows:
- Anxiety disorders
- Depressive disorders
- Posttraumatic stress disorder
- Dementia

Anxiety Disorders

Some level of anxiety is a normal human reaction to stressful events, experienced by all at some juncture. Anxiety disorders are different. Anxiety may become excessive and interfere with daily functioning. The *Diagnostic and Statistical Manual of Mental Disorders*, 5th edition (*DSM-5*; American Psychiatric Association [APA], 2013) considers anxiety disorders as those that are persistent and in general last more than 6 months and are accompanied by features of excessive fear, anxiety, and behavioral disturbances. Anxiety disorders are among the most common mental illnesses experienced by Americans and are twice as common in women as in men. Anxiety disorders are diagnosed when the symptoms are not attributable to the physiological effects of a substance/medication or to another medical condition and are not better explained by another medical disorder. Anxiety disorders include the following:

- Panic disorder (recurrent unexpected panic attacks)
- Specific phobia (fear of a particular object or situation)
- Social anxiety disorder/social phobia
- Agoraphobia (fear of being in public places)
- Generalized anxiety disorder (GAD)

TECHNICAL NOTE

Posttraumatic stress disorder (PTSD), although more common in women, is no longer classified as an anxiety disorder. PTSD is currently classified in the *DSM-5* (APA, 2013) as a trauma- and stressor-related disorder.

Epidemiology

According to the National Institutes of Health (NIH, 2016a) 18% of Americans experience anxiety disorders, and 60% of these are women.

Etiology

The exact cause of anxiety disorders is unknown. Research has shown that many of these disorders are caused by a combination of factors, including changes in the brain and environmental stress.

Risk factors include the following:

- Genetics
- Stressful life event or chain of events (e.g., family breakup or death)
- Biochemical changes
- Being female
- Personality (temperament that is timid or negative)

Signs and Symptoms

- Hot and cold flushes
- Tachycardia
- Tight feeling in chest
- Excessive worry
- Muscle tension and aches
- Headaches
- Sweating
- Nausea
- Concentration difficulties
- Irritability
- Restlessness
- Polyuria
- Sleep disturbances
- Numbness of extremities
- Hyperventilation

Diagnosis

Panic Disorder

- Panic disorder is characterized by recurrent unexpected panic attacks (i.e., abrupt surges of intense fear or discomfort that peak within minutes). Attacks may occur without a cue or trigger (unexpected attacks) or with a situational trigger (an expected attack).
- For most individuals, the frequency of the attacks varies, and the focus of the worry includes health concerns, concerns about peers, and issues with control.

> **CLINICAL PEARL**
>
> Panic disorders increase following puberty, peak in adulthood, and decline in older individuals.

Specific Phobia (Fear of a Particular Object or Situation)

- Specific phobia is diagnosed when there is intense fear or anxiety in the presence of a particular situation or object (the phobic stimulus) that occurs every time the person comes into contact with the stimulus and is out of proportion to the actual danger that the stimulus poses. The individual actively avoids the stimulus.

Social Anxiety Disorder (Social Phobia)

- Social anxiety disorder is diagnosed when there is intense fear or anxiety of social situations where the individual may be scrutinized by others occurring for over 6 months.
- Fear of being negatively evaluated by others and fear of offending others cause the individual to avoid the social situation or endure it with intense fear or anxiety. Concurrently, there is anticipatory anxiety sometimes far in advance of the upcoming situation that interferes significantly with the individual's normal routine.

> **CLINICAL PEARL**
>
> Some of these behaviors are considered appropriate in select cultural contexts.

Agoraphobia (Fear of Being in Public Places)

- Agoraphobia is diagnosed when the individual experiences persistent, intense fear or anxiety lasting for a minimum of 6 months, triggered by anticipated exposure to any two of the following situations:
  - Being in open spaces such as a parking lot, market, or bridge
  - Using public transportation
  - Being in enclosed spaces such as a theater or store
  - Being in a crowd or standing in line
  - Being outside of the home alone
- The person experiences fear or anxiety that is so out of proportion to the actual threat that he or she actively avoids the situation.

Generalized Anxiety Disorder

- GAD is diagnosed when there is excessive anxiety or worry about a number of events or activities. The focus of worry may shift from one concern to another. The worries are excessive and pervasive and followed by restlessness, feeling on edge, fatiguing easily, having trouble concentrating, disturbed sleep, and muscle tension.
- GAD comorbidities include autonomic hyperarousal, increased heart rate, somatic symptoms muscle aches or soreness, irritable bowel syndrome, and headaches.
- Diagnosis is based on results from the following:
  - Self-assessment tests
  - Medical history
    - Intensity and duration of symptoms

369

- Self-reports of being unable to complete everyday tasks
- Suicidal concerns in chronic cases
- Direct observation of the patient's behavior and attitude

CLINICAL PEARL

Nearly 18% of people with anxiety disorders may attempt suicide, and nearly 39% of people with anxiety disorders frequently harbor suicidal thoughts.

Management
Conventional

- Medications
  - Medications include serotonergic drugs (buspirone), benzodiazepines (alprazolam, lorazepam, clonazepam, diazepam), heterocyclic antidepressants (amitriptyline, clomipramine, doxepin), and selective serotonin reuptake inhibitors (SSRIs; fluoxetine, paroxetine, sertraline). SSRIs and tricyclic antidepressants have demonstrated the best efficacy.
- Cognitive behavioral therapy
- Other treatment approaches as recommended by trained mental health professionals

Complementary

Nutraceuticals

- Nutraceuticals to restore normal gut flora
  - Research studies have demonstrated that administering *Lactobacillus* and *Bifidobacterium* reduces anxiety in humans.
- Nutraceuticals used for mild to moderate anxiety, including the following:
  - Lemon balm (*Melissa officinalis*)

- Note: *M. officinalis* may pose a dependency risk and cause withdrawal symptoms if abruptly discontinued.
- Kava (*Piper methysticum*), which modulates glutamine acid decarboxylase autoantibodies (GABA) and is used for general anxiety
- Passionflower
- L-lysine
- L-arginine
- Ashwagandha
- Acupuncture
- Cognitive behavioral therapy
- Other treatment approaches as recommended by trained mental health professionals

Self-Care and Wellness

- Relaxation techniques, such as mindfulness meditation, progressive muscle relaxation, and deep-breathing exercises
- Diet: well rounded with frequent small meals, avoiding caffeine and alcohol
- Yogurt with live bacterial cultures
- Limiting or eliminating smoking
- Exercising regularly (i.e., 30 minutes most days of the week)
- Ensuring adequate sleep (i.e., 7 to 9 hours every night)

TECHNICAL NOTE

The specific mechanism by which microbes in the gut interact with mental illness remains unclear and is a promising area of research.

Fast Facts—Gut Bacteria

- Bacteria in the gut are known to produce neurotransmitters.
- Bacteria in the gut may generate neuroactive chemicals, such as butyrate, which may reduce anxiety and depression in humans.

- Bacteria in the gut are known to produce the chemical 4-ethylphenylsulphate (4EPS), which is produced in larger quantities in individuals with autism.
- Strains of *Lactobacillus* and *Bifidobacterium* reduce anxiety-like disorders.
- Human subjects who were given Prebiotics (carbohydrates that provide sustenance for gut bacteria) noted lower levels of cortisol and focused on more positive information.

Depression

Depression is a common mental disorder that is also called clinical depression or a major depressive disorder and is characterized by sadness, loss of interest, low self-esteem, sleep disturbances, and fatigue. It can be long lasting or intermittent, significantly weakening the ability to function. One measure of clinical depression is that an episode of sadness along with other symptoms lasts at least 14 successive days and disrupts daily life.

Epidemiology

According to the National Institutes of Health (2016b), 8% of the population has experienced a major depressive disorder, with the majority being women.

Etiology

The exact cause of depression is unknown. It is believed to be multifactorial. Neurological, hormonal, immunological, genetic and neuroendocrinological processes seem to contribute to the development of major depression, mostly by influencing a person's reaction to stressors and processing of emotional information. Of all these factors, studies have shown that approximately 40% to 50% are hereditary. Etiological processes are believed to be modified by gender, age, and developmental factors. Environmental interventions such as a positive family environment or the support of a good friend have been shown to have a positive impact on the outcome of depressive episodes.

TECHNICAL NOTE

Researchers have noted that some people with a history of depression have a smaller hippocampus than those without a history of depression. A smaller hippocampus has fewer serotonin receptors, which is significant because serotonin is a neurotransmitter that supports communication across circuits that connect different regions of the brain.

CLINICAL PEARL

Nearly 30% of people who misuse alcohol or other drugs experience at least one episode of major depressive disorder.

Signs and Symptoms

- Sadness and crying for no apparent reason
- Feelings of hopelessness
- No interest in activities previously enjoyed (anhedonia)
- Fatigue and lack of motivation
- Social isolation
- Low self-esteem, feelings of being unworthy
- Restlessness
- Major change in eating and/or sleeping patterns
- Expressions of irritability, anger, or hostility
- Frequent somatic complaints (e.g., headaches, generalized pain, stomachaches, and menstrual problems)
- Behavior problems such as frequent absences from work or school and being disruptive at home
- Poor concentration
- Thoughts or expressions of suicide or other self-destructive behaviors
- Behavioral changes in young people that demonstrate a sense of sadness, such as playing music with morbid themes, wearing black clothing, or writing stories and poetry that are gloomy
- Alcohol and drug abuse

CLINICAL PEARL

Depression and anxiety disorders are different, but people with depression often experience symptoms similar to those of an anxiety disorder, such as nervousness, irritability, and problems sleeping and concentrating. Each disorder has its own causes and its own emotional and behavioral symptoms.

Many people who develop depression have a history of an anxiety disorder earlier in life. There is no evidence that one disorder causes the other, but there is clear evidence that many people suffer from both disorders.

CLINICAL PEARL

Many bipolar illnesses begin with one or more depressive episodes, and a substantial proportion of individuals who initially appear to have major depressive disorder (especially when diagnosed in adolescence) will prove to instead have a bipolar disorder.

Diagnosis

There is no specific test to diagnose depression. Diagnosis is dependent upon symptomatology reported by the individual or by those in close contact.

According to the *DSM-5* (APA, 2013), for a diagnosis of major depressive disorder to be made, the individual must have experienced five or more of the following symptoms over a 2-week period for most of the day for most days, and at least one of the symptoms must be either a depressed mood or a loss of interest or pleasure:

- Depressed mood, such as feeling sad, empty, or tearful
- Significantly diminished interest or feeling no pleasure in almost all activities
- Significant weight loss, weight gain, or decrease or increase in appetite
- Insomnia or increased desire to sleep
- Either restlessness or slowed behavior as observed by others
- Fatigue or loss of energy

- Feelings of worthlessness or inappropriate guilt
- Trouble making decisions or concentrating
- Recurrent thoughts of death or suicide; planned or attempted suicide

These symptoms must be severe enough to cause noticeable problems in day-to-day activities, such as work, school, social activities, or relationships with others. A diagnosis of major depressive disorder may necessitate ruling out other conditions, such as thyroid anomalies that may be mimicking depression symptoms.

TECHNICAL NOTE

The *DSM-5* (APA, 2013) affirms that grief and major depressive disorders may coexist and advises practitioners to include notes in the patient records that delineate normal grieving from major depressive disorder.

CLINICAL PEARL

Practitioners may find it valuable to include a depression questionnaire, such as the Beck Depression Inventory (see the Appendix), in all intake materials.

Management

Conventional

Medications

- Antidepressants: SSRIs, such as Fluoxetine (Prozac), sertraline (Zoloft), escitalopram (Lexapro), paroxetine (Paxil), and citalopram (Celexa) are among the most common. Serotonin and norepinephrine reuptake inhibitors (SNRIs) are similar to SSRIs and include venlafaxine (Effexor) and duloxetine (Cymbalta).
- Tricyclics are older drugs that are powerful but have more serious side effects, such as suicidal ideation, low blood pressure, cardiac arrhythmias and tremors, and confusion in the elderly.

Included among the tricyclics are Tofranil (imipramine) and Pamelor (nortriptyline).

- Monoamine oxidase inhibitors (MAOIs) are the oldest class of antidepressants and are especially effective in cases of "atypical" depression, such as when a person experiences increased appetite. They also may help with anxiety or panic and other specific symptoms. Foods and beverages containing tyramine (including cheese and red wine) must be avoided, as must certain medications, including some types of birth control pills, some pain relievers, cold and allergy medications, and herbal supplements. These substances can interact with MAOIs and cause dangerous increases in blood pressure.

Procedures

- Psychotherapies, such as cognitive-behavioral therapy (CBT) and interpersonal therapy (IPT), are best suited for individuals with mild to moderate depression.
- Electroconvulsive therapy (ECT), formerly known as "shock therapy," can provide relief for people with severe depression who have exhausted other treatment options. The person, under general anesthesia, has small electric currents passed through the brain, intentionally triggering a brief seizure. ECT reverses symptoms of certain mental illnesses by causing changes in brain chemistry. Risks include memory loss and confusion.
- Brain stimulation therapies are used to treat severe depression. These include vagus nerve stimulation (VNS) and repetitive transcranial magnetic stimulation (rTMS). Although not yet commonly used, clinical trials suggest that these therapies show promise.

Complementary

- Therapies used to support individuals with depression include the following:
  - Acupuncture
  - Yoga and meditation

- Anecdotal reports and case studies support the following for easing the symptoms of depression in some individuals:
  - Homeopathic remedies such as sulfur, ignatia, and *Pulsatilla*
  - Aromatherapy ointments such as sage
  - Reflexology
  - Transcranial magnetic stimulation
  - Hypnotherapy where sleep disturbances compound depressive symptoms
  - Light therapy (exposure to bright light and the use of light boxes) for individuals suffering from seasonal affective disorder (SAD)
  - St John's wort

CLINICAL PEARL

St. John's wort should not be used by individuals on cardiovascular medications or those on oral contraceptives.

Self-Care and Wellness

- Avoid spending long periods alone.
- Evaluate the diet for nutritional deficiencies.
- Consider a whole-foods diet rich in vegetables.
- Engage in mild to moderate exercise for a minimum of 30 minutes most days of the week
- Practice diaphragmatic breathing.

CLINICAL PEARL

Population studies reveal that women with higher serum Mg and Zn levels had less depressive symptoms.

CLINICAL PEARL

Isotretinoin (Accutane and Roaccutane), drugs used in the treatment of acne, may cause or increase symptoms of depression in users.

TECHNICAL NOTE

The FDA placed a "black-box" warning label on all antidepressant drugs about the potential increased risk of suicidal thinking or attempts in children, adolescents, and young adults taking antidepressants. The warning emphasizes that patients of all ages taking antidepressants should be closely monitored, especially during the initial weeks of treatment.

Warning signs of severe depression/suicide include the following:

- Making comments about wanting to die, having nothing to live for, or committing suicide
- Looking for ways of killing oneself, such as stockpiling pills, searching online, or recent purchase of a gun
- Making comments about feeling hopeless or having no reason to live
- Having no plans for the future
- Talking about feeling trapped, having no way out of current problems, or being in pain that is overwhelming
- Talking about being a burden to others
- Increased use of drugs or alcohol
- Acting anxious or agitated; increased risk-taking behaviors/reckless behavior
- Change in sleeping pattern
- Withdrawal from social interactions or talking about feeling isolated
- Preoccupation with death
- Sudden change in mood to being happier/calmer
- Significant loss of interest in things/activities that person cared about previously
- Reaching out to people to say good-bye/have final conversations
- Making final personal arrangements or giving away prized possessions

Clinician responsibilities are to take all comments about suicidal thoughts or threats seriously:

- Acknowledge that the pain the person is experiencing is legitimate and offer to work together to get assistance.
- Don't assume that the person is only seeking attention.
- Seek help immediately by calling the local police emergency number or the National Suicide Prevention Lifeline.

Resources
- 911 or the local emergency number
- National Suicide Prevention Lifeline: 1-800-273-TALK (8255)

(continues)

- Community mental health resources, which can be identified by calling United Way—First Call for Help, toll-free: 1-800-543-7709.
  Look for red flags for suicidal behavior (IS PATH WARM):
- **I**deation: Threatened or communicated
- **S**ubstance abuse: Excessive or increased
- **P**urposeless: no reason for living
- **A**nxiety: agitation/insomnia
- **T**rapped: feeling there is no way out
- **H**opelessness
- **W**ithdrawing: from friends, family, society
- **A**nger: (uncontrolled) rage, seeking revenge
- **R**ecklessness: risk-taking behaviors
- **M**ood changes: dramatic fluctuation

CLINICAL PEARL

The QPR institute recommends the Question – Persuade – and Refer approach
  The premise of this approach is as follows:
Early Recognition of suicide: The sooner warning signs are detected and help sought, the better the outcome of a suicidal crisis will be.
Early QPR: Asking someone about the presence of suicidal thoughts and feelings opens up a conversation that may lead to a referral for help.
Early intervention and referral: Referral to local resources or calling 1-800-Suicide for evaluation and possible referral is critical (QPR Institute, 2016).

Premenstrual Dysphoric Disorder

Premenstrual dysphoric disorder (PMDD) is defined by the *DSM-5* (APA, 2013) as a specific and treatment-responsive form of depressive disorder that begins sometime following ovulation, remits within a few days following the onset of menses, and has a marked impact on functioning.

Epidemiology

- Among menstruating women, 1.8% to 5.8% experience PMDD.

Etiology

- Proposed causes of PMDD include the following:
- Increased sensitivity to normal cycling levels of estrogen and progesterone
- Increased aldosterone and plasma renin activity
- Neurotransmitter abnormalities, particularly serotonin
- Risk factors include the following:
  - Environmental stressors
    - Seasonal change
    - Sociocultural factors, including female gender roles and sociocultural aspects of female sexual behavior
  - History of personal trauma
  - Heredity factors

Signs and Symptoms

- Mood swings
- Marked irritability or anger
- Marked depressed mood
- Marked anxiety
- Decreased interest in usual activities
- Subjective difficulty in concentrating
- Lethargy, easily fatigued, marked lack of energy
- Significant change in appetite
- Hypersomnia or insomnia
- Feeling overwhelmed or out of control
- Breast tenderness, swelling, joint or muscle pain, bloating or weight gain

Diagnosis

The *DSM-5* (APA, 2013) criteria for a diagnosis of PMDD requires mood lability, irritability, dysphoria, and anxiety that occurs repeatedly during the menstrual phase of the cycle and remits around the onset of menses. Symptoms may be accompanied by behavioral and physical symptoms and must have adverse effects on work or social functioning. A minimum of five of the preceding symptoms must have been present for most of the menstrual cycles within the previous year.

Validated rating scales include the following (see the Appendix):

- Daily Record of Severity of Problems
- Visual analogue scales for premenstrual mood symptoms
- Premenstrual Tension Syndrome Rating Scale

CLINICAL PEARL

Differential diagnosis for PMDD includes the following:

- Premenstrual syndrome (PMS): Minimum of five symptoms is not required; less severe than PMDD.
- Dysmenorrhea: Varies in terms of onset of symptoms and symptom complexity.
- Bipolar disorder, major depressive disorder, persistent depressive disorder: Symptoms do not follow a premenstrual pattern.
- Hormonal treatments (substance-induced depressive disorder): May present with similar symptoms, but when the individual discontinues the hormones, the symptoms disappear.

Management

Conventional

Medications

- Serotonergic antidepressants such as citalopram, escitalopram, fluoxetine, sertraline, and venlafaxine

Complementary

Nutraceuticals

- Limited evidence supports supplementation with calcium, vitamin D, and vitamin B_6.

Cognitive-Behavioral Therapy

- Current evidence is insufficient in support of CBT as a treatment for PMDD.

Self-Care and Wellness

- Limited evidence supports exercise for improving symptoms of PMDD; however, regular exercise should be recommended for overall health and wellness.

CLINICAL PEARL

According to the *DSM-5* (APA, 2013), women who use oral contraceptives have fewer premenstrual complaints than those who don't.

CLINICAL PEARL

PMDD symptoms may worsen as menopause approaches and improve at menopause, but they may worsen again with hormone replacement therapy (HRT).

Posttraumatic Stress Disorder

PTSD is the development of characteristic symptoms following exposure to one or more directly experienced traumatic events. Traumatic events may include exposure to war as a combatant or civilian, threatened or actual physical assault, threatened or actual sexual violence, natural disasters, incarceration, and torture.

Epidemiology

- PTSD is more prevalent in females across the life span, and females experience PTSD for a longer duration than do males.
- Lifetime risk in the United States is 8%.

CLINICAL PEARL

Some of the increased risk for PTSD observed in women is attributable to a greater likelihood of exposure to traumatic events such as rape and other forms of interpersonal violence.

Etiology

- Exposure to one or more "directly experienced" traumatic events

Signs and Symptoms

- Recurrent, involuntary, and intrusive recollection of the event
- Recurrent distressing dreams related to the traumatic event
- Dissociative reactions in which the individual feels or acts as if the traumatic events are recurring
- Intense or prolonged psychological distress as a result of exposure to cues that mimic components of the traumatic event
- Persistent avoidance or efforts to avoid memories or thoughts associated with the event
- Efforts to avoid people, places, and situations that arouse distressing memories, thoughts, or feelings about the event
- Cognitive and mood changes associated with the event, such as dissociative amnesia, feelings of detachment and estrangement, and persistent negative emotional state

CLINICAL PEARL

PTSD symptoms may begin as early 3 months and up to several years after the trauma.

Diagnosis

- Signs and symptoms have occurred for more than 1 month.
- The symptoms are causing impairment in important areas of functioning.
- The disturbance is not attributable to the physiological effects of a substance or other medical condition.

Management

Conventional

Medications

- SSRIs and tricyclic antidepressants for anxiety and depression
- Hydrocortisone for prevention of PTSD development in adults

CLINICAL PEARL

Hydrocortisone administered early may reduce the risk for subsequent PTSD symptoms in adult patients with severe trauma.

Complementary

Nutraceuticals

- Nutraceuticals with research evidence supporting efficacy in PMS or PMDD include the following:
  - Chasteberry (Vitex)
  - Vitamin B_6
  - Calcium
  - Vitamin D

CLINICAL PEARL

A few anecdotal reports correlate spinal manipulation with improvement in PTSD symptomatology.

Self-Care and Wellness

- Engaging in practices that relieve stress, including the following:
  - Massage therapy
  - Yoga
  - Meditation
  - Support groups

CLINICAL PEARL

PTSD is associated with suicidal ideation and suicide attempts.

CLINICAL PEARL

Traumatic events such as childhood abuse increase a person's suicide risk.

Dementia

Dementia is a condition that broadly describes a range of cognitive symptoms that interfere with the ability to perform daily tasks.

Epidemiology

Alzheimer's accounts for 60% to 70% of reported cases of dementia. Vascular dementia, often caused by a stroke, is the second most common type. More women than men have Alzheimer's or other forms of dementia. Almost two-thirds of Americans with Alzheimer's are women.

Etiology

- Damage to the brain's nerve cells caused by a number of factors, including the following:
  - Alzheimer's disease is the most common cause of dementia in individuals over the age of 65.
  - Vascular dementia, as seen in individuals with stroke, is the second most common cause of dementia.
  - Lewy body dementia, in which proteins clump together in the brain of an affected individual, accounts for 10% of dementia cases.
  - Frontotemporal dementia is seen in younger older adults age 50 to 70. The nerve cells in the frontal and temporal lobes break down, causing problems with behavior, speech, and language.
- Other causes include the following:
  - Poor diet
  - Vitamin deficiency
  - Head trauma
  - Thyroid problems
  - Normal aging
  - Family history
  - Genetic mutations

Signs and Symptoms

- Memory loss affecting job skills
- Difficulty performing familiar tasks
- Language difficulties

- Disorientation of time and place
- Poor or impaired judgment
- Challenges with abstract thinking
- Mood swings
- Misplacing items
- Personality changes—confusion, phobias
- Loss of initiative

Diagnosis

- History and exam, including memory tests such as the Mini-Mental State Examination (MMSE)
- Psychological/psychiatric evaluation
- Computed tomography (CT) and magnetic resonance imaging (MRI) brain scans to rule out other possible problems
- Urine or blood levels of tau, beta-amyloid, or other biomarkers to look for changes
- Genetic testing for APOE-e4, a gene that increases risk for dementia

Management

Conventional

Medications

- Medications to delay symptomatology include cholinesterase inhibitors and glutamate regulators.
  - Cholinesterase inhibitors (donepezil [Aricept], galantamine [Razadyne], and rivastigmine [Exelon]) work by slowing down the process that breaks down a key neurotransmitter.
  - Glutamate regulators (memantine [Namenda]) work by regulating the activity of glutamate, an important neurotransmitter in the brain involved in learning and memory.

CLINICAL PEARL

Attachment of glutamate to cell surface "docking sites" called NMDA receptors permits calcium to enter the cell. This process is important for cell signaling and learning and memory. In Alzheimer's disease, excess glutamate can be released from damaged cells, leading to chronic overexposure to calcium, which can speed up cell damage.

Complementary

The research on complementary therapies in dementia is preliminary. Some studies indicate that the following may have efficacy, although further research is needed:

- Vitamin E
- Gingko
- Omega-3 fatty acids
- Coenzyme Q10
- Massage therapy
- Music therapy
- Pet therapy
- Aromatherapy

Self-Care and Wellness

- Task modification—breaking tasks into smaller, easier steps
- Environmental adaptions—removing distracting noises and clutter
- Training for caregivers
- Regular exercise
- Thought-stimulating activities and games
- Support groups

EATING DISORDERS

Female Athlete Triad

The female athlete triad consists of disordered eating (anorexia and bulimia nervosa), amenorrhea (primary, secondary, and oligomenorrhea), and osteoporosis.

Anorexia Nervosa

- Refusal to maintain body weight
- Body weight less than 85% of expected
- Intense fear of gaining weight

- Failure to make expected weight gain during period of growth
- Denial of seriousness of low body weight

Bulimia Nervosa

- Recurrent episodes of binge eating
- Lack of control over eating
- Eating excessive amounts during a discrete time period
- Recurrent compensatory behavior, such as self-induced vomiting; misuse of laxatives, enemas, or diuretics; and excessive exercise
- Self-evaluation that is heavily influenced by body shape and weight
- Behavior occurs at least twice a week over several months

Amenorrhea

Alterations of the rhythmic secretions of gonadotropin-releasing hormone (GNRH) leads to decreased levels of follicle-stimulating hormone (FSH) and luteinizing hormone (LH) and subsequently decreased levels of estrogen and progesterone, which results in amenorrhea.

- Primary amenorrhea
  - The absence of spontaneous uterine bleeding by the age of 14 without development of secondary sexual characteristics or the absence of spontaneous uterine bleeding by the age of 16 with otherwise normal development
- Secondary amenorrhea
  - Six-month absence of menstrual bleeding in a woman with regular menses or 12-month absence of menstrual bleeding in a woman with previous oligomenorrhea
- Oligomenorrhea
  - Infrequent menses

Osteoporosis

A primary function of estrogen is to inhibit osteoclastic activity. As a result of the hypoestrogenic state, osteoclast-mediated bone resorption is uninhibited, resulting in osteoporosis.

Epidemiology

The female athlete triad has historically been associated with athletes; however, it is now known that the condition is not limited to athletes and may be commonly found among age-matched females and males.

Etiology

- Participation in any sport that emphasizes lean physique or a specific body weight, including the following:
  - Gymnastics
  - Figure skating
  - Ballet
  - Distance running
  - Diving
  - Swimming
- Mental and psychosocial issues such as low self-esteem
- Parents and coaches who place undue expectations on the athlete
- Heavy energy expenditure
- Misinformation about nutrition
- Societal pressure to be thin
- Physical abuse, sexual abuse, and/or substance abuse

Signs/Symptoms

- Recurrent stress fractures
- Amenorrhea or oligomenorrhea

- Erosion of the tooth enamel from gastric acid produced with recurrent vomiting
- Very thin female
- Muscle injury
- Parotid swelling as a result of frequent stimulation of the salivary glands from recurrent vomiting
- Tooth marks on the back of the hand from induced vomiting
- Fatigue and decreased ability to concentrate
- Presence of lanugo hair
- Sensitivity to cold
- Palpitations
- Chest pain
- Endothelial dysfunction
- Reduced cardiovascular dilatation response to exercise
- Increased risk of cardiovascular disease
- Urinary incontinence
- Binge eating
- Eating alone
- Frequent trips to the bathroom during and after meals

Diagnosis
- Comprehensive history and exam
- Menstrual history
- History of amenorrhea
  - This is often the first sign; however, it is also important to remember that there are many reasons for amenorrhea.
- Delayed onset of menarche
- History of oligomenorrhea
- Absence of physical signs of ovulation such as mittelschmerz
- Previous or current use of hormonal therapy
- Diet history
  - Less threatening to inquire about past disordered eating rather than current
  - Record of what was eaten during the last 24 hours
  - Extensive list of "forbidden foods"
  - Happiness with current weight

- Ideal weight according to patient and highest/lowest weight since menarche
- Use of diet pills or laxatives
- Exercise history
  - Exercise patterns
  - Training intensity
- History of previous fractures
- History of overuse injuries
- Additional exam protocols (see the Appendix for descriptions and screening tools):
  - Height
  - Weight
  - Body mass index (BMI)
  - Sexual maturity rating
  - Scoliosis
  - Neglect/abuse screening
  - Blood pressure
  - Pelvic ultrasound
  - Electrocardiography (ECG)
  - Bone mineral density (BMD)
    - BMD should be evaluated if the athlete has been amenorrheic for over a year or has a history of stress fracture or a BMI of less than 18.
- Laboratory tests
  - Complete blood count (CBC) to assess for anemia, especially iron-deficiency anemia
  - Complete metabolic panel to evaluate liver function, serum electrolytes, and kidney function
  - Thyroid panel to rule out hyper- or hypothyroidism
  - Pregnancy test (urine or plasma)
  - Erythrocyte sedimentation rate (ESR) and/or C-reactive protein (CRP) to assess for infection or inflammation
  - Enzymes such as amylase and lipase
  - Hormone panel, including estradiol, testosterone, and dehydroepiandrosterone (DHEA), to assess for ovarian or adrenal pathology

Management

The primary health-care provider needs to be astute and willing to work collaboratively with a multidisciplinary team that includes psychologists, dietitians, coaches, teachers, and parents.

The dietitian facilitates the design of healthy nutritional choices, the plan for attaining and maintaining an ideal weight, and education regarding the prevention of caloric deficit and maintenance of a positive energy balance.

Conventional

- Birth control pills or estrogen supplementation is often necessary, especially if a progesterone challenge does not result in the onset of menses.
- Care from a psychiatrist or psychologist is needed to manage eating disorders and esteem concerns.
- Coaches should modify exercise intensity. Typically, a 10% to 20% decrease in exercise intensity is needed.
- Teachers and parents should monitor progress, assess for compliance, and provide support and encouragement.

Complementary

Nutraceuticals

- Daily calcium intake of a minimum 800 mg and as much as 1,500 mg/day of elemental calcium to prevent osteoporosis

> **TECHNICAL NOTE**
>
> Studies conducted on female athletes with osteoporosis demonstrated a lack of improvement in bone density with calcium supplementation in the presence of amenorrhea. Bone density improved with calcium supplementation only with the return of menses or the addition of estrogen therapy.

- Boron—1 mg a day to aid utilization of calcium
- Vitamin D—800 to 1,000 units/day to aid calcium absorption

- Vitamin C—up to 2 g a day in split doses to aid development of the collagen portion of bone
- Folic acid
  - Folic acid in 10-mg daily dosage has been found to improve endothelial function; however, no large studies have specifically included amenorrheic female athletes.

CLINICAL PEARL

- High-phosphate substances, such as artificially carbonated beverages, tend to increase bone loss of calcium and should be avoided.
- Red meats should be eaten sparingly because the uric acid from protein synthesis can increase calcium loss.
- High-protein diets cause larger-than-normal calcium excretion, thereby increasing the potential for bone loss.

CLINICAL PEARL

Orthorexia Nervosa

According to the National Eating Disorders Association (Kratina, 2016) Orthorexia Nervosa is a disorder, thus far not classified as a clinical disorder in the DSM-5.

Orthorexia Nervosa or fixation on righteous eating as described by Dunn and Bratman (2016), is an unhealthy obsession with otherwise healthy eating. Orthorexia begins as an attempt to eat a healthy diet , but results in a fixation on food quality, quantity and purity. The self esteem of the person with Orthorexia is directly linked to the purity of the diet, and feelings of superiority to others with regards to food intake. Food choices ultimately become so restricted that the individuals health (and the health of their wards) suffers. Eventually, the obsession with healthy eating impairs relationships, and becomes physically dangerous. Orthorexia is best treated by a specialist in eating disorders (Kratina, 2016; Dunn & Bratman, 2016)

CHAPTER 10

Metabolic and Endocrine Disorders in Women

ADRENAL DYSFUNCTION

Addison's Disease (Adrenal Insufficiency)

Addison's disease is a potentially life-threatening endocrine disorder marked by inadequate production of cortisol by the adrenal glands. Addison's disease is primary adrenal insufficiency. Secondary adrenal insufficiency is caused by the failure of the pituitary gland to produce enough adrenocorticotropic (ACTH) hormone.

Epidemiology

- Rare condition that is more common in women and children
- Presenting age between 30 and 50

Etiology

- Primary adrenal insufficiency caused by autoimmune disorders in which the adrenal cortex is destroyed as part of the pathological process
- Infection such as tuberculosis that destroys the adrenal gland
- Cancer of the adrenal glands

Signs and Symptoms

- Extreme fatigue
- Prolonged fatigue
- Loss of appetite
- Abdominal pain
- Low blood pressure
- Fainting
- Hyperpigmentation (occurs only in Addison's, not in secondary adrenal insufficiency)
- Hypoglycemia
- Weight loss
- Musculoskeletal pain, especially in the lower back and legs
- Salt craving

- Hyponatremia
- Hyperkalemia
- Oligomenorrhea
- Amenorrhea

Diagnosis

- Serologic analysis
  - Cortisol
  - ACTH
  - Sodium
  - Potassium
  - ACTH stimulation test
  - Corticotropin-releasing hormone (CRH) stimulation test if ACTH stimulation test is normal
- Procedures
  - Magnetic resonance imaging (MRI) of the pituitary gland to rule out pituitary tumor
  - Computed tomography (CT) scan of the abdomen to check the size of the adrenal gland and evaluate for other anomalies
  - Insulin-induced hypoglycemia test

Management

Conventional

Medications

- Corticosteroids
- Corticosteroid injections

Complementary

Nutraceuticals

- Dehydroepiandrosterone (DHEA) supplementation

Self Care and Wellness

- High-sodium diet

Adrenal Crisis (Addisonian Crisis, Acute Adrenal Insufficiency)

Adrenal crisis is a life threatening group of symptoms brought on by low cortisol levels

Epidemiology

Adrenal crisis is frequently associated with adrenal insufficiency. Forty two percent of patients with adrenal insufficiency report at least one episode of adrenal crisis.

Etiology

- Damage to any of the glands involved in cortisol production to include the adrenals and the pituitary gland
- Gastrointestinal infection
- Physiologic stress such as major pain, surgery, psychic distress
- Untreated adrenal insufficiency
- Steroid Therapy—specifically rapid withdrawal of long-term steroid therapy

Risk Factors

- Abrupt termination of glucocorticoid medications
- Physiologic stressors such as heat, and pregnancy
- Adrenocorticotrophin therapy
- Conditions such as HIV/Aids, and tuberculosis
- Infection from staph aureus, streptococcus and hemophilus influenza
- Meningococcemia
- Long-term use of steroids
- Use of topical steroids over a large area of the body as occurs in burn therapy

Signs and Symptoms

- Unexplained shock
- Nausea/Vomiting

- Abdominal/flank pain
- Confusion, loss of consciousness, Coma
- Dizziness/light-headedness
- Headache
- Dehydration
- Fatigue
- Fever
- Changes in heart or respiratory rate
- Excessive sweating on face or palms
- Hyperthermia or hypothermia

Diagnosis

Lab Testing

- ACTH stimulation test: A small amount (250 mcg) of ACTH is injected, and the amount of cortisol that the adrenals produce in response is measured 30 and 60 minutes after ACTH administration. An increase of less than 9 mcg/dL of cortisol is considered diagnostic of adrenal insufficiency.
- Serum Cortisol (< 20mcg/dL)
- Complete blood count (CBC) to assess for anemia, inflammation and infection
- Serum potassium, sodium, blood sugar and pH to assess for hyponatremia, hyperkalemia, metabolic acidosis, and hypoglycemia

Management

Conventional

Adrenal crisis is a medical emergency. Treatment includes immediate injection of hydrocortisone, intravenous fluids and treatment of infection, shock or other presentation.

CLINICAL PEARL

The ACTH test is diagnostic.

> **CLINICAL PEARL**
>
> According to Hahner et al. (2010), Adrenal crisis incidence in adrenal insufficiency is not influenced by BMI, DHEA treatment, educational status, age at diagnosis, hypothyroidism, hypogonadism, or glucocorticoid dose.

> **CLINICAL PEARL**
>
> Recognition and treatment of adrenal crisis in trauma centers reduces trauma patient mortality by ~50% (Hahner et al., 2010).

Cushing's Syndrome

Cushing's syndrome is a condition marked by overproduction of cortisol.

Epidemiology

- Occurs three times as often in women as in men
- Occurs with a higher incidence (2% to 9%) in high-risk populations, such as patients with diabetes, hypertension, or osteoporosis

Etiology

- Glucocorticoids used in the treatment of cancer, asthma, rheumatoid arthritis, and autoimmune conditions
- Glucocorticosteroids such as prednisone
- Cushing's disease (primarily a condition of overproduction of ACTH by the pituitary gland)
- Adrenal gland tumors
- Distal tumors causing the release of CRH

Signs and Symptoms

- Round, full face, also known as moon face
- Central obesity

- Purple marks or striae on the abdomen, thighs, and breasts
- Bruising easily
- Oligomenorrhea/amenorrhea
- Hirsutism
- Musculoskeletal changes, including bone pain, muscle weakness, and fractures of the spine and ribs
- Depression, anxiety, and fatigue

Diagnosis
- Physical exam findings as noted previously
- Lab tests:
  - Blood cortisol
  - Blood sugars
  - Salivary cortisol
  - 24-hour urine for cortisol and creatinine
  - Dexamethasone suppression test
  - Bone mineral density (BMD)
  - ACTH levels and ACTH stimulation test
  - Pituitary MRI

Management
Conventional
- Change/decrease in medications contributing to the syndrome
- Surgery if a tumor is involved
- Radiation
- Cortisol replacement therapy following surgical resection
- Depending on the cause, medications to block cortisol release

Complementary
- Nutraceuticals
  - Ginseng, which can function as an adaptogen, is anecdotally reported as a stress-reducing strategy.
  - Magnolia bark is anecdotally reported to relieve anxiety.

> **CLINICAL PEARL**
>
> Herbs with adaptogenic effects should only be used in consult with experts because the net effect on the hormonal milieu may be deleterious, especially when these herbs are used in conjunction with other medications.

- Massage therapy

Self-Care and Wellness

- Nutritious, healthy diet
- Hot baths
- Mental and physical exercises
- Tai chi
- Support groups

Subclinical Hypoadrenalism

Subclinical hypoadrenalism (also known as adrenal fatigue) is a term used to describe symptoms correlated to suboptimal functioning of the adrenal glands. Subclinical hypoadrenalism is different from Addison's disease. Addison's disease is manifested by insufficient production of cortisol and aldosterone.

Epidemiology

- Individuals who have been subject to intense or prolonged physical, emotion, or mental stress
- Individuals who have had acute or chronic infections such as pneumonia, influenza, or bronchitis

> **TECHNICAL NOTE**
>
> Other terms sometimes affiliated with subclinical hypoadrenalism include non-Addison's hypoadrenia, subclinical hypoadrenia, neurasthenia, adrenal neurasthenia, adrenal apathy, and adrenal fatigue.

Etiology

- The demands of work, family, children, aging parents, and society at large may place undue stresses on many women. The result is a perpetual fight-or-flight cycle. The adrenal glands, which were designed to function only in times of danger, function constantly, releasing norepinephrine and epinephrine from the adrenal medulla and corticoids, mineral corticoids, and androgens from the adrenal cortex.

- The mineral corticoids (primarily aldosterone) regulate the balance of minerals (sodium, potassium, and magnesium) in the cells. Stress triggers the release of aldosterone, which raises blood pressure by its action on cells to hold on to sodium and lose potassium. Long-term release of stress levels of mineral corticoids can cause a potassium deficiency, magnesium imbalance, chronic water retention, and high blood pressure. The resultant magnesium insufficiency as noted by red blood cell magnesium levels can affect many of the enzyme-driven metabolic pathways in the body.

- The adrenal cortex makes all of the sex hormones in small amounts and DHEA in large amounts. DHEA is important in the growth and repair of protein tissues and is a precursor to androstenediol, testosterone, and the estrogens. It is not a precursor to progesterone, aldosterone, pregnenolone, or the cortisols. Alterations to the normal production of the hormones of the adrenal cortex can predispose to multiple symptoms, including aggression and anger from too much testosterone, passivity, oversensitivity, mental confusion and agitation from too much or too little estrogen, and depression from too little estrogen or progesterone.

Signs and Symptoms

- Generalized fatigue that is not significantly improved by rest
- Generalized feelings of malaise
- Chronic fatigue
- Increasing blood pressure
- Depression
- Loss of libido
- Total exhaustion

Diagnosis

- Blood hormonal assays and salivary tests
  - Morning and afternoon salivary or serum cortisol
  - Urinary cortisol
  - Plasma ACTH
- Tests to rule out other potential causes of chronic fatigue

Management

Conventional

- Currently, there are no known conventional treatments for subclinical hypoadrenalism.

Complementary

- Short-term use of DHEA
- Licorice root
- Ashwagandha
- *Melissa officinalis* leaf tea (when sleep disorders are a factor. Note: Long term use of Melissa officinalis is associated with dependency risk)
- Bioidentical hormones
  - Caution: DHEA converts to testosterone, which converts to estrogen and may result in an increased estrogen load. The potential negative impact of the increased estrogen load on estrogen-related cancers cannot be minimized. Recommendations are for the lowest dosage possible, and levels should be monitored with blood analysis.

> **CLINICAL PEARL**
>
> DHEA supplementation may cause or worsen symptoms of acne.

Self-Care and Wellness

- Exercise—low- to medium-intensity exercise program
- Coping mechanisms such as biofeedback, yoga, and meditation

- Dietary management—including legumes and phytoestrogens; avoiding sources of xenoestrogens
- Managing for insulin resistance
- A good multivitamin with adequate dosages of calcium, magnesium, and the essential fatty acids
- Psychosocial and psychological factors such as decreasing stress and developing and nurturing support systems

DIABETES

Insulin Resistance, Metabolic Syndrome/Syndrome X, Adult and Juvenile Diabetes

Insulin resistance is caused by the failure of the cells to respond adequately to stimulus from insulin; this initiates a vicious cycle in which blood sugar levels rise, and in response, the pancreas accelerates insulin production. The cells eventually respond, and glucose in the blood enters the cells en masse, resulting in a corresponding rapid drop in blood sugar levels and a hypoglycemic state. As simple carbohydrates and high-glycemic-index foods are ingested, the cycle repeats until eventually the pancreas is overextended and is no longer able to produce sufficient amounts of insulin, resulting in diabetes. Insulin resistance is marked by simultaneous elevations of blood sugars and blood insulin. The liver responds to the elevated blood sugar levels by rapidly converting the excess sugars to fat. Glucose from sugars is converted to energy in the cells; in the absence of this critical source of energy, fatigue and food cravings result.

The excess fat cells result in increased hormone load as more estrogen is stored in fatty tissue and synthesized via the aromatase enzyme. Aromatase enzyme synthesizes estrogen via the androstenedione pathway, which may ultimately result in excess testosterone. Insulin resistance is a prediabetic condition.

Syndrome X, also known as **metabolic syndrome** is a cluster of symptoms that predispose to heart disease and is defined by the National Cholesterol Education Program as the presence of any three of the following:

- Excess weight around the waist (waist measurement of more than 40 inches for men and more than 35 inches for women)
- High levels of triglycerides (150 mg/dL or higher)
- Low levels of high-density lipoprotein (HDL) cholesterol (below 40 mg/dL for men and below 50 mg/dL for women)
- High blood pressure (130/85 mm Hg or higher)
- High fasting blood glucose levels (110 mg/dL or higher)

Adult-onset **diabetes**, also known as type 2 diabetes, is caused by the inadequate response of the body to insulin and inadequate production of insulin by the pancreas.

Diabetes in Women

The burden of diabetes can be tough on women because the condition can affect both mothers and their unborn children. Diabetes can cause added difficulties during pregnancy, including miscarriage and birth defects. According to the American Diabetes Association (ADA), other challenges experienced by women with diabetes include the following:

- Recurrent yeast infections—glucose is a trigger for candidal growth
- High blood pressure, ocular disease, and kidney disease as a consequence of taking oral contraceptives, which cause increases in blood sugar levels
- Premature menopause
- Cardiovascular disease
- Increased risk of heart attack at a younger age
- Loss of libido resulting from changes in blood glucose levels that can cause feelings of fatigue and irritability
- Depression

Epidemiology

According to the Centers for Disease Control and Prevention (CDC), 29 million Americans are living with diabetes, and

86 million are living with prediabetes. Type 2 diabetes accounts for 90% to 95% of all diagnosed cases of diabetes, and type 1 diabetes accounts for approximately 5%.

Etiology

- Stress
- Diet
- Being overweight
- Family history of diabetes
- Low HDL and high triglycerides
- High blood pressure
- History of gestational diabetes
- Genetics/hereditary factors

Risk Factors

- History of giving birth to babies weighing over 9 pounds
- Being from one of the following minority groups:
  - African American
  - American Indian
  - Hispanic/Latino
  - Asian American/Pacific Islander

Signs and Symptoms

- Excessive thirst
- Fatigue following high-carbohydrate meals
- Increased abdominal weight gain
- Extreme fatigue after eating-high-glycemic index foods

Diagnosis

- Blood tests used to diagnose diabetes include the following:
  - Fasting glucose levels of 126 mg/dL or higher on more than one test are evidence of diabetes. Levels of 100 to 125 mg/dl indicate impaired fasting glucose and suggest a prediabetic or insulin-resistance state.
  - In the glucose tolerance test, the patient is required to fast overnight and be evaluated 2 hours after drinking a sweet

liquid. Insulin resistance or a prediabetic state is suspected if the blood glucose is between 140 and 199 mg/dL 2 hours after drinking the sweet liquid, and diabetes is indicated if the levels are over 200 mg/dL.

- Hemoglobin A1C assay readings over 7% indicate diabetes or poor diabetic control.
- The euglycemic clamp, which is a complicated and expensive test, is a measure of tissue insulin sensitivity that is used to assess insulin resistance. Glucose infusions are used to maintain plasma glucose concentration, and insulin infusions are used to maintain plasma insulin concentration.

Management

Conventional

Medications

- Biguanides, such as metformin (Glucophage), which improve insulin responsiveness
- Alpha-glucosidase inhibitors, such as acarbose, which restrict or delay the absorption of carbohydrates after eating, resulting in a slower rise in blood glucose levels
- Sulfonylureas and meglitinides, which increase insulin production
- Intensive insulin management, which includes continuous subcutaneous insulin infusion or daily injections

CLINICAL PEARL

Insulin pens make injection easier and more discreet because the insulin and injecting device are in one unit. Some come prefilled with insulin and are disposed of once used; others are reusable and can be refilled with separate insulin cartridges. Insulin pens may be used for both long-acting and short-acting insulin.

Screening/Monitoring

- Blood pressure (<140/80)
- Lipid management

- Ocular examination
- Screening for renal disease
- Peripheral vascular examination and a foot exam, including evaluation for and management of foot ulcers and infections.

CLINICAL PEARL

Blood pressure upper limits for diabetics are lower than those for nondiabetics. For diabetics without complications, the upper limit is 140/80. For diabetics with complications, such as kidney disease, the recommended upper limit is 130/80.

CLINICAL PEARL

Studies have found that to reduce the risk of developing complications from diabetes, control of blood pressure is more important than control of blood sugar.

Complementary

Nutraceuticals

- Vitamin E (400 mg/day) and evening primrose oil (500 to 1,000 mg/day): Small-scale studies found that these can relieve the symptoms of diabetic neuropathy.
- Eicosapentaenoic acid (EPA)/docosahexaenoic acid (DHA): Several meta-analyses have confirmed that the most consistent action of omega-3 polyunsaturated fatty acid (PUFA) in insulin resistance and type 2 diabetes is the reduction in triglycerides. The evidence on the effects of omega 3-PUFA on hemoglobin A1c is inconclusive.
- Chromium picolinate: Chromium has positive effects on insulin sensitivity and induces glucose tolerance in cases of insulin resistance. However, it remains unclear whether there is a significant benefit to supplementing patients with type 2 diabetes with chromium.

CLINICAL PEARL

Annona squamosa (sugar apple/custard apple), a tropical tree native to South America, is known for its nutrient-dense leaves and seeds. Laboratory studies have demonstrated that a tea made from the leaves of the plant can significantly decrease lipid levels and blood sugar levels.

Self-Care and Wellness

A diet based on the ADA recommendations and a low-fat vegan diet have been demonstrated to improve glycemic and lipid control in type 2 diabetics. Whole grains and foods high in magnesium are important components of the diet. Select recommendations include all legumes, most vegetables, brown rice instead of white rice, whole fruits instead of fruit juices, blackstrap molasses or sugar substitutes instead of white sugar, low-glycemic-index foods, garlic, onions, olives, mangoes, and nuts.

Exercise

Researchers at the National Institutes of Health Diabetes Prevention Program found that lifestyle changes reduced the risk of diabetes by 58%—far better than the 31% improvement noted with pre-diabetic drugs such as metformin.

Maintain a Healthy Body Mass Index (See Appendix)

BMI is an assessment of overweight and obesity that is calculated from height and weight. It is an estimate of body fat and a gauge of risk factors that can occur with increased body fat. The higher the BMI, the higher the risk for type 2 diabetes.

BMI
Underweight = <18.5
Normal weight = 18.5–24.9
Overweight = 25–29.9
Obesity = BMI of 30 or greater

CLINICAL PEARL

BMI may underestimate body fat in older persons and others who have lost muscle.

CLINICAL PEARL

Patients who are very athletic may have a high body mass index (BMI) but have low body fat. These individuals may benefit from body-fat analysis. Conversely, a low BMI does not necessarily mean low body fat. BMI and waist-to-hip ratio should be utilized concurrently.

CLINICAL PEARL

Nutrition therapy recommendations from the ADA are as follows. With regard to fat, the quality of fat is more important than the quantity. Leaner protein sources and meat alternatives are preferred. With regard to carbohydrates, nutrient-dense, high-fiber foods should be chosen in place of processed foods with added fat, sugars, and sodium. Soft drinks, fruit drinks, iced tea, energy drinks, vitamin water, and other beverages sweetened with high-fructose corn syrup should be avoided.

CLINICAL PEARL

According to the ADA, the majority of lifestyle weight-loss interventions observed in overweight or obese adults with type 2 diabetes resulted in weight loss of less than 5%. As such, current systematic reviews recommend that if the goal is glycemic control, weight loss should not be used as a primary strategy. The rationale is based on the fact that for most individuals, achieving the degree of weight loss that provides beneficial effects on hemoglobin A1c, lipids, and blood pressure (i.e., weight loss greater than 5%) requires significant interventions, including frequent contact with health professionals, energy restriction, and regular physical activity. Most individuals are not compliant with these interventions.

> **CLINICAL PEARL**
>
> Current recommendations for nutrition therapy for individuals with type 2 diabetes encourage a healthful eating pattern (emphasis on nutrient-dense foods and appropriate portion sizes), reduced energy intake, regular physical activity, education, and support as primary treatment strategies.

Juvenile Diabetes

Type 1 diabetes, also known as juvenile diabetes, is an autoimmune disease that destroys the insulin-producing cells of the pancreas.

Epidemiology

- Juvenile diabetes is commonly diagnosed in children and young adults.
- Type 1 diabetes accounts for 5% of all diabetes diagnoses.
- Of all women diagnosed with diabetes, 10% have juvenile diabetes.

Etiology

The pancreas does not produce sufficient insulin to regulate blood glucose levels, and the body is unable to mobilize glucose from the blood into the cells, which are then forced to rely on other forms of energy, such as ketones. Ketones are produced by the liver and can cause ketoacidosis. Diabetic ketoacidosis is a life-threatening condition that requires hospitalization.

> **CLINICAL PEARL**
>
> Worldwide, juvenile diabetes diagnosis in children aged 14 and younger has risen by 3% every year since 1989. In the United States, about 15,000 children and 15,000 adults are diagnosed with type 1 diabetes each year.

Signs and Symptoms

- Excessive thirst
- Unexplained weight loss
- Loss of muscle

- Fatigue
- Increased urinary frequency
- Additional symptoms might include the following:
  - Vaginal itching
  - Blurred vision
  - Cramping
  - Skin infections

CLINICAL PEARL

Women with diabetes are at increased risk for vaginal dryness, decreased libido, and urinary tract infections.

Diagnosis

- History and physical exam
- Fasting blood glucose and hemoglobin A1c
- Urinalysis
- Assessments for ketoacidosis
- Antibody screening, including glutamine acid decarboxylase autoantibodies (GADA) and insulin autoantibodies

Management

Conventional

- Daily insulin is administered by injection or with an insulin pump.
- Complications from insulin administration can include the following:
  - Changing insulin requirements because of exercise, stress, or diet
  - If poorly managed, can cause heart disease
  - Hypoglycemia—sweating, nausea, irritability, confusion, unconsciousness, and death

CLINICAL PEARL

Changing hormone levels as occur across the menstrual cycle place women at higher risk for complications from diabetes than men. This is because the fluctuating female hormonal environment makes blood sugar regulation more challenging.

> **CLINICAL PEARL**
>
> Women with type 1 diabetes have a 35% greater risk of dying from stroke compared with men with type 1 diabetes.

> **CLINICAL PEARL**
>
> Women with type 1 diabetes have a 40% greater risk of dying from kidney disease than men with type 1 diabetes.

OSTEOPOROSIS AND POLYCYSTIC OVARIAN SYNDROME

Osteoporosis

- Osteoporosis is a decline in the mass of bone.
- Osteoblasts make bone.
- Osteoclasts resorb (dissolve) bone.
- A primary function of estrogen is to inhibit osteoclastic activity. During menopause, estrogen levels decline, osteoclast-mediated bone resorption is uninhibited, and osteoblastic function declines, resulting in osteoporosis.

Epidemiology

Osteoporosis is influenced by the following factors:

- Heredity/genetics
  - Asian women and Caucasian females with a slight frame are at higher risk.
- Lack of or inadequate weight-bearing exercises
- Dietary factors, including inadequate calcium intake and excessive phosphate intake
  - The phosphates found in many soft drinks compete with calcium and can force the expulsion of calcium.
- Inadequate exposure to sunlight, which can impede vitamin D synthesis
  - Vitamin D is necessary for calcium absorption.

CLINICAL PEARL

Deficiencies in vitamin D can be compounded by living in a Nordic climate, being dark-skinned, and wearing clothing that covers the entire body.

- Prolonged use of medications such as blood thinners, thyroid hormone, glucocorticoids, antiseizure medications, and gonadotropin-releasing hormone (GNRH) agonists
- Use of aluminum-containing antacids.
- Early-onset menopause as a result of a hysterectomy or an oophorectomy
- Illnesses such as celiac and Crohn's disease, which interfere with gastric absorption of calcium and other minerals
- Hormonal imbalances brought on by conditions such as hyperthyroidism, Cushing's syndrome, female athlete triad, and hyperparathyroidism

Signs and Symptoms

- Dowager's hump
- Hip pain from fracture
- Spinal pain as a result of compression fractures and microfractures
- Loss of height
- Stooped posture

Diagnosis

Screening Procedures

- BMD screening/assessment is a noninvasive procedure that can also be used to monitor treatment efficacy. The BMD measurement is given as a T-score and a Z-score. The T-score is the deviation from the mean bone density of healthy young adults of the same gender and ethnicity, and the Z-score is the deviation from the mean bone density of adults of the same age and gender.
- Dual-energy x-ray absorptiometry (DEXA) scans the entire body and measures BMD. From the results, physicians assess the risk for fracture in the hip, spine, and wrist. Radiation exposure

is low, and the time commitment is minimal (approximately 5 minutes). DEXA can be used to monitor changes in bone density during treatment.

- Quantitative computed tomography (QCT) measures bone density in the hip and spine and produces a three-dimensional image that shows true volume density. The radiation level in QCT is 10 times higher than that in DEXA.
- Peripheral bone density testing uses ultrasound to identify bone loss in a localized area, such as the heel or hand.
- X-ray is also used, although osteoporosis does not show up on regular spinal x-rays until there is a 30% loss of bone.

CLINICAL PEARL

DXA is currently the recommended imaging technique for the diagnosis of osteoporosis. It demonstrates the best predictive value for fracture risk.

Management

Conventional

The following guidelines are summarized from the US Preventative Services Task force, the American Association of Family practice, the bone and joint decade, the American Society for Bone and Mineral Research, the National Osteoporosis Society, and the North American Menopause Society:

- For women under the age of 65 dual-energy X-ray absorptiometry (DEXA) is neither valuable, nor cost effective for screening for osteoporosis.
- The Bisphonates ((Alendronate (Fosamax), Risedronate (Actonel), Ibandronate (Boniva), Zoledronic acid (Reclast)) remain the first choice for treatment when the goal is to reduce vertebral and extravertebral fracture risk.
- Bisphonate therapy may be continued up to ten years in high risk individuals when there are no osteoporotic fractures

during the course of bisphonate therapy. Women who experience osteoporotic fractures while using bisphonate therapy should undergo reassment every two to three years and may either continue with bisphonate therapy or consider alternative therapies. Note: According to the American Society for Bone and Mineral Research, (2017), the benefits of switching to an alternative anti-fracture therapy after prolonged bisphosphonate treatment have not been adequately studied.

- The selective estrogen-receptor modulators (SERM's) raloxifene (Evista) may reduce vertebral fracture risk and prevent bone loss.
- Daily injections of Parathyroid hormone (Teriparatide) (used for no more than two years) may stimulate bone formation and improve bone density in those with high fracture risk. Teriparatide may increase risk of osteosarcoma
- Systemic hormonal replacement therapy (Estrogen and Progesterone) may be indicated when the benefits are indicated for other menopausal symptoms such as hot flashes.
- Calcitonin may be indicated for women who are more than 5 years post menopause or those with bone pain from vertebral compression fractures

Complementary

Nutraceuticals
- Calcium—1,000 to 1,500 mg/day
- Vitamin D—minimum of 400 to 800 IU/day for those up to age 64; minimum of 800 IU/day for those older than 65

Manual Therapies
- Falls risk assessment in the intake of all patients over the age of 65 (see the Clinical Pearl)
- Balance training
- Postural reeducation
- Spinal extensor strengthening
- Core muscle strengthening
- Pelvic-floor training

- Weight-bearing exercises
- Hip flexor, erector spinae, and abdominal muscle stretching

Pain Management in the Presence of Fractures

- Hydrotherapy once a day for 1 to 2 weeks when the patient has pain from recent vertebral fracture and/or postural and balance problems
- Transcutaneous electrical nerve stimulation (TENS)
- Interferential therapy (high-frequency signals of interferential current; used to relieve pain)
- Heat therapies
- Acupuncture
- Aromatherapy
- Reflex therapy
- Relaxation techniques
- Bracing

For Falls Prevention

- Tai chi and qigong

CLINICAL PEARL

For the screening and management of osteoporosis, consider the CDC's Stopping Elderly Accidents, Deaths, and Injuries (STEADI):

- ASK patients if they've fallen in the past year, feel unsteady, or worry about falling
  - Have you fallen in the past year?
  - Do you feel unsteady when standing or walking?
  - Do you worry about falling?
- REVIEW Medications
  - If permitted within the scope of practice, stop, switch, or reduce the dosage of drugs that increase fall risk.
- RECOMMEND
  - Recommend vitamin D supplements of at least 800 IU/day with calcium.

Data from Centers for Disease Control and Prevention. (2016). STEADI–Older adult fall prevention. Retrieved from https://www.cdc.gov/steadi/stories/ehrs.html

Self-Care and Wellness

- Recognizing and managing the factors that contribute to osteoporosis, including the following:
  - Get adequate sunlight.
  - Consume adequate amounts of calcium in the diet.
  - Avoid excessive intake of calcium-depleting products, such as the phosphates found in some sodas.
  - Initiate weight-bearing exercise at an early age. (Bones mineralize fully only when placed under stress.)

Diet

- Consume a diet rich in fruits and vegetables, especially green vegetables.
- Consume whole grains, such as brown rice, millet, buckwheat, whole-wheat triticeal, quinoa, and rye; legumes; and leafy vegetables that are rich in calcium. Whole grains and legumes also are rich in magnesium, which helps bone to incorporate calcium.
- Minimize high-protein diets because they can cause larger-than-normal calcium excretion, thereby increasing the potential for bone loss.

CLINICAL PEARL

Most adults lose the ability to make the enzyme lactase by age 45 and at younger ages in some ethnic populations. Most people of African descent, for example, lose the ability to make the enzyme by age 18; as such, milk is not an ideal source of calcium in adults. Yogurt and buttermilk are suitable sources of calcium for adults because they are fermented products made with cultures that break down the lactose. Cheese is a protein curd that does not contain lactose and also is appropriate.

TECHNICAL NOTE

Summary information on calcium supplements is as follows:

Type of Calcium Supplement	Easily Absorbed?	Calcium Content (%)	Other Benefits	Disadvantages
Calcium ascorbate	Yes	10		
Calcium aspartate	Yes	20		
Calcium carbonate	Not always Should be taken with food for maximum absorption	40	Inexpensive source of calcium Has antacid effect	Has antacid effect Can interfere with digestion May not be well absorbed in people with insufficient output of stomach acid Can cause gas
Calcium citrate	Yes	24	Can be absorbed by those with poor digestion Reduces risk for kidney stones	Larger molecule is bulkier than calcium carbonate, thus requiring more tablets/capsules to achieve the same dosage as calcium carbonate
Calcium lactate	Yes	15		May contain milk or yeast by-products Larger molecule is bulkier than calcium carbonate, thus requiring more tablets/capsules to achieve the same dosage as calcium carbonate

Amino acid chelate	Yes	10–20	May be used by individuals who are lactose intolerant	May be incorrectly made as a soy blend
Bone meal		39	Contains many of the minerals needed for healthy bone formation	May contain lead, arsenic, cadmium and other unidentified minerals. Some of the organic constituents are destroyed by heat during processing
Microcrystalline hydroxyapatite concentrate (MCHC)	Yes/No. Depends on individual	25	Contains collagen and several of the other minerals needed for healthy bone formation, including phosphorous, fluoride, magnesium, iron, zinc, and copper	More expensive
Calcium phosphate	No			Least likely to cause constipation
Coral calcium, oyster shell, and calcium dolomite			Essentially unpurified calcium carbonate	May contain high levels of lead and other impurities

Polycystic Ovarian Syndrome (PCOS)

Polycystic ovarian syndrome (PCOS) is an umbrella term used to label a group of symptoms that all appear to be connected to the menstrual cycle and have a strong correlation with insulin sensitivity. Symptoms associated with PCOS include hirsutism, obesity, menstrual irregularities, infertility, and acne.

Epidemiology

PCOS occurs primarily in the menstruating female. It is commonly diagnosed in females in their 20s but frequently begins during adolescence. PCOS is currently the most common hormonal disorder among women of reproductive age in the United States, affecting 5% to 10% of women

Etiology

Insulin Resistance (see section on Insulin Resistance)

In insulin resistance, the cells fail to respond adequately to stimulus from insulin; this initiates a vicious cycle in which blood sugar levels rise, and the pancreas accelerates insulin production in response. The increased insulin levels ultimately result in an en masse entry of blood sugars into the cells, a corresponding rapid drop in blood sugar levels, and a hypoglycemic state. As the cycle repeats, the pancreas eventually becomes overextended and is no longer able to produce sufficient amounts of insulin, resulting in diabetes. Insulin resistance is marked by simultaneously elevated levels of blood sugars and blood insulin. Ingesting simple carbohydrates and high-glycemic-index foods can compound the problem because they cause a rapid rise in blood sugars. Glucose from sugars is converted to energy in the cells; in the absence of this critical source of energy, fatigue and food cravings result. The liver responds to the elevated blood sugar levels by rapidly converting the excess sugars to fat. The excess fat results in increased hormone load as more estrogen is synthesized via the aromatase enzyme.

Metabolic Syndrome

See the section on metabolic syndrome.

Androgen Excess

- Aromatase enzyme synthesizes estrogen via the androstenedione pathway, which may ultimately result in excess testosterone.
- Excess testosterone levels cause male-distribution hair growth (on the chest and chin) and acne.

Ovarian Failure

- The ovarian follicles mature but do not release an egg, resulting in cyst formation on and around the ovaries, which can subsequently cause infertility and amenorrhea.

Abnormal Gonadotrophin Dynamics

Gonadotrophin abnormalities observed in PCOS can include any of the following:

- Elevated levels of testosterone and LH
- Elevated LH-to-FSH ratio
- Increased LH pulse frequency
- Altered diurnal rhythm of LH secretion

CLINICAL PEARL

Not all patients with PCOS have metabolic syndrome or impaired glucose tolerance.

Signs and Symptoms

- Amenorrhea or oligomenorrhea
- Obesity
- Infertility
- Acne

- Hirsutism
- Polycystic ovaries
- Pelvic pain
- Thinning hair
- Hair loss
- Insulin resistance
- Type 2 diabetes
- Elevated cholesterol and other lipid abnormalities
- Elevated blood pressure
- Cardiovascular disease

CLINICAL PEARL

- PCOS remains a challenging condition, in part because of the varying presentations of patients with the condition.
- When infertility is the presenting complaint, the patient's history reveals the following:
  - Of patients, 37% concurrently present with comorbid symptoms of amenorrhea.
  - Of patients, 90% concurrently present with comorbid symptoms of oligomenorrhea.
  - Of patients, 73% concurrently present with anovulatory cycles
- When hirsutism is the presenting complaint, 87% of patients have regular menses.

CLINICAL PEARL

Not all patients with PCOS are overweight or obese.

Diagnosis

- Diagnostic workup for PCOS includes the following:
  - Careful gynecological history
  - Vaginal or abdominal ultrasound of the ovaries to evaluate for multiple cysts
  - Progesterone challenge (progesterone withdrawal test)

TECHNICAL NOTE

The progesterone challenge test is also known as the progesterone withdrawal test. The patient is given medroxyprogesterone acetate (Provera) orally for 5 to 10 days or by injection.

Bleeding will typically occur 2 to 7 days after the last dose of Provera but may not occur for up to 2 weeks. A withdrawal bleed indicates anovulation; estrogen is present, and there is a buildup of the uterine lining.

- Blood chemistries may reveal the following:
  - Elevated levels LH
  - Low normal levels of FSH
  - Elevated blood glucose
  - Hyperandrogenism
  - Elevated blood lipids
- Testing may include monitoring of the ovary's response to either a stimulatory dose of a GNRH agonist such as leuprolide or a suppressive dose of medications such as dexamethasone (a glucocorticoid class of steroid hormones).

CLINICAL PEARL

PCOS may be diagnosed when any two of the following are present:
- Polycystic ovaries visible on ultrasound
- Oligomenorrhea, amenorrhea, or anovulation
- Hyperandrogenism as demonstrated by the presence of acne, hirsutism, or central obesity

CLINICAL PEARL

A typical diagnostic workup includes a pelvic ultrasound, a lipid panel, hemoglobin A1c, and the 2-hour glucose test.

> **TECHNICAL NOTE**
>
> Metabolic syndrome may be diagnosed when three or more of the following are present:
> - Abdominal obesity (waist over 35 inches)
> - Triglyceride levels of 150 mg/dl or above
> - HDL levels less than 50 mg/dl
> - Fasting blood sugar (FBS) of 110 to 126 mg/dl
> - 2-hour glucose of 140 to 199
> - Blood pressure of 130/85 or above

Management

- Treatment for PCOS is based on symptomatology, taking into consideration whether the patient wants to conceive or needs contraception.
- The focus of current treatment is on the management of insulin resistance.

Conventional

Medications

- Metformin (Glucophage), a diabetes drug, is used to manage insulin resistance in PCOS. Metformin and other anti-insulin drugs are concurrently used to regulate the cycle, improve hirsutism, facilitate weight loss, and improve acne.
- Birth control pills or vaginal rings that are a combination of estrogen and progestin are used to produce monthly bleeding, to protect against endometrial cancer, and to decrease testosterone concentrations. Further birth control medications are recommended when other treatments may cause birth defects.
- Progestin-only shots or pills are used for women who cannot tolerate estrogen.
- Fertility medications such as clomiphene (Clomid, Serophene) and LH and FSH injections are used if conception is a concern.
- Antiandrogenic medications such as spironolactone (Aldactone) are used for hirsutism and acne.

- Retinoids (tretinoin [Avita], adapalene [Differin], tazarotene [Tazorac], and Retin-A), antibiotics, and antibacterials (clindamycin and erythromycin [Erythrocin]) are used to treat acne.

CLINICAL PEARL

Although they are not approved to treat PCOS, metformin and the antiandrogens are approved by the U.S. Food and Drug Administration (FDA) to treat the specifically identified symptoms associated with PCOS.

CLINICAL PEARL

Some of the retinoids are known to cause birth defects.

CLINICAL PEARL

Metformin may adversely affect fertility.

Complementary

Dietary Recommendations

- To improve overall health and mitigate systemic inflammation, the following are recommended:
  - Avoiding trans fats
  - Avoiding known food allergens
  - Considering a gluten- and dairy-free diet

Nutraceuticals

- EPA/DHA for symptomatology related to the menstrual cycle
- Chasteberry extract for oligomenorrhea
- Nutraceuticals for liver and systemic detoxification

- Vitamin D (5,000 IU/day)
  - Vitamin D deficiency is common in women with PCOS.
- Inositol
  - Inositol acts as a second messenger in the insulin-signaling pathway. Inositol deficiency in insulin-resistant women with PCOS has been observed in several studies. Inositol is found in fruits such as cantaloupe and oranges and in plants as a phytate (which, depending on the plant, may not be easily digestible).
  - There remains controversy as to whether inositol should be considered a B vitamin. Inositol; formerly known as vitamin B_8, is not considered an essential nutrient because it is metabolized from glucose by the body.

CLINICAL PEARL

Administration of inositol in PCOS has been shown to improve metabolic and hormonal parameters, ovarian function, and the response to assisted reproductive technology (ART).

CLINICAL PEARL

In some studies, a combination of myoinositol (MI) and D-chiro-inositol (DCI) was found to work better than MI alone for glycemic control.

CLINICAL PEARL

Studies comparing the efficacy of metformin and inositol in PCOS suggest similar beneficial effects from metformin (1,500 mg/day) and MI (4 g/day). These benefits include improvement in insulin sensitivity, a significant decrease in BMI, and normalization of the menstrual cycle. No significant changes have been observed for acne and hirsutism.

Progesterone

- Application of progesterone creams to the inner wrist and upper chest during the luteal phase to initiate menstrual bleeding

Chiropractic Spinal Manipulation

- Chiropractic approaches to managing PCOS focus on spinal manipulation, with emphasis on spinal segments that influence the inferior mesenteric plexus.

Massage Therapy

- Full-body relaxation massage
- Trigger-point therapy to the abdominal and pelvic muscles
- Muscle-stripping techniques to the adductor muscles
  - Muscle stripping has been anecdotally reported to restore monthly bleeding

Naturopathy

- Vitamins, herbs, homeopathics, and lifestyle changes are recommended to restore gonadal function, improve insulin sensitivity, facilitate weight loss, and enhance fertility.
- Dairy-free, gluten-free, and sugar-free diets are often recommended.

Acupuncture

- Multiple studies have demonstrated positive effects of acupuncture alone, electroacupuncture, and acupuncture and herb combinations in infertility management; infertility is a common occurrence with PCOS.

Self-Care and Wellness

Diet

- Follow the recommended diet for insulin resistance: increased complex carbohydrates, high-fiber foods, and low-glycemic-index foods, such as mung beans, soybeans, and other legumes; nuts, artichokes, garlic, onions, and mangoes; whole-grain breads and cereals; barley; and brown rice.

- Avoid/decrease intake of simple carbohydrates, including sodas, cookies, and candy.

CLINICAL PEARL

The Mediterranean diet, fiber intake, and isoflavones intake have been linked to luteal-phase deficiency (i.e., luteal phases less than 10 days). Selenium has been negatively associated with luteal-phase deficiency.

CLINICAL PEARL

Some research studies suggest that diet and exercise improve body composition, hyperandrogenism, and insulin resistance in women with PCOS but do not improve lipid profiles and glucose tolerance.

Exercise

- Mild to moderate exercise is recommended, following the U.S. Preventative Services Task Force recommendation of 30 minutes of exercise most days a week.
- Intense exercise training may increase the symptoms of PCOS.
- Exercise improves the body's sensitivity to insulin. Including a combination of cardio training (lowers the risk of cardio-vascular disease in women with PCOS) and strength training (to raise the basal metabolic rate) is recommended.

Hair Removal

- Manage the excess hair growth with laser hair removal treatments, electrolysis, depilatories, bleaching, tweezing, shaving, or waxing.
- Waxing may lead to scarring, skin irritation, and skin damage, which may affect self-image.

TECHNICAL NOTE

Depilatories are chemical hair-removal products that are directly applied to the skin.

TECHNICAL NOTE

Multiple studies confirm a correlation between vitamin D, metabolic syndrome, and insulin sensitivity. Specific to PCOS, patients with PCOS and vitamin D deficiency more commonly exhibit dysglycemia. The current evidence does not demonstrate improved symptoms of metabolic syndrome in PCOS patients who use vitamin D supplements.

TECHNICAL NOTE

The correlation between vitamin D (25-OH) and insulin resistance observed in PCOS patients who were overweight or obese has not currently been observed in underweight or normal-weight women with PCOS.

CLINICAL PEARL

There is an association between hyperinsulinemia and hyperandrogenism in lean women with PCOS. Women who are not overweight but exhibit chronic anovulation and hyperandrogenism should be screened for metabolic disorders.

THYROID DISORDERS

Hyperthyroid—Graves' Disease

Graves' disease is an autoimmune condition that manifests with hyperthyroidism. It is the most common cause of hyperthyroidism.

Epidemiology

- Graves' disease is primarily a disease of younger women; however, it may occur at any age.
- The typical age range is 20 to 40 years.
- The female-to-male ratio is 8:1.

Etiology

Graves' disease is the most common cause of hyperthyroidism. It results from an abnormal immune system response (autoantibodies) that causes the thyroid gland to produce too much thyroid hormone. Thyroid-stimulating immunoglobulins bind to and activate thyrotropin receptors; this causes growth of the thyroid gland and increased synthesis of thyroid hormone by the follicles.

Signs and Symptoms

- Anxiety/nervousness
- Heat intolerance/sweating
- Tachycardia
- Weight loss
- Frequent bowel movements
- Difficulty concentrating and other cognitive impairments
- Double vision, dry eyes, tearing, and irritation of the eyes
- Exophthalmos
- Fatigue
- Oligomenorrhea
- Musculoskeletal complaints
- Mood swings

Diagnosis

- History and physical exam (exophthalmos, goiter, arrhythmia, etc.)
- Lab testing of thyroid-stimulating hormone (TSH), T4 and T3 (low TSH, high T4 and T3), and autoantibodies (see Table 10-1)
- Radioactive iodine uptake

Table 10-1 Serologic Assessment for Thyroid Function

	Hyperthyroid	Euthyroid	Hypothyroid
T4, T3	Elevated	Normal	Decreased
TSH	Decreased	Normal	Elevated

T4 = thyroxine

T3 = triiodothyronine

TSH = thyroid-stimulating hormone

- Thyroid ultrasound (used in pregnancy in lieu of radioactive iodine uptake)
- CT/MRI of the eyes and eye sockets to determine the effect, if any, of the disease on the eyes

Management

Conventional

Medications

- Antithyroid medications such as methimazole (Tapazole) and propylthiouracil
- Beta blockers, including propranolol (Hemangeol, Inderal, and InnoPran), for cardiovascular symptoms

Procedures

- Radioactive iodine therapy
- Radiation therapy
- Surgery
  - If surgery is warranted in Graves' disease, it is commonly a total thyroidectomy.

CLINICAL PEARL

Thyroid surgery, radiation therapy, and radioactive iodine cause hypothyroidism. Thyroid hormone replacement is required.

Complementary

Nutraceuticals

- Herbs: Bugleweed (*Lycopus virginicus*), motherwort (*Leonurus*), and lemon balm (*Melissa officinalis*) have documented evidence to support utility in hyperthyroidism. Herbs should be not be discontinued abruptly.
- L-carnitine: This amino acid is known to prevent thyroid hormones from entering the cell nucleus, thereby limiting the symptoms of hyperthyroidism. Note that L-carnitine does not directly influence the overactive thyroid gland.
- Acupuncture: Acupuncture has been used along with medications or with traditional Chinese herbs to normalize thyroid hormone levels and decrease the eye disease seen in Graves' disease.

Self-Care and Wellness

- Stress management
  - Stress is a known contributor to many autoimmune disorders.
- Diet
  - Limited iodine intake
  - Addition of cruciferous vegetables, which theoretically work as goitrogens and may help to block iodine absorption
  - Avoidance of known food allergens

CLINICAL PEARL

Anecdotal reports suggest that gluten-free, dairy-free, sugar-free, and vegan diets may reduce some of the symptoms of autoimmune disorders.

Hypothyroid

Hypothyroidism, or underactive thyroid, is a failure of the thyroid gland to produce enough hormones.

Epidemiology

- An estimated 4.6% of the U.S. population has hypothyroidism.
- Hypothyroidism is more common in women and most common in women over the age of 60.

Etiology

- Autoimmune disorders such as Hashimoto's thyroiditis are the most common cause of hypothyroidism.
- Iatrogenic causes such as the treatment for hyperthyroidism/Graves' disease with radioactive iodine or surgery can result in hypothyroidism.
- Medications with negative side effects on the thyroid gland that can cause hypothyroidism include the following:
  - Lithium, which is used to treat psychiatric disorders
  - Antithyroid medications
  - Interferon alpha, which is used in cancer treatment
  - Amiodarone, which is used in cardiovascular treatment
- Genetic mutations account for 15% to 20% of cases of congenital hypothyroidism; however, the most common cause of congenital hypothyroidism worldwide is dietary iodine deficiency.
- Pituitary adenomas, although slow growing and commonly benign, may compress the portion of the pituitary gland that influences TSH production. Diminished TSH could result in hypothyroidism.
- Postpartum hypothyroidism occurs when antibodies are produced by the female to her own thyroid gland.
- Inadequate or excessive dietary iodine, which is necessary for the synthesis of the thyroid hormones, can cause hypothyroidism.

Signs and Symptoms

- Increased sensitivity to cold
- Lethargy
- Fatigue
- Thinning hair
- Peripheral neuropathies
- Weight gain
- Gastrointestinal concerns such as constipation
- Dry skin
- Musculoskeletal complaints, including joint swelling and muscle fatigue
- Puffy face

- Hypercholesterolemia
- Cognitive changes, forgetfulness, and depression
- Changes in heart rate

Diagnosis

- Serologic testing of TSH, T4, and T3, which reveals elevated TSH and decreased T3 and T4 (see Table 10-1)

Management

Conventional

- Medications: Daily use of medication such as levothyroxine (Synthroid, Levothroid, Tirosint) is indicated. The level of TSH is checked at 6 weeks to 3 months to ensure correct dosage.

CLINICAL PEARL

Iron supplements, aluminum hydroxide (found in antacids), calcium supplements, soy products, and cholestyramine may all affect the body's ability to absorb levothyroxine.

CLINICAL PEARL

Signs of excessive dosage of levothyroxine include shakiness, heart palpitations, lack of sleep, and an increased appetite.

CLINICAL PEARL

Complications of untreated hypothyroidism include the following:
- Goiter
- Preeclampsia in pregnancy
- Infertility
- Myxedema
- Cardiovascular disease

CLINICAL PEARL

Hashimoto's thyroiditis is a common cause of goiter.

Hashimoto's Thyroiditis (Hashimoto's, Hashimoto's Disease)

Hashimoto's thyroiditis is an autoimmune disorder whereby the immune system attacks the thyroid gland, causing hypothyroidism.

Epidemiology

- Hashimoto's affects seven times as many women as men.
- Hashimoto's is the most common cause of hypothyroidism.

Etiology

- Unknown
- Pregnancy and delivery: Many women develop Hashimoto's following pregnancy and delivery.
- Genetic/hereditary factors: People with Hashimoto's frequently have other family members with Hashimoto's or other genetic disorders.
- Excessive iodine: Certain medications and too much iodine can trigger thyroiditis in some people.
- Radiation exposure: There is an increase in the incidence of Hashimoto's in people who are treated with radiation for cancers such as Hodgkin's disease.

Signs and Symptoms

- Generalized fatigue
- Joint and muscle pain
- Hair loss
- Thinning hair
- Irregular menses
- Menorrhagia
- Weight gain
- Constipation
- Paleness or puffiness of the face
- Depression
- Bradycardia

Management

Management is as described for hypothyroidism.

Conventional

- Wait-and-see approach when there is no evidence of thyroid hormone imbalance
- Medication
  - Levothyroxine (Synthroid)

Thyroiditis

Subacute thyroiditis is a self-limiting condition that involves three phases: hyperthyroidism, hypothyroidism, and normal thyroid function. The most common types are as follows:

- Subacute granulomatous thyroiditis (de Quervain's thyroiditis)
- Subacute lymphocytic thyroiditis
- Subacute postpartum thyroiditis

The clinical course of subacute thyroiditis is as follows:

- Phase 1—Hyperthyroid (1 to 3 months): Thyroid follicle destruction => preformed thyroid hormone released (not new thyroid hormone synthesis) => thyrotoxicosis and hyperthyroidism
- Phase 2—Hypothyroid (~2 months): Thyroid is depleted of colloid and cannot produce thyroid hormone => mild hypothyroidism.
- Phase 3: Follicles regenerate, the euthyroid state is restored, and return to normal thyroid function occurs.

Subacute Granulomatous Thyroiditis

Subacute granulomatous thyroiditis is the most common cause of a painful thyroid gland. It is a transient inflammation of the gland. It is not an autoimmune condition. It commonly occurs in the summer and fall following viral epidemics.

Etiology
- Unknown
- Viral illness: Most episodes follow a respiratory infection.
- Genetic: HLa-B35 has been observed in more than half of all patients assessed.

Epidemiology
- Most commonly affects ages 40 to 50

Signs and Symptoms
- Pain over the thyroid gland
- Dysphagia
- Symptoms associated with hyper- and hypothyroid
- Symptoms associated with a viral/respiratory infection

Management
- Self-limiting

Subacute Lymphocytic Thyroiditis

Subacute lymphocytic thyroiditis is thought to be an autoimmune condition and is often associated with goiter.

Etiology
- Medications, including amiodarone, interferon alpha, and lithium

Epidemiology
- Any age group

Signs and Symptoms
- Painless, firm, and enlarged thyroid gland

Diagnosis
- Elevated thyroid hormone levels

Management

- Removal of the iatrogenic cause
- Self-limiting

Subacute Postpartum Thyroiditis

Subacute postpartum thyroiditis is thought to be an autoimmune condition. Patients may develop an autoimmune goiter.

Epidemiology

- Women in the reproductive phase

Etiology

- Pregnancy
- Cigarette smoke
- Unknown

Signs and Symptoms

- Enlarged, firm, and painless thyroid gland
- Symptoms that occur within 6 months of childbirth
- Other signs and symptoms associated with hyperthyroidism

Diagnosis

- Elevated thyroid hormone levels

Management

- Self-limiting

CLINICAL PEARL

Medications for subacute thyroiditis may be prescribed based on symptoms and severity. They include the following:
- Beta blockers for tachycardia
- Antithyroid drugs for severe cases
- Glucocorticoids in rare cases

Thyroid Cancer

Thyroid cancer is an umbrella term for a number of different presentations, of which the two most common are follicular and papillary cancer, also known as well-differentiated thyroid cancer.

Epidemiology
- Most commonly occurs in women.

Etiology
- Unknown
- Risk factors such as exposure to ionizing radiation and some genetic syndromes

Signs and Symptoms
- Lump, nodule, or mass in the thyroid gland
- Lymphadenopathy
- Cervicalgia
- Dysphagia

Diagnosis
- History and physical exam
- Blood tests, including thyroglobulin
- Needle biopsy
- Thyroid scan
- CT/MRI
- Genetic testing

Management
- Conventional therapies include the following:
  - Thyroidectomy—surgery to remove the nodule, a lobe, or the entire thyroid gland; amount removed dependent on the pathological analysis
  - Lymphadenectomy
  - Radioactive iodine capsule or liquid
  - External beam radiation therapy

- Less common management strategies for thyroid cancer include the following:
  - Chemotherapy
  - Alcohol ablation
- Targeted drug therapy is used in advanced thyroid cancer.
- Thyroid hormone replacement therapy in the form of levothyroxine follows treatment for the cancer.

Prognosis

- Very good

CLINICAL PEARL

Suppressing TSH production improves survival in patients with thyroid cancer.

CHAPTER 11

Pain Syndromes (Musculoskeletal)

ARTHRITIS

Osteoarthritis
Rheumatoid Arthritis

OTHER CHRONIC CONDITIONS

Fibromyalgia

PELVIC PAIN SYNDROMES

Coccydynia
Chronic Pelvic Pain

ARTHRITIS

Arthritis is an umbrella term used to describe a group of conditions that manifest with inflammation of one or more joints and irritation of the surrounding tissue. The most common forms of arthritis in women are rheumatoid arthritis and osteoarthritis. Rheumatoid arthritis is an autoimmune condition that affects several organ systems; osteoarthritis is primarily a degenerative joint disease (DJD).

Epidemiology

According to the Centers for Disease Control and Prevention (CDC, 2016) one in four women has some form of arthritis, 16% of underweight and normal weight adults report doctor-diagnosed arthritis, 23% of overweight report doctor-diagnosed arthritis, and 31% of obese U.S. adults report doctor-diagnosed arthritis.

CLINICAL PEARL

According to the CDC (2010) weight loss of as little as 11 pounds results in a 50% reduction in the risk of developing knee osteoarthritis among women.

Etiology

There are a number of proposed causes for arthritis, including the following:

- Genetic susceptibility
- Environmental factors
- Systemic hormones
- Obesity
- Cigarette smoke
- Bone overuse

Osteoarthritis

Osteoarthritis is primarily a DJD.

Signs and Symptoms

- Joint stiffness in the morning or following a period of inactivity (specifically in the hips, knees, and low back)
- Tender and painful joints
- Loss of flexibility in the joints that improves with movement
- Mild swelling around a joint
- Clicking or cracking sounds when the joint is used
- Grating sensation in the joint

Diagnosis

- History and physical exam
- Blood analysis to rule out rheumatoid arthritis (rheumatoid factor (RA) on serum analysis) and other causes
  - There are no specific blood markers for osteoarthritis.
- Joint aspiration to assess for inflammation and infection and to evaluate for monosodium urate (uric acid) crystals, as seen in gout, or calcium pyrophosphate crystals, which could further damage the joint
- X-ray to reveal bone spurs and loss of intervertebral disc space
- Magnetic resonance imaging (MRI) for a higher level of soft tissue evaluation

Management

- Therapies are geared toward pain relief and limiting disability.

Conventional

- Medications
  - Nonsteroidal anti-inflammatory drugs (NSAIDs), such as aspirin (Bayer), naproxen (Aleve), and ibuprofen (Advil, Motrin), to decrease inflammation and relieve pain
  - Cortisone shots (local corticosteroid injections) to relieve joint pain
- Physical and occupational therapy to increase range of motion and strengthen muscles
- Assistive devices
- Surgery—joint replacement

Complementary

- Manipulation and mobilization of the joints with chiropractic or osteopathic techniques
- Acupuncture
- Massage therapy
- Nutraceuticals
  - Glucosamine and chondroitin: Research shows improved symptoms when taken for a minimum of 3 months.
- Topicals
  - Vegetable extract (avocado/soybean unsaponifiables)

Self-Care and Wellness

- Physical activity—strengthening and stretching exercises, such as swimming, walking, yoga, and tai chi
- Maintenance of an ideal weight
- Over-the-counter analgesics and NSAIDs for pain control
- Hot and cold compresses
- Diets purported to reduce inflammation, such as the Mediterranean diet
- Hydrotherapy

Rheumatoid Arthritis

Rheumatoid arthritis is an autoimmune condition that affects the joints, causing erosion and deformity; it also affects several organ systems.

Signs and Symptoms

- Joint stiffness in the morning or following a period of inactivity
- Tender and painful joints
- Bilateral symptoms
- Fatigue
- Loss of appetite
- Low-grade fever
- Warm, swollen joints

Diagnosis

- History and physical exam
- Blood analysis
  - Erythrocyte sedimentation rate (ESR)—a marker of inflammation
  - C-reactive protein (CRP)—a marker of inflammation
  - RA
  - Anticyclic citrullinated peptide (anti-CCP)
- X-ray to evaluate for DJD
- MRI for a higher level of soft tissue evaluation

Management

- Therapies are geared toward decreasing inflammation, providing pain relief, and limiting disability.

Conventional

- Medications
  - NSAIDs, such as aspirin (Bayer), naproxen (Aleve), and ibuprofen (Advil, Motrin), to decrease inflammation and relieve pain
  - Cortisone shots (local corticosteroid injections) to relieve joint pain
  - Disease-modifying antirheumatic drugs (DMARDs), such as abatacept (Orencia), methotrexate (Rasuvo), and infliximab (Remicade)
  - Biologic agents, a subset of DMARDs
- Physical and occupational therapy to increase range of motion and strengthen muscles
- Assistive devices
- Arthrocentesis (joint aspiration)
- Surgery—tendon repair, synovectomy, joint replacement

Complementary

- Manipulation and mobilization of the joints with chiropractic or osteopathic techniques

- Acupuncture
- Massage therapy
- Nutraceuticals
  - Turmeric
  - Omega-3 and omega-6 fatty acids

Self-Care and Wellness

- Physical activity—strengthening and stretching exercises, such as swimming and walking
- Balance of activity and rest
- Maintenance of an ideal weight
- Over-the-counter analgesics and NSAIDs for pain control (aspirin [Bayer], naproxen [Aleve], and ibuprofen [Advil, Motrin])
- Hot and cold compresses
- Diets purported to reduce inflammation, such as the Mediterranean diet
- Relaxation techniques
- Support systems
- Tai chi
- Hydrotherapy
- Yoga

OTHER CHRONIC CONDITIONS

Fibromyalgia

Fibromyalgia is a common chronic condition characterized by fatigue, widespread pain, and sleep disruption. The pain of fibromyalgia is in the muscles, joints, bones, tendons, and other soft tissues; is commonly bilateral; and occurs in areas above and below the waist.

Epidemiology

- Fibromyalgia occurs primarily in women in their late 20s through 50s.

Etiology

The cause of fibromyalgia syndrome is unknown, but proposed causes include the following:

- Autoimmune dysfunction
- Sleep disorders
- Abnormal central nervous system functioning
- Autoimmune disorders such as lupus
- Rheumatoid arthritis
- Hypothyroidism
- Aluminum toxicity
- Stress
- Repetitive use
- Physical trauma
- Emotional trauma
- History of bacterial infection

Signs and Symptoms

- Widespread pain above and below the waist and on both sides of the body
- Pain and tenderness in at least 11 of 18 tender-point sites, which are as follows (Figure 11-1):
  - Base of the occiput at the insertion of the suboccipital muscles
  - Anterior neck at the lower cervical spine from C5 to C7
  - The midpoint of the upper trapezius muscle
  - Supraspinatus muscle near its medial border above the spine of the scapula
  - Thoracic paraspinal muscles at T4 to T8 between the shoulder blades
  - Second rib at the second costochondral junction
  - Pectoral muscles at the fourth rib at the anterior axillary line
  - Medial epicondyle and lateral epicondyles (the elbow joint)
  - Gluteal muscles at the upper outer quadrant of the buttocks
  - Greater trochanter of the hip
  - Medial knee
  - Skin-fold tenderness

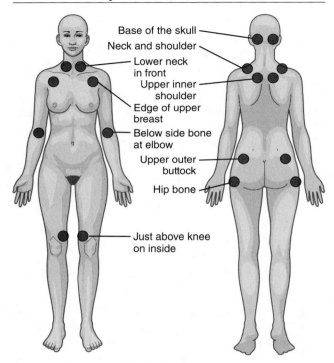

Figure 11-1 Pain points in fibromyalgia

- Symptoms which worsen in cold or damp weather
- Associated symptoms, including headaches, fatigue, sleep disturbances, morning stiffness, numbness in the hands and feet, anxiety disorders, facial pain, irritable bowel syndrome, painful menses, dizziness, mood changes, dry eye, difficulty concentrating, and depression

Diagnosis

- It is important to separate true fibromyalgia syndrome from the numerous conditions that may manifest with similar symptoms. These include hypothyroidism, Lyme disease, chronic fatigue syndrome, rheumatoid arthritis, vitamin and mineral deficiencies, and side effects from medications such as the cholesterol-lowering statin drugs.

- The classic fibromyalgia patient presents with increased sensitivity to pain (hyperalgesia) and the perception of pain in response to a normally nonpainful stimulus (allodynia).
- Blood tests are conducted to rule out conditions such as hypo- or hyperthyroidism, Graves' disease, and rheumatoid arthritis
- Chest x-rays are conducted to rule out other pathology.
- Fibromyalgia is diagnosed if the patient has a minimum of 3 months of widespread pain above and below the waist, on both sides of the body, and a minimum of 11 of 18 identified tender points.

CLINICAL PEARL

Lab test results in fibromyalgia are frequently normal.

- Note: Current diagnostic criteria recommended by the American College of Rheumatology are to use the Widespread Pain Index and symptom severity scale score in lieu of the tender-point assessment (see Table 11-1).

Management

Currently, there is no known treatment that benefits all fibromyalgia patients. Patients may need to try several types of modalities (e.g., acupuncture, chiropractic care, massage therapy, biofeedback, hydrotherapy) to find the one that provides them with the greatest relief and symptomatic benefit. Current research indicates that the most effective treatments for fibromyalgia are aerobic exercise, cognitive-behavioral therapy, amitriptyline, and multicomponent therapy. NSAIDs as a single intervention and corticosteroids are not recommended. Acupuncture and trigger-point injections are also recommended (Ablin et al., 2013; Menzies, 2016).

Table 11-1 Fibromyalgia Diagnosis Criteria Recommended by the American College of Rheumatology

A patient satisfies diagnostic criteria for fibromyalgia if the following 3 conditions are met:
1) Widespread pain index (WPI) ≥7 and symptom severity (SS) scale score ≥5 or WPI 3–6 and SS scale score ≥9.
2) Symptoms have been present at a similar level for at least 3 months.
3) The patient does not have a disorder that would otherwise explain the pain.

Ascertainment
1) WPI: note the number areas in which the patient has had pain over the last week. In how many areas has the patient had pain? Score will be between 0 and 19.

Shoulder girdle, left	Hip, left	Jaw, left	Upper back
Shoulder girdle, right	Hip, right	Jaw, right	Lower back
Upper arm, left	Upper leg, left	Chest	Neck
Upper arm, right	Upper leg, right	Abdomen	
Lower arm, left	Lower leg, left		
Lower arm, right	Lower leg, right		

2) SS scale score:
Fatigue
Waking unrefreshed
Cognitive symptoms

For the each of the three symptoms above, indicate the level of severity over the past week using the following scale:
0 = no problem
1 = slight or mild problems, generally mild or intermittent
2 = moderate, considerable problems, often present and/or at a moderate level
3 = severe: pervasive, continuous, life-disturbing problems

Considering somatic symptoms in general, indicate whether the patient has:
0 = no symptoms
1 = few symptoms
2 = a moderate number of symptoms
3 = a great deal of symptoms

The SS scale score is the sum of the severity of the three symptoms (fatigue, waking unrefreshed, cognitive symptoms) plus the extent (severity) of somatic symptoms in general. The final score is between 0 and 12

Reproduced from Wolfe, F. et al. (2010). The American College of Rheumatology preliminary diagnostic criteria for fibromyalgia and measurement of symptom severity. *Arthritis Care & Research, 62*(5), 600–610. Reprinted by permission of Wiley.

Self-Care and Wellness

- Support groups
- Massage therapy
- Yoga
- Tai chi
- Qigong
- Whole-foods diet
- Guided imagery
- Good sleep health
- Pain diary
- Hypnosis
- Biofeedback

PELVIC PAIN SYNDROMES

Coccydynia

Coccydynia is pain in the coccyx.

Epidemiology

- Coccydynia can affect women of all ages; however, the mean age of onset is approximately age 40.
- Coccydynia is five times more common in women than men and accounts for 1% of all back complaints.

Etiology

- Direct trauma to the tailbone, typically from a fall resulting in irritation or inflammation to the ligaments of the sacrococcygeal articulation, disarticulation of the sacrococcygeal articulation, and/or fracture of the tailbone

- Childbirth, which can cause irritation, inflammation, or disarticulation of the sacrococcygeal articulation as the infant's head travels through the birth canal

Signs and Symptoms

- Moderate to severe pain at the sacrum, coccyx, and surrounding tissues.
- Pain that worsens with prolonged sitting

CLINICAL PEARL

Women may experience more pain than men when sitting because the broader female pelvis necessitates that women sit on the ischial tuberosities and the coccyx, whereas men sit primarily on the ischial tuberosities.

Diagnosis

- History and exam
- History of pratfall or birth
- Digital rectal exam that reveals localized tenderness over the sacrococcygeal articulation or a misaligned coccyx
- Complete physical exam to rule out referred pain from the lumbosacral spine, lumbar disc herniation, tumors, and other pathology
- X-rays of the pelvis and lumbosacral spine to rule out fracture or tumor
- MRI of the pelvis to rule out smaller tumors or localized infectious processes and aid in diagnosis, particularly in adolescents

Management

Conventional

Medications

- NSAIDs (aspirin [Bayer], naproxen [Aleve], and ibuprofen [Advil, Motrin])

Procedures
- Local injection of steroids, such as cortisone
- Local injection of a numbing agent, such as lidocaine
- Surgery—coccygectomy

Physical Therapy
- Ultrasound over the sacrococcygeal articulation and ligaments

Complementary

Massage Therapy
- Trigger-point therapy to the levator ani muscle and surrounding muscles
- Massaging or stretching of the muscles attached to the coccyx

Chiropractic Manipulation
- Manipulation of the coccyx—internal and external coccygeal maneuvers
- Manipulation of the sacrum and other pelvic structures

Self-Care and Wellness
- Donut pillow
- Ice applied directly over the area of complaint several times a day
- Avoidance prolonged sitting
- Stool softeners as needed if pain is complicated by bowel movement

Chronic Pelvic Pain

Chronic pelvic pain is defined as noncyclical pelvic pain lasting for more than 6 months.

Epidemiology
- It is estimated that worldwide prevalence is from 5% to 26%.
- In the United States, chronic pelvic pain accounts for 10% of all gynecological referrals, and estimates are that 1 in 7 women is afflicted.

Etiology

- Endometriosis
- Fibroids
- Pelvic inflammatory disease (PID)
- Pelvic-floor muscle tension/spasms
- Scars from an episiotomy
- Trigger points in the pelvic musculature
- Pelvic structural imbalances caused by the following:
  - Pelvic misalignments
  - Leg-length imbalance
  - Muscle tension
  - Lumbar spine misalignments
- Ovarian cysts or ovarian remnants
- Bladder syndromes
- Irritable bowel syndrome
- Psychosocial and psychological factors, including the following:
  - History of abuse
  - Trauma
  - Anxiety
  - Chronic stress

Signs and Symptoms

- Constant or intermittent pelvic pain that is dull or sharp and may or may not be associated with a specific pelvic pathology
- A feeling of heaviness in the pelvis
- Dyspareunia
- Dysmenorrhea

Diagnosis

- History and physical exam
- Pelvic exam
- Abdominal exam
- Laboratory testing
  - Sexually transmitted disease (STD) screening
  - Complete blood count (CBC) and ESR to rule out systemic inflammation and malignancy

- Hormone panel—thyroid-stimulating hormone (TSH), follicle-stimulating hormone (FSH), and estradiol—to rule out hypothyroidism and ovarian remnant syndrome
- Additional tests may include the following:
  - X-ray of the pelvis and abdomen to rule out fracture or other structural abnormalities
  - Hysterosalpingogram (x-ray with contrast) to rule out obstructional endometriosis
  - Sonography or ultrasound to evaluate for pelvic masses
  - MRI of the lumbopelvic region and abdomen to rule out pelvic masses, disc lesions, and other structural anomalies
  - Computed tomography (CT) scan of the pelvis, which is less commonly used in lieu of or in addition to ultrasound to evaluate for pelvic masses
  - Laparoscopy to rule out endometriosis, scar tissue, PID, postoperative peritoneal cysts, or other pathology

CLINICAL PEARL

Fibromyalgia should be considered whenever a female patient presents with multiple regions of chronic pain and multiple somatic symptoms.

Management

- Where a cause is found, management is targeted at the specific cause.
- Absent an identified cause, the primary goal of treatment is to reduce pain.

Conventional

Medications

- Pain relievers and anti-inflammatories, including acetaminophen (Tylenol), ibuprofen (Advil), and naproxen (Aleve)
- Birth control pills or other hormone therapies
- Antidepressants, such as nortriptyline (Pamelor)
- Antibiotics if the workup reveals STD, PID, or other infection (see Chapter 6)

Physical Therapy

- Stretching/strengthening exercises
- Dilators
- Transcutaneous electrical nerve stimulation (TENS)
- Pelvic-floor strengthening

Surgery

- Surgical procedures range from minimally invasive to significant dependent on the suspected triggers for the chronic pain syndrome:
  - Trigger point injections
  - Sacral nerve ablation
  - Total hysterectomy
  - Surgeries for endometriosis, ovarian cysts, and ovarian remnant syndrome
  - Various nerve-blocking procedures

Therapy

- Counseling by a mental health professional for the depression that often accompanies chronic pain syndrome

Complementary

- Massage therapy
- Trigger-point therapy
- Craniosacral therapy
- Chiropractic manipulation and other forms of manual therapy
  - These have demonstrated efficacy in small case studies of chronic pelvic pain, indicating that for some patients, the etiology is an osteo-myofascial disruption.
- Acupuncture
  - Multiple studies affirm the efficacy of acupuncture for the treatment of chronic pelvic pain either as a primary modality or in conjunction with other therapies.

Self-Care and Wellness

- Exercise, including yoga and Pilates
- Deep breathing
- Stress Management
- Diet that minimizes systemic inflammation by avoiding food allergens, increasing fruits and vegetables, and minimizing red meats

CLINICAL PEARL

Gluten-free, dairy-free, and sugar-free diets are anecdotally reported to aid in the relief of some pelvic pain syndromes.

CLINICAL PEARL

Chronic pelvic pain is a challenging condition that is best managed with an integrated team of conventional and complementary practitioners.

TECHNICAL NOTE

The incidence of ovarian remnant syndrome (ORS), a condition in which ovarian tissue remains following laparoscopic bilateral salpingo-oophorectomy, is increasing. ORS is considered to be a primary cause of chronic pelvic pain because in addition to scar tissue formation in the pelvis and its ligaments, the residual ovarian tissue that remains is influenced by and responsive to systemic hormones.

CHAPTER 12

Skin Disorders

COMMON SKIN CONDITIONS

Acne
Urticaria (Hives)
Sunburn
Atopic Dermatitis
Contact Dermatitis
Perioral Dermatitis
Rosacea

SKIN MALIGNANCIES

Basal Cell Carcinoma
Squamous Cell Carcinoma
Melanoma

COMMON SKIN CONDITIONS

Acne

Acne is a chronic disorder that primarily involves increased sebum secretions that result in plugged pores. In fewer cases, acne is caused by the rapid production of the bacteria *Propionibacterium acnes*. Lesions may be open (i.e., blackheads) or closed (i.e., whiteheads). Lesions occur primarily on the face but also on the back, chest, neck, and shoulders. Mild acne is noninflammatory. Moderate acne involves papules (or inflamed pimples) filled with pus. Severe acne involves multiple papules, pustules (inflamed pimples filled with yellow pus), and nodules.

Epidemiology

Acne is the most common of the skin diseases, accounting for 22% to 32% of all dermatologic diagnoses. In women, acne peaks in the teenage years, affecting almost 100% of adolescents in the United States and the United Kingdom. In addition, acne affects 45% of women aged 21 to 30, 26% of women aged 31 to 40, and 12% of women aged 41 to 50.

CLINICAL PEARL

Some parts of the world, such as rural Brazil, report no cases of acne.

Etiology

- Hormonal changes
- Medications, including antiepileptics, such as carbamazepine and phenobarbital; antidepressants, such as amoxapine and lithium; and immunosuppressants, such as cyclosporine
- Nutraceuticals, such as vitamin B_{12}
- Increased sebum secretions
- Bacteria

CLINICAL PEARL

Acne may substantially impact self-esteem and quality of life.

Signs and Symptoms

- Presence of acne lesions

Diagnosis

- History and physical exam
- Swab/scrape from the acne lesion to examine for and rule out bacteria, such as *Staphylococcus aureus*, or fungi, such as *Microsporum canis*
- Assessment for contributing factors, such as exacerbating medications
- Evaluation of endocrine dysfunction, as seen in polycystic ovarian syndrome (PCOS), including pelvic ultrasound to rule out cysts and x-ray or magnetic resonance imaging (MRI) to rule out pituitary tumor
- Hormonal assays to rule out conditions such as Cushing's syndrome, hyperprolactinemia, hyperandrogenism, and pregnancy
  - Testosterone
  - Sex-hormone-binding globulin (SHBG)
  - Dehydroepiandrosterone sulfate (DHEAS)
  - Free androgen index (FAI)
  - Adrenocorticotrophic hormone (ACTH)
  - Prolactin
  - Cortisol
  - Luteinizing hormone (LH)
  - Follicle-stimulating hormone (FSH)
  - 17-hydroxyprogesterone

Management

Conventional

- Topical retinoids, such as tretinoin and adapalene, which decrease the number of comedones and minimize inflammation
  - These retinoids may cause erythema and scaling and require application for a minimum of 3 months.
- Topical antimicrobials, including the antibiotics erythromycin and clindamycin, and benzoyl peroxide
  - Note: The risk for antibiotic resistance is high with the topicals. Use is restricted to 1 month or in combination with benzoyl peroxide.
- Combination of retinoids and antibiotics
- Oral antibiotics, including minocycline, erythromycin, and tetracycline
  - Note: Minocycline is known to increase the risk for autoimmune disorders such as lupus.
- Isotretinoin (Accutane)
  - This vitamin A derivative has demonstrated significant efficacy in the treatment of acne; however, the side effects are also significant.
  - Note: Common isotretinoin side effects include anemia, thrombocytopenia, back pain, arthralgia, and increased triglycerides. Less common side effects include suicidal ideation and attempts. Blood work should precede oral isotretinoin therapy.
  - Isotretinoin is a known teratogen.
- Hormonal therapies, including oral antiandrogens and estrogen-containing oral contraceptives such as Ortho Tri-Cyclen, Yaz, and Estrostep
  - Note: Yaz contains drospirenone. According to the U.S. Food and Drug Administration (FDA), the risk of venous thromboembolism (VTE) in women taking drospirenone is approximately two times greater than the risk from taking other hormonal contraceptives.

CLINICAL PEARL

Nodules on the lower face and neck are especially responsive to hormonal therapy.

CLINICAL PEARL

The over-the-counter treatment Proactive contains a low dosage of benzoyl peroxide.

CLINICAL PEARL

Progesterone-only contraceptives may worsen acne.

TECHNICAL NOTE

Estrogen-containing oral contraceptives decrease the levels of free testosterone by increasing SHBG. In some cases, this is a benefit to women who suffer from acne.

Complementary

- The following have demonstrated efficacy in single trials:
  - Tee tree oil
  - Bee venom
  - Low-glycemic-load diets
- Anecdotal evidence supports the following
  - Herbal medicine
  - Acupuncture
  - Cupping
- Scar treatments include the following:
  - Steroids
  - Dermabrasion
  - Surgery
  - Laser resurfacing

Urticaria (Hives)

Urticaria is an outbreak of swollen, pale red bumps or wheals on the skin. The lesion is sudden and causes itching.

Epidemiology

- Approximately 60% of all persons afflicted with urticaria are female.

Etiology

- Immunoglobulin E–mediated reactions
  - Allergens (food, medications including antibiotics such as penicillin)
  - Parasitic infections
  - Insect venom
- Non-immunoglobulin E–mediated reactions
  - Autoimmune diseases
  - Cryoglobulinemia
  - Lymphoma
  - Vasculitis
  - Fungal, viral, and bacterial infections
- Nonimmunologically mediated causes
  - Food allergens
  - Medications
  - Light
  - Elevation of core temperature
  - Physical stimuli such as cold, local heat, pressure, and vibration
  - Water

Signs and Symptoms

- Presence of lesion (Figure 12–1)

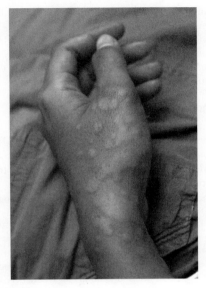

Figure 12-1 Urticaria
© konmesa/Shutterstock

Diagnosis

- History and physical exam
- Laboratory analysis for recurrent or chronic symptoms, including complete blood count (CBC), erythrocyte sedimentation rate (ESR), thyroid-stimulating hormone (TSH), and antinuclear antibodies

Management

Conventional

- None: Symptoms typically self-resolve.
- Antihistamines: A nonsedating H1 antihistamine is the first line of therapy.
- Diphenhydramine (Benadryl)

- Histamine H1 blockers, such as loratadine (Claritin) and cetirizine (Zyrtec)
- Leukotriene receptor antagonists (LTRAs): LTRAs, such as montelukast, zafirlukast, and pranlukast, are not recommended as monotherapy and are most effective if used in conjunction with antihistamines.

Self-Care and Wellness

- Avoidance of known triggers
- Cold compresses
- Cold compresses of oatmeal paste or cornstarch
- Consumption or topical application of red alder tea
- Quercetin
- Avoidance of aspirin, nonsteroidal anti-inflammatory drugs (NSAIDs), and alcohol

---

CLINICAL PEARL

High-dose short-term vitamin D_3 (4,000 IU/day) is considered a safe and potentially beneficial immunomodulator in patients with chronic urticaria.

Sunburn

Sunburn refers to damage to the skin's layers caused by exposure to sunlight.

Epidemiology

- Most fair-skinned individuals will experience at least one episode of sunburn.

Etiology

- Overexposure to ultraviolet (UV) rays from the sun

Signs and Symptoms

- Fair skin that has turned red

- Painful skin following sun exposure
- Subsequent flaking and itching as the body attempts to rid itself of the damaged tissue

Management
Conventional
- Medications and ointments
  - NSAIDs for the pain, including Naproxen (Aleve), aspirin (Bayer), and ibuprofen (Advil)
- Increased fluids to counter dehydration

Self-Care and Wellness
- Avoid excessive sun exposure.
- Avoid being in the sun during the hours that UV light is most intense (i.e., between the hours of 10 a.m. and 4:00 p.m.).
- Apply cold compresses over the skin.
- Apply cold compresses of oatmeal, fat-free milk, or cornstarch.
- Apply compresses of witch hazel.
- Apply compresses of aluminum acetate.
- Apply aloe vera.
- Add baking soda to a lukewarm bath (baking soda soak).

Atopic Dermatitis

Atopic dermatitis is a common form of eczema that affects people who have a personal or family history of eczema, asthma, or hay fever. It is the most common form of eczema.

Epidemiology
- Can manifest at any age

Etiology
- Susceptibility
- Skin defects
- Exposure to environmental irritants such as household chemicals

Management

Conventional

- Anti-inflammatories such as hydrocortisone (Cortaid)
- Antibiotics
  - The choice of antibiotic is dependent on the type of pathogen identified and may include cephalosporin (cephalexin [Keflex]), penicillin, clindamycin (Cleocin), or trimethoprim (Bactrim).
- Antihistamines, such as diphenhydramine (Benadryl)
- Immunomodulators, such as cyclosporin (Neoral), in severe cases
- UV light
- UV light and psoralen

Self-Care and Wellness

- Skin lotion and other lubricants

CLINICAL PEARL

Supplementation with probiotics (*Lactobacillus rhamnosus*) and gamma linolenic acid may reduce the development and severity of atopic dermatitis.

Contact Dermatitis

Contact dermatitis is dermatitis caused by contact with allergy-triggering substances.

Epidemiology

- Can affect anyone

Etiology

- Contact with allergy-triggering substances, including cosmetics

Management

Conventional

- Topical steroids, such as triamcinolone 0.1% (Kenalog, Aristocort), clobetasol 0.05% (Temovate), and desonide ointment (Desowen), are indicated; daily prednisone may be used for severe cases.
- Antibiotics may be needed if an infection develops.

Self-Care and Wellness

- Removal of causative factor
- Symptom relief
  - Cool compresses
  - Oatmeal baths
  - Calamine lotion
  - Moisturizers

Perioral Dermatitis

Perioral dermatitis is a facial rash that primarily affects the area around the mouth.

Epidemiology

- Most commonly seen in young women

Etiology

- Allergic reaction to a topical ointment

Signs and Symptoms

- Bumps and a burning sensation around the mouth

Diagnosis

- Bacterial culture to rule out infection

Management
Conventional
- Oral or topical antibiotics, including tetracycline and doxycycline

Self-Care and Wellness
- Discontinue use of all facial creams.

Rosacea

Rosacea (adult acne) is a chronic inflammatory skin condition and is incurable. There are four subtypes, and each has its own set of symptoms; however, the trademark is flushing of the skin of the cheeks, forehead, and nose accompanied by small, red, pus-filled bumps on the skin. Flare-ups often occur in cycles.

Epidemiology
- Rosacea is three times more common in women than men.
- Onset is between the ages of 30 and 60.
- Rosacea appears to be more common among fair-skinned people of northern European ancestry and affects 5% of Americans, or 1 in 20.
- Hot flashes during menopause may instigate the first appearance of rosacea.

Etiology
- Unknown
- Abnormalities in facial blood vessels
- Light skin color
- *Demodex folliculorum* (microscopic mites): These mites live on normal skin and cause no problems. People with rosacea have much higher numbers of these mites, which may be a cause or a consequence of rosacea.
- *Heliobacter pylori*: These bacteria reside in the gut and stimulate the production of bradykinin, which plays a role in the dilatation of blood vessels.

- Genetic predisposition to rosacea: Up to 40% of people with rosacea have a close relative with the condition.
- Vitamin B_3 (niacin)
- Medications, including vasodilator antihypertensives

Signs and Symptoms
- Facial flushing and redness
- Visible broken blood vessels (spider veins)
- Swollen red bumps
- Skin that may burn, sting, and feel very sensitive.
- Eye problems, such as dryness, irritation, and eyelids that are reddish.

Diagnosis
- History and exam

Management

Conventional
- Medications
  - Topical brimonidine (Mirvaso) for rapid (12- to 24-hour) symptom relief— improves redness by constricting the blood vessels
  - Topical metronidazole—demonstrates improvement in redness within 1 month
  - Topical azelaic acid and sulfacetamide products—improvement following 1 month of use
  - Topical acne medications
  - Topical retinoids, such as tretinoin—thought to be as effective in some instances as oral isotretinoin
  - Oral acne medications, such as isotretinoin
    - Note: Isotretinoin is known to cause birth defects and is contraindicated in pregnancy (see the Clinical Pearl).
  - Oral antibiotics, such as doxycycline
  - Immunosuppressants, such as pimecrolimus and tacrolimus, which are topical calcineurin inhibitors

> **TECHNICAL NOTE**
>
> Pimecrolimus and tacrolimus inhibit T-lymphocyte activation and prevent the release of cytokines, thereby decreasing the immune response at a local level.

- Vascular laser (commonly referred to by the manufacturer name "V-Beam"): This procedure involves brief, intense, targeted heat pulses to destroy the dilated blood vessels commonly seen in rosacea. A dye may be used to generate laser beams of different colors.
- Anecdotal reports suggest that a positive side effect of some medications is improved rosacea symptomatology. These medications include oral contraceptives, some beta blockers, and some selective serotonin reuptake inhibitors.

> **TECHNICAL NOTE**
>
> To avoid injury to the surrounding tissue, the pulses in vascular laser treatment are calibrated to allow for heat only to the affected tissue, such that the surrounding tissue doesn't receive enough heat to sustain damage. Further, the color of laser light is selective for the hemoglobin within the targeted tissue.

Complementary

- Relaxation techniques, yoga, and other mind–body techniques for managing stress and anxieties
- Gentle facial massage
- Counseling when there are self-esteem concerns
- Dietary changes: Anecdotal reports suggest that limiting foods with a high acidity potential, such as meats, dairy, and processed foods, while increasing foods with a high alkalinity potential, such as fruits, vegetables, and olive oil, may improve the intensity of rosacea symptomatology.

Self-Care and Wellness

- Sunscreen that protects against both UV-A and UV-B light
- Avoidance all known triggers, including some or all of the following:
  - Hot, spicy foods and drinks
  - Foods and drinks containing caffeine
  - Dairy products
  - Alcohol
  - Extremes in temperature
  - Sun, wind, and high humidity
  - Anxiety and stress
  - Embarrassment, anger
  - Vigorous exercise
  - Hot baths or saunas

SKIN MALIGNANCIES

Basal Cell Carcinoma

Basal cell carcinoma (BCC) is a type of skin cancer caused by a DNA mutation originating from the basal cells of the epidermis.

Epidemiology

- Currently, there are no registries that collect data on BCC; however, estimates are that 2 to 3 million cases are treated annually in the United States.
- An estimated 1/1000 women are diagnosed with BCC.
- BCC is the most common of the skin cancers.

Etiology

- Exposure to UV light, primarily from the sun

Signs and Symptoms

- Waxy whitish-brown or black bump on the face or neck
- Nonhealing sore
- Growing area of patchy skin on the back or chest

Diagnosis

- Skin biopsy: The type of biopsy is dependent on factors such as the location, size, and type of cancer and may include a punch, incisional, excisional, or shave biopsy. The shave biopsy is typically all that is required for BCC diagnosis.

TECHNICAL NOTE

The types of skin biopsies are described as follows:

Shave (tangential) biopsy—removal of the most superficial layer (dermis) of the skin with a surgical blade

Punch biopsy—allows for samples from the deeper layers of the skin

Incisional biopsy—removes a portion of a tumor that may have grown into the deeper layers

Excisional biopsy—removes all of a tumor that involves the deeper layers of the skin

Management

Conventional

- Cryosurgery
- Surgical excision
- Electrodesiccation and curettage
- Mohs surgery—layer-by-layer removal and examination
- Topical medications, creams, and ointments applied over a few weeks, with the following indications:
  - Topical 5% imiquimod for nonfacial BCC that is less than 2 cm in diameter is applied 5 days a week for 6 to 12 weeks.
  - Topical fluorouracil is used two times daily for 3 to 6 weeks for lesions on the trunk or extremities.

CLINICAL PEARL

The risk of recurrence is high with BCC. Approximately 40% of patients who have had one BCC will develop another lesion within 5 years.

Squamous Cell Carcinoma

Squamous cell carcinoma (SCC) is a type of skin cancer originating from the superficial squamous cells of the skin.

Epidemiology

- Very common type of skin cancer
- Second most common of the skin cancers (second to BCC)

Etiology

- Exposure to UV rays, primarily from the sun

Signs and Symptoms

- Sore with a scaly crust
- Reddish or brownish nodule that is firm

Diagnosis

- Skin biopsy: The type of biopsy is dependent on factors such as the location, size, and type of cancer and may include a punch, incisional, excisional, or shave biopsy.
- Incisional or punch biopsies are most commonly the first steps in diagnosis of SCC.

Management

Conventional

- Cryosurgery: This inexpensive method involves the application of liquid nitrogen with either a cotton-tipped applicator or spray to the lesion and does not require anesthesia. Multiple treatments may be necessary. The lesion falls off within weeks. This method is generally not used for invasive SCC.
- Surgical excision
- Electrodesiccation and curettage: This treatment is reserved for small lesions; the growth is scraped off with a curette. Cure rates are approximately 90%.
- Mohs surgery: This technique involves layer-by-layer removal and examination of the sample and is used in areas that are

hard to access, such as around the eyes or the nose, and with recurrent SCC. It has a 94% to 99% cure rate and should be performed by a designated Mohs surgeon.

- Topical medications, creams, and ointments applied over a few weeks
  - 5-FU is a recent example.
- Photodynamic therapy: This treatment is of value for lesions on the face and scalp. Topical agents that react to light, such as topical 5-aminolevulinic acid (5-ALA) or methyl aminolevulinate (MAL), are applied to the lesion. The lesion is subsequently exposed to a light, and the agents destroy the SCC.
- Laser therapy
- Radiation therapy: This is a nonsurgical procedure in which x-ray beams are aimed at the lesion. It does not require anesthesia and is reserved for those for whom surgery is not advisable. The cure rate is 85% to 95%.
- Prevention: Limit sun exposure.

Melanoma

Melanoma is the most serious of the skin cancers; it develops within the melanocytes.

Epidemiology

- Melanoma accounts for 1% of skin cancers but causes the majority of skin cancer deaths. Melanoma is the third most common cancer among women aged 20 to 39.
- Incidence rates are higher in women than in men before the age of 50, but by age 65, rates in men double those in women.

CLINICAL PEARL

Of people with melanoma, 1 in 10 has a family history of melanoma.

CLINICAL PEARL

Worldwide, Caucasian populations have the highest risk of developing melanoma, and Asian populations have the lowest risk.

Etiology
- Exposure to UV light

CLINICAL PEARL

Melanomas are known to occur in areas that are not exposed to the sun.

CLINICAL PEARL

Because of the connection between indoor tanning and skin cancer, several states in the United States and several countries worldwide prohibit indoor tanning for people younger than age 18.

Signs and Symptoms
- New and unusual skin growth
- New changes in an old mole

CLINICAL PEARL

The mnemonic ABCDE can be used to alert patients to possible melanoma or other skin cancer; it refers to the characteristics of a suspicious mole, as follows:

A—asymmetrical

B—borders that are irregular

C—changes or irregularities in color

D—diameter larger than 6 mm

E—evolving (changes in size, shape, color, or symptoms)

Diagnosis

- Biopsy (punch, excisional, incisional)

Management

Conventional

- Depending on staging and sentinel node involvement, management may include one or several of the following:
  - Surgery
  - Chemotherapy
  - Radiation
  - Targeted therapy: In this approach, drugs target the abnormal aspects of tumor cells without harming the normal cells. Treatment is personalized based on the genetic profile, or subtype, of the tumor.
  - Immunotherapy: Systemic therapy is commonly used if the risk for recurrence is high or if the melanoma has metastasized. These therapies activate the individual's immune system to facilitate the destruction of system-wide melanoma cells.

Complementary

- Nutrition therapy, such as fermented wheat germ extract (Avemar)
- Acupuncture
- Herbal therapies
- Manual therapy

Self-Care and Wellness

- Limit sun exposure.

CLINICAL PEARL

Patients receiving chemotherapy for melanoma who were supplemented with fermented wheat germ extract (Avemar) for 1 year noted significant improvement in progression and overall survival.

CHAPTER 13

Urinary Tract Disorders

Bladder Syndrome/Painful Bladder Syndrome/Interstitial Cystitis (Bladder Pain Syndrome)

Painful bladder syndrome/interstitial cystitis (PBS/IC), also known as bladder pain syndrome, is a chronic condition of unknown etiology marked by irritation or inflammation of the lining of the bladder wall. It includes all cases of urinary pain not attributable to a specific cause, such as an infection or kidney stones.

Epidemiology

- Bladder pain syndrome occurs primarily in middle-aged women; however, it can occur in women as young as 18 years of age.
- Estimates are that 2.7% to 6.6% of women in the United States aged 18 years or older (3.3 to 7.9 million women) have bladder pain syndrome/interstitial cystitis.

Etiology

The cause of bladder pain syndrome is unknown. Proposed causes include the following:

- Autoimmune response following an acute bladder infection
- Allergic reaction to urinary substrates
- Irritation to the nerves of the sacral plexus
- Fibromyalgia
- Irritable bowel syndrome
- Hereditary factors

Signs and Symptoms

- Urinary frequency
- Urinary urgency
- Pain in the bladder ranging in intensity from mild pressure to severe pain
- Pain in the lower abdomen and pelvis
- Sensation of increased pressure in the lower abdomen

- Dyspareunia
- Dysmenorrhea

Diagnosis

- Ruling out of conditions such as urinary tract infections (UTIs), sexually transmitted infections (STIs), reproductive tract malignancy, and endometriosis
- Presence of the signs and symptoms listed in the previous section
- Urinalysis
  - In PBS/IC, there is an absence of infection indicators, such as bacteria and white and red blood cells.
- STI screening
- Pelvic examination
- Cystoscopy for definitive diagnosis, either alone or with biopsy
  - Cystoscopy is used to detect signs of inflammation and bleeding, determine bladder capacity and bladder wall flexibility, and rule out bladder cancer.
  - Cystoscopy in PBS/IC is painful and is performed under anesthesia.

Management

Conventional

- Treatments are focused on symptom relief and include those described in the following subsections.

Medications

- Elmiron
- Nonsteroidal anti-inflammatories (NSAIDs)
- Pain medications
- Antidepressants

Physical Therapy

- Biofeedback for bladder training, pain control and muscle, relaxation
- Transcutaneous electrical nerve stimulation (TENS) for pain modification

Procedures
- Bladder instillation
  - This procedure involves catheterization with dimethyl sulfoxide (DMSO/Rimso-50) solution. The solution is retained for 15 minutes and then expelled. Treatments are self-administered or clinician administered weekly for up to 2 months. According to the National Institute of Diabetes and Digestive and Kidney Diseases (NIDDM, 2016) patients report symptom relief 3 to 4 weeks after completing a 6- to 8-week cycle of treatments.
- Sacral nerve stimulation implants
- Bladder distention

Surgery

Surgery does not guarantee improved outcomes and is considered when more conservative methods have been exhausted. Surgical procedures include the following:

- Fulguration—laser or electrical therapy applied to the (Hunner) ulcers within the bladder
- Resection to cut and remove any ulcers
- Augmentation using tissue from the colon to replace and enlarge the diseased bladder tissue
- Cystectomy (bladder removal) and urostomy (rerouting of the ureters, typically to the colon) to allow for emptying through the stoma into an external bag

Self-Care and Wellness

- Evaluate for diet and other lifestyle factors that increase the sensation of frequency and urgency. Suspected triggers include the following:
  - Dairy
  - Caffeine
  - High-acid foods
  - Artificial sweeteners

- Some spices
- Chocolate
- Tobacco
- Bladder training that combines scheduled voiding with relaxation techniques
- Support groups

> **CLINICAL PEARL**
>
> There is no clear scientific evidence directly linking diet to PBS/IC; however, anecdotal reports suggest that for some patients, certain foods contribute to bladder irritation and inflammation.

> **CLINICAL PEARL**
>
> Symptoms of PBS may flare up during stressful circumstances.

> **CLINICAL PEARL**
>
> The pain associated with PBS is intermittent; it increases and decreases with the amount of urine in the bladder. PBS symptoms may spontaneously regress for a time (weeks or months) and then return.

Cystitis

Cystitis is inflammation of the bladder, most commonly caused by a urinary tract infection.

Epidemiology

- Women are eight times more likely to develop cystitis than men because the female urethra is shorter than the male urethra and opens closer to the anus.
- Up to 15% of women have cystitis each year, and approximately 50% of women have at least one bout of cystitis in their lifetime.

Etiology

The majority of cases of cystitis are caused by *Escherichia coli*. Other causes include the following:

- Chemotherapy drugs (cyclophosphamide and ifosfamide)
- Radiation to the pelvic region
- Long-term use of a catheter
- Hypersensitivity to chemicals such as those found in some bubble bath solutions and feminine hygiene sprays
- Complications of other disorders, such as Crohn's disease, gynecologic cancers, pelvic inflammatory disorders, and endometriosis

Risk Factors

- Diabetes
- Pregnancy
- Sexual activity
- Middle age
- Irritable bowel syndrome
- Fibromyalgia

Signs and Symptoms

- Strong, persistent urge to urinate
- Burning sensation when urinating
- Passing frequent, small amounts of urine
- Hematuria
- Strong-smelling or cloudy urine
- Dull ache in the pelvic area
- Feeling of pressure in the lower abdomen
- Low-grade fever
- Back pain
- Nausea and vomiting

CLINICAL PEARL

Daytime wetting accidents in young girls may be an indication of a urinary tract infection.

Diagnosis

- Medical history that includes any of the risk factors
- Urinalysis that reveals bacteria, blood, and other inflammatory exudates
- Pelvic exam
- Imaging tests when other tests are negative
- Cystoscopy

Management

Conventional

Medications

- Antimicrobials targeted for the type of bacteria found in the urine, including the sulfonamides (Bactrim), the fluoroquinolones (Cipro), and the cephalosporins (Cefaclor)

TECHNICAL NOTE

The risk of antibiotic resistance is significant. Antibiotics should only be taken if urinalysis reveals the presence of bacteria in the urine.

Complementary

- Pure cranberry juice or capsules
- Pure blueberry juice or capsules

Self-Care and Wellness

- Elimination of causative factors
- Fluids, including 6 to 8 glasses of water daily
- Careful feminine hygiene with each voiding
- Elimination of all sugary drinks

CLINICAL PEARL

If the cause of cystitis is thought to be sexual, it is recommended that the individual take a single dose of antibiotics after intercourse.

Symptoms from first-time infections typically improve within a couple of days. Repeat infections may necessitate referral to a urologist.

Urinary Incontinence

Urinary incontinence (UI) is the inability to control urine flow. The different types of UI are as follows:

- Stress incontinence: Loss of urine with coughing, sneezing, laughing, and other activities that increase intra-abdominal pressure.
- Urge incontinence or overactive bladder (OAB): Sudden urge to urinate, frequently followed by an involuntary loss of urine.
- Mixed incontinence: Combination of stress and urge incontinence.
- Overflow incontinence: Inability to empty the bladder completely, resulting in involuntary loss of urine. This loss of urine is postulated to be caused by overdistention, which is facilitated by outlet obstruction or an underactive detrusor muscle.
- Functional incontinence: Nonurogenital UI caused by factors such as mental and physical compromise resulting in inability to void independently.

Epidemiology

- UI affects women of all ages.
- Many women report incontinence during pregnancy and the postpartum period.

Etiology

- Pelvic-floor compromise as a result of childbirth and other causes
- Urinary muscle spasms
- Nerve damage caused by factors such as injury, childbirth, stroke, multiple sclerosis, and diabetes

- Bladder storage capacity
  - Conditions such as irritable bowel syndrome and treatments such as bladder radiation can cause irritation and scarring.
- UTIs

Risk Factors
- Overweight or obesity
- Genetic weaknesses
- Multiple pregnancies

Signs and Symptoms
- The main symptom of incontinence is the inability to control urination.
- In stress incontinence, there is an involuntary leakage of urine, especially when a person coughs, sneezes, or laughs.
- In urge incontinence, there is a frequent and sudden uncontrollable need to urinate.
- Complete loss of bladder control can occur in severe cases.

Diagnosis
- Careful history and physical, including urinary postvoid residual, which assesses the amount of urine that remains in the bladder after urination, and pad test, which uses the weight of a saturated pad to assess leakage
- Cystoscopic exam
- Pelvic/abdominal ultrasound
- Contrast studies of the kidneys and bladder
- Electromyogram (EMG)

CLINICAL PEARL

Urinary incontinence often goes unreported for years because many women are either embarrassed by the condition or feel there is no cure.

TECHNICAL NOTE

Bladder control problems require attention for several reasons:
- They may indicate a serious underlying medical condition, such as diabetes or kidney problems.
- They may cause restriction in physical activities.
- They may cause the individual to withdraw from social interactions.

CLINICAL PEARL

There is an increased risk of falling when rushing to the bathroom to avoid urine leakage.

Management

Conventional

Bladder Training

- Timed voiding—urinating on specific schedule every day
- Pelvic-floor (Kegel) exercises with or without vaginal cones (see the Appendix)
- Pessaries and bladder neck support devices to manage prolapse
- Urethral-opening occlusion devices, such as tampons, Reliance, CapSure, and FemAssist

Physical Therapy

- Bladder training/timed voiding
  - The patient is trained to empty the bladder at a specific time of day. In addition, the patient relearns how to control the bladder and strengthen the involved muscles. Biofeedback and pelvic-floor exercises are typically included.
- Biofeedback to strengthen and coordinate the pelvic-floor muscles, often coordinated with pelvic-floor (Kegel) exercises
- Pelvic-floor stimulation (InterStim therapy), in which electrical therapies are applied directly over the pelvic-floor muscles

Medications

- Tolterodine (Detrol)
- Tolterodine extended release (Detrol LA)

- Trospium (Sanctura)
- Oxybutynin patch (Oxytrol) for overactive bladder
- Antibiotics if bacterial infection is identified as a cause
- For dosages and contraindications, see the links in the Appendix

Procedures

- Sacral nerve stimulation by direct placement of a pulse generator after testing confirms treatment efficacy (see the Appendix)
- Periurethral bulking injections
  - Durasphere or collagen is injected into the tissue around the urethra to add bulk and retard leakage. Results are expected to last up to 1 year. Sometimes more than one treatment is required.
- Botulinum toxin (Botox)
  - Botox is sometimes injected into the bladder muscles to relieve muscle spasms. It can provide symptom relief for up to 1 year.

Surgery

- Pubovaginal, tension-free vaginal tape (TVT), and other sling procedures
- Burch urethropexy procedures (bladder neck suspension surgery)

TECHNICAL NOTE

Urethropexy involves suturing the tissue of the vagina to the pubic bone to reposition the bladder and provide additional support to the urethra.

Complementary

Spinal Manipulation

- Spinal manipulation to ensure optimal sacral nerve functioning and to correct pelvic misalignments

Acupuncture

- Randomized trials suggest that acupuncture can have effects similar to those of medications.

CLINICAL PEARL

Chiropractic manipulative therapy and lumbosacral flexion distraction techniques have demonstrated efficacy in the management of UI. Case-series reports indicate long-term symptom improvement.

Self-Care and Wellness

- Diet
    - Avoid triggers. For some women, these include certain foods, caffeine, and alcohol.
    - Keep a daily food/symptom diary to identify other potential triggers.
- Pelvic-floor (Kegel) exercises (see the Appendix)

TECHNICAL NOTE

Systemic estrogen therapy is not approved by the U.S. Food and Drug Administration for the treatment of incontinence; however, local estrogen therapy may help some women with bladder and vaginal symptoms.

TECHNICAL NOTE

The American College of Physicians (ACP) recommends the following clinical practice guidelines for the nonsurgical management of urinary incontinence in women.

Stress UI

- Pelvic-floor muscle training (PFMT) increases continence rates and improves UI and quality of life in women with stress UI.
- Vaginal estrogen formulations improve continence and stress UI, but transdermal estrogen patches worsen UI.
- The ACP recommends against treatment with systemic pharmacologic therapy.

Urgency UI

- Bladder training
    - Note: In clinical trials, the addition of PFMT to bladder training did not improve continence compared with bladder training alone for urgency UI.

- Pharmacologic treatment (see previous list) is recommended in women with urgency UI if bladder training was unsuccessful.

Mixed UI
- PFMT with bladder training

For all women with UI, nonpharmacologic therapy with PFMT should be the first-line treatment.

Data from Qaseem, A., Dallas, P., Forciea, M. A., Starkey, M., Denberg, T. D., & Shekelle, P. (2014). Nonsurgical management of urinary incontinence in women: A clinical practice guideline from the American College of Physicians. *Annals of Internal Medicine, 161*(6), 429–445.

TECHNICAL NOTE

Recommended nursing care protocols and assessments for incontinence care include the following:

Type of Incontinence	Protocol
Stress	Pelvic-floor muscle training (PFMT) Toileting assistance and bladder training as needed Pharmacological and surgical referral if needed
Urge/ overactive bladder	Bladder training and urge inhibition strategies PFMT Pharmacological and surgical referral if needed
Overflow	Allowance of sufficient time for voiding Instruction in Credé's maneuver Pharmacological and surgical referral if needed Sterile intermittent catheterization preferred over indwelling
Functional	Assistance with scheduled toileting and timed voiding Adequate fluid intake Physical and occupational therapy referral if needed

Data from Dowling-Castronovo, A., & Bradway, C. (2012). *Nursing standard of practice protocol: Urinary incontinence (UI) in older adults admitted to acute care.* Retrieved from https://consultgeri.org/geriatric-topics/urinary-incontinence; Boltz, M., Capezuti, E., Fulmer, T.T., Zwicekr, D., & O'Meara, A. (Eds.) (2012). *Evidence-based geriatric nursing protocols for best practice.* New York, NY: Springer.

Fecal Incontinence

Fecal incontinence (bowel incontinence) involves loss of control of bowel movements and leakage of stool; in extreme cases, total loss of bowel control occurs. It is an underreported and undertreated condition that results in isolation and poor quality of life.

Epidemiology

- Fecal incontinence occurs in both sexes and in all ages; however, it is more prevalent in older women.
- Overall, it is estimated that approximately 9% of women have some form of fecal incontinence (liquid stool, solid stool, or mucus) weekly.
- Estimates range from 2.6% in women between the ages of 20 and 30 to 15.3% in women over age 70.

Etiology

- Muscle damage—damage of the muscles of the anal sphincter during childbirth as a result of a difficult delivery, episiotomy, or use of forceps
  - The younger female can compensate for this damage; however, as women age and muscle laxity occurs, the changes in anal sphincter pressure may result in fetal incontinence. Some women notice fetal incontinence immediately after a birth.
- Pelvic-floor compromise as a result of childbirth
- Rectocele as a result of aging
- Constipation
  - Hardened stools become lodged in the rectum, and watery stools leak around the hardened stool. The impacted stools cause the muscles of the rectum to stretch and weaken.
- Damage to the sensory nerves to the anal sphincter, which can cause the individual to lose the sensation of stools in the rectum
- Rectal storage capacity
  - Conditions such as irritable bowel syndrome can cause irritation and scarring, which affect the ability of the rectum to stretch. As a result, rectal volume is compromised.

- Diarrhea
  - Looser stools are more difficult to control.

Signs and Symptoms

- Urgency
- Loss of bowel control

Diagnosis

- History and physical exam, including a digital rectal exam
- Additional diagnostic tests
  - Anal manometry assesses the integrity of the anal sphincter and rectum. The rectum is distended with a balloon, and a sensor assesses for the rectosphincteric reflex.
  - Anorectal ultrasound
    - Proctography (defecography) shows how much stool the rectum can hold, how well the rectum holds it, and how well the rectum can evacuate the stool.
    - Anal electromyography evaluates for nerve damage, which is often associated with obstetric injury.
    - Proctosigmoidoscopy evaluates for inflammation, tumors, scar tissue, and other disease processes.

Management

Conventional

Medications

The specific drugs used depend on the cause and include the following:

- Bulk laxatives such as psyllium (Metamucil) and methylcellulose (Citrucel)
- Stool softeners
- Anti-diarrheals such as loperamide hydrochloride (Imodium)
- Medications for irritable bowel syndrome, which may include injectable bulking agents such as dextranomer microspheres/hyaluronate sodium in 0.9 % NaCl (Solesta) injected directly into the anal canal

Physical Therapy
- Bowel training
  - The patient learns to empty the bowels at a specific time of day. In addition, the patient relearns how to control the bowels and strengthen the involved muscles.
- Biofeedback to strengthen and coordinate the pelvic-floor muscles, often coordinated with pelvic-floor (Kegel) exercises
- Pelvic-floor (Kegel) exercises (see the Appendix)

Procedures
- Sacral nerve stimulation via a pulse generator (see the Appendix)

Surgery

Surgical recommendations depend on the cause and severity of the condition and the response to other modes of treatment. Options include the following:
- Colostomy for severe conditions
- Sphincteroplasty to repair a weakened anal sphincter
- Procedures to manage for rectal prolapse

Complementary

- Chiropractic treatment: Case reports indicate that low-force chiropractic treatment (activator adjustments) followed by shortwave diathermy to the lumbar spine and sacrum can enhance bowel control.

Self-Care and Wellness

Diet

- Identify food triggers by keeping a food diary. Common triggers include caffeine, dairy products, alcohol, spicy foods, pork, sweeteners, fatty foods, and some fruits.
- Eat smaller meals.
- Avoid drinking fluids with meals.
- Keep well hydrated.

- Modulate fiber intake. Depending on whether constipation or diarrhea is the cause of the incontinence, it may take a course of trial and error to reach the right amount of fiber. Soluble-fiber foods, such as bananas, smooth peanut butter, oatmeal, yogurt, and rice, are recommended in most cases over insoluble fiber because they slow gastric transit time.

Urinary Tract Infections

UTIs are infections of the urinary tract, most commonly caused by *E. coli* bacteria.

Epidemiology

- One out of every two American women will experience at least one UTI over the course of their lifetime.
- One-third of all UTIs recur within 6 months.

> **CLINICAL PEARL**
>
> The epidemiology of UTI varies worldwide. Women in some parts of the world rarely experience UTIs.

Etiology

- In 90% of cases of true UTI, *E. coli* bacteria are causative.
- *E. coli*, which normally inhabits the digestive tract, may be introduced into the urinary tract as a result of poor hygiene, sexual activity, susceptibility, and other factors.

Risk Factors

- Multiple sexual partners
- A new sexual partner
- Diabetes
- Pregnancy
- Birth control pills
- Prior history of UTI

Signs and Symptoms

- Pain or burning with urination
- Increased urinary frequency
- Increased urinary urgency
- Fever, chills, generalized malaise
- Hematuria
- Lower abdominal pain or cramping
- Foul- or strong-smelling urine

Diagnosis

- History and physical exam
- Urinalysis to elicit the presence of excessive white blood cells and/or bacteria

Management

Conventional

- Antibiotics, such as trimethoprim/sulfamethoxazole (Bactrim, Septra)

Complementary

- Pure unsweetened blueberry juice
- Pure unsweetened cranberry juice or capsules
- Various homeopathics, such as *Arnica montana*, *Sepia*, *Aconite*, and *Pulsatilla*, as recommended by a licensed homeopath

Self-Care and Wellness

- Drinking copious amounts of filtered water
- Drinking herbal teas, including goldenseal and *Arctostaphylos uva-ursi*, during the infection
- Eliminating known food allergens
- Consuming foods rich in antioxidants, such as blueberries
- Minimizing refined foods
- Avoiding stimulants, including coffee
- Emptying the bladder frequently

PART THREE

Special Topics

The special topics in this section influence patient care because they affect patient compliance and patient outcomes. They should be taken into consideration as early as possible during the patient encounter and prior to the physical assessment.

CHAPTER 14

Cultural Considerations

Awareness
Knowledge
Skills

Cultural competence has many definitions; however, at the core is the ability of providers and organizations to effectively deliver health-care services that meet the social, cultural, and linguistic needs of patients (Betancourt et al., 2002). Cultural competence implies that providers will examine their own attitudes and values and acquire knowledge, skills, and attributes that enable them to work appropriately in cross-cultural situations (National Center for Cultural Competence, 2016), including working within the patient's values system and reality conditions (U.S. Department of Health and Human Services [USDHHS], 2016).

The lack of cultural competency in women's health care is known to influence some of the health disparities experienced by many women. Factors such as unconscious bias, stereotyping, gender bias, limited English proficiency, and limited health proficiency are all factors in the health disparities experienced by women (Hayman & Wilkes, 2016).

In addition, broader factors also influence women's health care, including ethnicity, culture, class, sexuality, race, marginalization, invisibility, and sexual discrimination (Núñez, 2000). Cultural competence in women's health care involves increasing awareness, knowledge, and skills, with the goal of optimizing patient outcomes.

Awareness

Awareness involves appreciation and acceptance of the various interacting cultures and cultural belief systems that exist in any patient–provider encounter, some of which are as follows:

- The culture of different health-care systems, for example, allopathy, complementary and integrative medicine, oriental medicine, chiropractic, naturopathy, and homeopathy
- Patients' cultural beliefs about the health-care system, about their own health, and about the cause, management, and outcomes of the condition or circumstance for which they are presenting
- The provider's personal and professional cultural beliefs, including a code of ethics, which influence his or her decisions in health-care delivery

Knowledge

The basis of the provider's interest in and knowledge of some of the differing cultural norms commonly encountered in health-care settings is the assumption that the patient-centered approach to health care warrants respectful consideration of the patient's belief systems even when they are in conflict with the provider's. It also involves acknowledging the potential for mutual learning that exists in the patient–provider encounter and purposefully learning the perspectives of various worldviews. Examples of differing cultural views on health care include the following:

- Cultural views on weight management
  - Obesity as evidence of affluence versus obesity as a cause of illnesses
- Cultural views on disease
  - One disease–one cure versus one disease–multiple cures
  - Only Allah or God has the cure for disease versus medication may cure the disease
  - There is a cure for every disease versus many diseases are terminal
- Cultural views on exercise
  - Exercise is scheduled, deliberate, and purposeful versus exercise happens as a result of daily activities
- Cultural views on preventative care
  - A visit to a health-care provider is necessitated by illness versus a visit to a health-care provider is necessary for prevention
- Cultural views on health disclosure
  - Full disclosure is mandated by law versus delivering bad news is taboo and terminal outcomes are never spoken of

Skills

The provider's failure to acknowledge differing worldviews has the potential to affect patient compliance and patient outcomes, and skill development is therefore essential. Skill development, as with all aspects of health-care practice, is an ongoing process. Seeking out differing cultural encounters and recognizing the limitations inherent in some encounters are useful strategies. Interpreters, cultural brokers, community leaders, chaplains, and other healers are valuable resources.

> **CLINICAL PEARL**
>
> Unconscious, automatic racial bias contributes to racial disparities in medical care. Research has shown that completion of measures such as the Black–White Implicit Association Test can decrease unconscious racial bias (Understanding Prejudice, 2017).

> **CLINICAL PEARL**
>
> According to research, cultural competence among health-care professionals is acquired partly through leadership; however, culturally competent individuals are not necessarily the formal leaders within an organization (Dauvrin and Lorant, 2015).

One means of enhancing cultural competence skills is by performing a cultural assessment, such as the LEARN model (Table 14-1).

Table 14-1 LEARN Model of Cultural Assessment

L	Listen sympathetically to the patient's and family's perception of the problem and their concepts of illness
E	Explain your perceptions of the problem and your strategies for management (visual aids are useful)
A	Acknowledge and discuss the differences and similarities between the patient and provider perspectives, emphasizing common ground
R	Recommend your management strategy, and listen carefully to the patient's response
N	Negotiate agreement in a manner that accommodates (where possible) the cultural beliefs and practices of the patient and family

Data from Berlin, E.A., & Fowkes, Jr. W.C. (1983). A teaching framework for cross-cultural health care: Application in family practice. *The Western Journal of Medicine, 139*(6), 934–38.

In addition, cultural competence skills can be enhanced by considering factors that might influence the patient's ideas about disease and illness. Areas to consider include the following:

- Level of ethnic identity
- Use of informal network and supportive institutions in the ethnic/cultural community values orientation
- Language and communication process
- Migration experience
- Self-concept and self-esteem
- Influence of religion/spirituality on belief systems and behavior patterns
- Views and concerns about discrimination and institutional racism
- Views about the role that ethnicity plays
- Educational level and employment experiences
- Habits, customs, and beliefs
- Importance and impact associated with physical characteristics
- Cultural health beliefs and practices
- Current socioeconomic status

CLINICAL PEARL

Clinician empathy enhances patient empowerment, and the ultimate goal of cultural competency in health care is that the provider is effective in interactions that involve individuals of different cultures and that neither the provider nor the patient culture is considered the preferred view (Betancourt et al., 2002).

TECHNICAL NOTE

Engaging in community health field experiences, learning another language, engaging in a cultural competence/awareness experience, becoming more aware of the perspectives of individuals from different backgrounds, and attending schools with higher social mission scores have been associated with enhanced desire to engage in clinical practice in underserved areas Boscardin et al. (2014).

CLINICAL PEARL

According to the Institute of Medicine (2014), lesbian and gay individuals face discrimination from health-care providers. Favorable and increased contact were found to enhance positive attitudes.

CLINICAL PEARL

The presence of an advanced practice nurse in long-term care settings has been found to enhance markers such as the health status and behaviors of older adults and family satisfaction with the care provided (Donald et al., 2013).

Domestic Violence/ Intimate Partner Violence

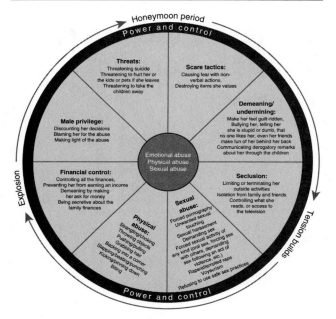

Figure 15-1 Domestic violence cycle of abuse

Data from Domestic Abuse Intervention Programs.

Domestic violence or intimate partner violence is abuse and violence experienced in intimate relationships. The abuse can be physical, mental, or emotional (see Figure 15-1).

Epidemiology

- Intimate partner violence (IPV) occurs across all socioeconomic, gender, racial, ethnic, age, ideological, cultural, and spiritual barriers.
- IPV occurs in opposite-sex and same-sex relationships.
- IPV affects both men and women; however, more women are abused than men.
- Data from the Bureau of Justice Statistics (2016) suggest that women in their late teens to early 20s are more likely to be

victims of domestic violence from a husband, boyfriend, or former partner than older women, and that women between the ages of 35 and 45 are more likely to be murdered by their intimate partners because they have been in abusive relationships for longer periods of time.

- IPV can escalate during pregnancy.
- Abuse and violence experienced by women in intimate relationships is a health concern that affects approximately 1 in 9 American women and as many as 1 in 4 pregnant women.

Etiology

- There are many causes for IPV, including issues with control and a historical failure in society to acknowledge IPV as a health-care concern and not solely as a private matter.

Signs and Symptoms/Presenting Complaints

- Migraines
- Chronic headaches
- Bruises
- Neck pain
- Back pain
- Anxiety disorders
- Muscle tension
- Digestive complaints
- Dysfunctional menstrual bleeding caused by stress
- Depression
- Eating disorders
- Chest pain
- Tingling and numbness
- Pelvic pain
- Arrhythmia
- Urinary tract infections and vaginitis
- Ear pain or evidence of a ruptured tympanic membrane
- Dyspareunia or evidence of rectal or genital injury
- Bruises on the face, neck, or abdomen
- Bruises on the arm

- Centrally located injuries involving the buttocks, breasts, abdomen, and genital region, also known as the "bathing suit pattern"
- Injuries involving the head and neck
- Defensive-posture injuries, which may involve the palms, the fingers, and the forearm

Diagnosis

- Signs and symptoms
- History and physical exam

IPV Screening

- Health-care providers are uniquely positioned to screen for domestic violence in a private setting and to provide information on resources that can empower their patients to work their way out of the domestic violence cycle.
- It is recommended that health-care providers screen all adult female patients for IPV and incorporate IPV screening into the general intake.
- Health-care providers should also screen for IPV in the following situations:
  - Patients report to the emergency room for complaints associated with trauma.
  - The cause given for the injury does not support the type of injury.
  - Fractures and injuries in various stages of healing are observed.
  - A delay has occurred in the patient seeking medical attention.
  - The patient demonstrates visible signs of depression.
- IPV should be suspected in the following situations:
  - The partner appears controlling.
  - The partner attempts to answer all questions for the patient.
  - The partner insists on being present while care is being provided to the patient.
  - The patient fails to make eye contact.

CLINICAL PEARL

Some of the aforementioned behaviors are cultural norms and are not necessarily indicative of IPV. The health-care provider should attempt to ask the patient when her partner is not close by if she would like her partner to be present during the office visit. IPV screening should never occur in the presence of the partner.

- Sample screening questions include the following:
  - How are things at home?
  - Do you feel safe at home?
  - Has your partner ever physically hurt you?
  - Are you afraid of your partner?
  - Do you feel your partner tries to control you?
  - Has your partner ever forced you into a sexual act that you did not wish to participate in?
  - Are you in danger?
  - Does your partner hit you when he or she is angry?

CLINICAL PEARL

Facilitators for screening for IPV include IPV posters in the health-care environment.

- Screening questions may be preceded by a framing statement, such as the following:
  - We've started talking to all of our patients about safe and healthy relationships because they can have a large influence on your health.
  - There are certain questions that I ask all my patients because we know from the data that many women are or have been victims of domestic violence.
  - There are certain questions that I ask all my patients because some of my patients are in relationships where they are afraid their partners may hurt them.

CLINICAL PEARL

Commonly used standardized screening tests for IPV include the following:

- Intimate Partner Violence Screening, available at http://www.us preventiveservicestaskforce.org/Page/Document/UpdateSummaryFinal /intimate-partner-violence-and-abuse-of-elderly-and-vulnerable -adults-screening
- Woman Abuse Screening Tool (WAST), available at http://www .healthyplace.com/psychological-tests/woman-abuse-screening-tool/oc

Once domestic violence has been identified, it is important that the provider validates the victim as the victim and not the perpetrator. It is equally important that the provider does not minimize the victim's experience.

Appropriate sample responses to disclosures of IPV include the following:

- I believe you.
- You are not alone.
- This situation must be very difficult for you.
- The violence is not your fault, and only [name of abuser] can choose to stop this behavior.
- Your safety concerns me.
- I am concerned for your safety.
- No one deserves to be abused.
- You have options.
- There are resources available.

The health-care provider should educate the patient regarding available resources, assist as needed in following up with selected resources (e.g., domestic violence shelters, advocacy groups), and encourage and facilitate the preparation of an exit plan. The exit plan involves identifying resources—such as friends, family, and neighbors—who can be called upon to assist in the event of an imminent exit from the home and locating a safe place to store critical items, such as medications, cash, family documents, and children's favorite toys.

Management

Once domestic violence has been identified, appropriate health-care provider actions include the following:

- Validate the individual's story.
- Remind the victim that she is not at fault and that no one deserves to be abused.
- Ascertain if there are children involved and if they are at risk.
  - Follow all state guidelines for reporting if there are children at risk (health-care providers are mandated to report if they are made aware of violence involving children).
- Provide information on resources, such as domestic violence shelters, reading materials, local advocacy agencies, and even the police.
- Follow state guidelines for reporting abuse when the victim is an adult. Most states do not mandate reporting if the abuse is perpetrated against an adult (some states make an exception if there are weapons involved or the adult is classified as a vulnerable adult), and many advocacy groups do not recommend the provider reporting on behalf of the victim.
- Document in as much detail as possible all examination findings.

CLINICAL PEARL

What can be done to prevent domestic violence? The following strategies can help:

- If abuse is suspected, ask the individual about her safety.
- If abuse is confirmed, voice concern, listen to the woman's story, and validate her experience.
- Discretion is critical. The abuse should not be discussed with others without permission.
- Empower the patient by commenting on the courage and strength that it takes to survive domestic violence.
- Provide resources.
- Be mindful of personal safety.
- Be clear about the role of the health-care provider, and avoid crossing patient–provider boundaries.

Why do women remain in abusive relationships? The reasons why women stay are varied and include the following:

- Finances
- Fear of the abuser
- Concern about the welfare of the children
- Commitment to the abuser
- Love for the abuser
- Lack of self-esteem
- Fear that the abuser might hurt himself
- Fear that the abuser might hurt the children or the victim herself

Why do abusers abuse? The reasons are varied and include the following:

- Learned behavior in abusers who were themselves abused as children
- Lack of self-esteem
- Poor coping skills
- Substance abuse
- The need to control

TECHNICAL NOTE

Reported barriers to screening for IPV include personal barriers, resource barriers, perceptions and attitudes, fears, and patient-related barriers. Provider-related barriers are reported more often than patient-related barriers.

CLINICAL PEARL

Provider personal discomfort with IPV is the most consistently reported barrier to screening.

CHAPTER 16

Health Literacy and Health-Care Access

Health literacy is the ability to obtain, process, and understand the basic health information needed to make informed health decisions. Limited health literacy is associated with poorer health outcomes and higher health-care costs.

Health literacy is dependent on the following:

- Communication skills of laypeople
  - Ability to read, write, and work with numbers
  - Ability to comprehend
  - Oral communication skills
- Communication skills of health-care practitioners
  - Ability to relate health information in a manner appropriate to the context
- The individual's knowledge of health topics
  - Understanding of health, disease, and lifestyle factors and how these are related
  - Recognition of when to seek care
- The health practitioner's knowledge of health topics
- The individual, societal, and health-care culture
  - How does the individual define health?
  - How does society define health?
  - How does the health-care system define health?
- When and where people seek care
- Situational and contextual demands
  - Health-care settings and systems are often unfamiliar to the individual, thereby creating undue stress and fear.
  - Physical, mental, and other impairments create additional barriers to accessing health-care setting.
- Demands of the public health and health-care systems

Epidemiology

Individuals and groups at greater risk for limited health literacy include the following:

- Older adults with hearing and/or vision loss
- Individuals with limited financial wealth
- Individuals with limited education
- Minority populations/immigrants
- Individuals with limited English proficiency
- Individuals who are incarcerated
- Disabled and mentally ill individuals

Consequences of Limited Health Literacy

- Studies have correlated limited health literacy with an increase in preventable hospital visits and admissions and higher health-care costs.
- Persons with limited health literacy skills are more likely to skip important preventive measures, enter the health-care system when they are sicker, have chronic conditions, and manage their conditions less effectively.
- Persons with limited health literacy skills are significantly more likely than persons with adequate health literacy skills to report their health as poor.

CLINICAL PEARL

Studies have found that people with limited health literacy skills reported a sense of shame about their skill level; as result, these individuals may hide reading or vocabulary difficulties to maintain their dignity.

Modified from U.S. Department of Health and Human Services. (n.d.). Quick guide to health literacy. Retrieved from https://health.gov/communication/literacy/quickguide/factsliteracy.htm

Strategies for Improving Health Literacy

- Assess all health information for appropriateness.
- Identify the intended user and decide on the most effective channels.

- Acknowledge cultural differences.
- Practice respect.
- Use plain language, break down complex information, and organize information so that the most important information is first.
- Speak clearly.
- Listen attentively.
- Ask open-ended questions.
- Check for understanding.
- Consider using other patients as content and delivery experts.
- Identify and use new and emerging delivery methods

Tips for Providers

The following provider health literacy tips are summarized from Robinson, White, and Houchins (2006), USDHHS (2015b), Hersh, Salzman and Snyderman, (2015), and Hartzler and Pratt (2011):

- Assess all patients for health proficiency using a health literacy tool.
- Make a connection with each patient physically and emotionally.
- Allow extra time—do not appear rushed or uninterested.
- Avoid distractions. Give your patients your undivided attention in the first 60 seconds.
- Sit face to face.
- Maintain eye contact where culturally appropriate.
- Listen attentively.
- Speak slowly, clearly, and loudly when working with older patients.
- Use short, simple words and sentences that are familiar to the patient.
- Avoid information overload by addressing one topic at a time.
- Simplify and write down instructions. Provide an information sheet that summarizes the most important points of the visit in a list format.
- Use charts, models, and pictures.
- Frequently summarize the most important points.
- Allow ample opportunity for questions.

- Consider alternate information delivery methods, including patient experts, cell phones, and other electronic devices.
- Follow up.

Assessment tools from the Agency for Health Care Research and Quality (2016) include the following:

- Short Assessment of Health Literacy–Spanish and English
- Rapid Estimate of Adult Literacy in Medicine–Short Form
- Short Assessment of Health Literacy for Spanish Adults

CLINICAL PEARL

According to Hartzler and Pratt (2011), there are significant differences in mechanisms of health information delivery between patient experts and clinician experts. Clinician experts focus on facts and opinions tied to the health-care system, whereas patient experts focus on the lived experience and confer more actionable strategies.

CLINICAL PEARL

Providing patients with access to their own electronic health records enhances patients' understanding of their health.

Overweight, Obesity, and Underweight

The Centers for Disease Control and Prevention (CDC, 2016) defines overweight as a body mass index (BMI) over 25, obesity as a BMI over 30, and underweight as a BMI under 18.5.

Epidemiology

- According to the National Center for Health Statistics (2016) 1.7% of people in the United States are underweight, and 69% are overweight or obese.

Etiology

- Societal influences on weight remain a challenging component of the overall health of women and girls.
- Much of the research on weight has focused on obesity; however, the health causes and consequences of being underweight are no less significant than those associated with overweight or obese.

Underweight

- Societal norms and expectations
- Illnesses
  - Hyperthyroidism/Graves' disease
  - Cancer
  - Tuberculosis
  - Diabetes
  - HIV/AIDS
- Genetics
- Eating disorders
  - Many women develop eating disorders as a result of sports participation and societal expectations.
- Depression
  - Many women struggling with depression experience loss of appetite.
- Sports and athletics
  - Certain sports place strict boundaries on body weight, thereby predisposing athletes to abnormal eating or exercise habits.

Overweight and Obesity

- Energy imbalance
  - Imbalance between energy intake from the diet and energy output through physical activities and bodily functions can result in overweight when energy intake exceeds output.
- Genetics and environment
  - Research suggests that when one or both parents are overweight or obese, there is increased likelihood that the children will also be overweight or obese.
  - Children often adopt the lifestyle habits of their parents, including eating and exercise patterns.
  - Environmental factors such as lack of access to healthy food and safe places for recreation can lead to overweight.
- Lifestyle factors
  - Sedentary lifestyle
- Illnesses
  - Hypothyroidism
  - Polycystic ovarian syndrome (PCOS)
  - Cushing's disease
- Psychosocial factors
  - Emotional eating
  - Smoking cessation
  - Insomnia or lack of adequate sleep
- Medications (Note: See the Appendix for a list of drugs that may cause weight gain.)
  - Antidepressants—tricyclics (TCAs), such as amitriptyline (Elavil), imipramine (Tofranil), and nortriptyline (Pamelor); monoamine oxidase inhibitors (MAOIs), such as phenelzine (Nardil); some selective serotonin reuptake inhibitors (SSRIs), such as paroxetine (Paxil, Pexeva) and mirtazapine (Remeron)
  - Antiseizure medications, such as valproic acid (Depakote, Depakene) and lithium (Lithobid)

- Antihistamines, such as cetirizine (Zyrtec) and fexofenadine (Allegra)
- Antihypertensives, including the beta blockers metoprolol (Lopressor) and atenolol (Tenormin)
- Corticosteroids—oral corticosteroids including prednisone, methylprednisolone, and hydrocortisone
- Diabetes medications—oral medications, such as glyburide (DiaBeta) and glipizide (Glucotrol), and injectable insulin.
- Pregnancy
  - Weight gain is needed to sustain a healthy pregnancy. Many women struggle to lose the weight gain of pregnancy, which may be compounded by subsequent pregnancies.

CLINICAL PEARL

Nicotine raises the rate at which the body burns calories.

The muscle loss that occurs in aging decreases the rate at which the body burns calories.

CLINICAL PEARL

Adequate sleep facilitates the balance between the "hunger hormones" ghrelin and leptin. Ghrelin causes a sense of hunger; leptin causes a sense of fullness. With lack of sleep, ghrelin levels rise, and leptin levels decrease. Lack of sleep further affects the body's response to insulin. Lack of sleep is associated with increased blood sugar levels.

Signs and Symptoms

Underweight

- Compromised immune system
- Low muscle mass
- Hair loss

- Irregular hormone regulation
- Osteoporosis
- Anemia
- Pregnancy complications (or inability to get pregnant)
- Menstrual irregularities
- Nutritional deficiencies

CLINICAL PEARL

Increased severity of maternal underweight BMI is associated with increased risk of preterm birth. Achieving the gestational weight gain recommended by the Institute of Medicine (IOM, 2009) is essential for preventing adverse maternal and infant outcomes.

IOM Recommendations for Gestational Weight Gain

Prepregnancy Weight Category	BMI	Total Weight Gain (lb)
Underweight	<18.5	28–40
Normal weight	18.5–24.9	25–35
Overweight	25–29.9	15–25
Obese	≥ 30	20

Data from Institute of Medicine. (2009). *Weight gain during pregnancy: Reexamining the guidelines.* Retrieved from http://www.nationalacademies.org/hmd/~/media/Files/Report%20Files/2009/Weight-Gain-During-Pregnancy-Reexamining-the-Guidelines/Report%20Brief%20-%20Weight%20Gain%20During%20Pregnancy.pdf

Overweight and Obesity

- Hypertension
- Insulin resistance
- Hyperglycemia
- Hyperlipidemia
- Cardiac failure
- Ischemic stroke
- Nonalcoholic fatty liver disease

CLINICAL PEARL

- Obesity is a contributing factor to cardiac failure in 10% of patients.
- Overweight/obesity plus hypertension is associated with increased risk of ischemic stroke.
- A neck circumference of more than 40.5 cm in women is associated with obstructive sleep apnea.
- Of all cancer deaths among nonsmokers, 10% are related to obesity.
- Of all endometrial cancers, 30% are related to obesity.
- Obesity is a causative factor in 6% of cases of primary infertility in women.

CLINICAL PEARL

Excessive weight gain is shown to be protective for small-for-gestational-age infants but increases the risks for large-for-gestational-age infants.

Tips for the Provider

- Provide patients with resources that identify the consequences of overweight and underweight.
- Help the patient establish healthy goals for weight management.
- Facilitate understanding of the patient's optimal weight for mental and physical health.
- Avoid shaming—both for underweight and overweight.

CHAPTER 18

Spirituality and Health

Why Address Spirituality?
Tips for Providers

Spirituality and *religion* are synonymous terms to some and distinct and separate entities to others. For this reason, the definition of religion and spirituality adopted in this handbook are as follows: Religion is a system of faith and worship that stems from a belief in a superhuman power, and spirituality (derived from the root word *spiritus*) is that which gives life, breath, or the essence of life—a sense of connection to something bigger than ourselves. Specific religious practices are not discussed in this handbook except to the extent that religion and spirituality are considered synonymous.

Why Address Spirituality?

- According to the research, when patients feel that spiritual needs are neglected in the health environment, they may not continue to seek or receive care.
- Ethical concerns may arise when patients rely on faith healing instead of medical care for themselves or their children.
- Anxiety and hope are factors in health outcomes.
- Spirituality provides a framework for coping with pain, chronic illness, and disability.
- An emerging body of evidence supports the significant health benefits associated with religious and spiritual practices.
- Spirituality is an important resource for coping with illness.

CLINICAL PEARL

Case law allows treatment refusal in competent adults for religious reasons.

Tips for Providers

- Screen all patients. Sample screening questions include the following:
  - Do you consider yourself spiritual or religious?
  - How important are these beliefs to you?
  - Do these beliefs influence how you care for yourself?
  - Do you belong to a spiritual community?

- How might we as health-care providers best address any needs in this area?
- Permit patients to express their spirituality should they wish to do so.
- Refer patients to spiritual leaders.
- Support autonomy.
- Do not encourage patients to "get" religious
- Avoid stepping into the role of pastoral caregiver or spiritual leader. Even when the provider is, cross-trained as both a clinician and a pastoral caregiver/spiritual leader; professional boundaries encourage separation of roles. The rationale for separating the role of health-care provider from the role of spiritual leader or pastoral caregiver include the following:
  - Certain components of the patient's health might be better disclosed to the spiritual leader rather than the health-care provider.
  - The provider taking on the role of spiritual leader might encourage a paternalistic view of the provider.
  - The provider taking on the role of spiritual leader mystifies the provider.

CLINICAL PEARL

Lack of appropriate spiritual referral may be construed as negligence.

CLINICAL PEARL

Research suggests that certain religious and spiritual practices may affect health outcomes as follows:
- Reduce depression
- Reduce stress
- Aid in substance abuse prevention and recovery
- Reduce high blood pressure
- Prevent heart disease
- Mitigate pain
- Aid in adjusting to disability

Vulnerable Populations

Vulnerable populations that may experience disparate care in the U.S. health-care system, along with some of their specific issues, include the following:

- Adolescents
- Older adults
  - Sexual health and the elderly
- Disabled/mentally ill individuals
  - Rehabilitation of mentally ill women
- Lesbian, gay, bisexual, and transgender (LGBT) individuals
- Immigrants/non-English-speaking individuals
  - Female genital cutting

Adolescents

Adolescence is a time of significant physical, mental, and emotional change. Allowing for modesty at every opportunity and providing reassurance that the changes accompanying adolescence are normal are essential practices. Major causes of morbidity and mortality in adolescence include trauma, sexually transmitted diseases (STDs), and pregnancy, all of which have a psychosocial component.

Guidelines for effective communication with adolescents include the following:

- Time spent in the first visit is time well spent to establish trust and rapport.
- Relate directly and respectfully to the client, not through the parent.
- Assure confidentiality.
- Listen attentively.
- Avoid lecturing and preaching.
- Use open-ended questions to avoid yes/no or head-shaking responses.
- Maintain a nonjudgmental attitude and tone of voice.
- Give patients permission to be honest and forthcoming, and encourage disclosure by introducing topics the adolescent may be reluctant or embarrassed to bring up—for example, "Some

clients your age are concerned about the changes in their bodies that are starting to occur," or "Some clients your age are interested in learning about different methods of birth control."

- Appeal to their current concerns (e.g., body image) rather than future health risks.

Key points to remember include the following:

- Emotional development lags behind biological/sexual development.
- Values and behaviors are frequently incongruent.
- Teenagers often feel invincible, invulnerable, and immortal, which can lead to their engagement in risky behavior.

CLINICAL PEARL

Teenagers have the legal right to obtain birth control, STD testing and treatment, drug rehabilitation and counseling, and pregnancy tests without parental consent, regardless of age. Parental consent or court waiver is required for an abortion.

CLINICAL PEARL

There remains a disconnect between what adolescent females want to discuss with their providers (e.g., STDs, acne, weight concerns, fear of cancer) and what they do discuss with their providers (e.g., menses).

Older Adults

According to the IOM (2012) within the next decade, adults over the age of 65 will account for 20% of the population of the United States. The needs of the older adult are unique, and although many older adults will continue to remain active and experience good health, declining health as a component of aging predisposes the older adult to many areas of vulnerability. These include the following:

- Access to care
- Socioeconomic factors and their correlation with independence
- Polypharmacy

- Self-care concerns
- Depression
- Falls risk
- Mobility concerns
- Cognitive decline
- Potentially diminishing social support systems
- Comorbid and chronic health conditions
- Increased diversity and longevity

Tips for providers include the following:

- Elicit the presence (or absence) of a main support person.
- Assess other social support systems.
- Assess sleep patterns.
- Assess self-care and skin care.
- Assess for wandering.
- When appropriate, encourage self-management and independence.
- Connect the patient to community resources.
- Elicit acute and chronic health concerns.
- Explore potential concerns with sensitive topics, such as incontinence and sexuality.
- Provide education on personal safety.
- Provide education on disease prevention.
- Facilitate care coordination.
- Assess for chronic pain.
- Assist family and friends with the knowledge and skills needed to provide care.
- Assist family and friends with resources to manage personal stress.
- Focus on improving quality of life.

Perform screening protocols for the following (see Appendix for screening tools):

- Dementia/wandering and other cognitive function
- Falls/mobility
- Depression
- Self-care
- Medications/polypharmacy

Sexual Health and the Elderly

The level of sexual interest and activity among older women is as diverse as those who make up that population. Many older women desire and enjoy an active sex life.

Epidemiology

- Of married women in the age range of 60 to 64, 89% are sexually active.
- Of women over the age of 80, 25% are sexually active.

Tips for Providers

Physical changes that can affect sexuality include the following:

- The tissues covering the pubic bone and labia lose firmness.
- The walls of the vagina become less elastic, and the vagina itself becomes drier.
- The clitoris can become highly sensitive, even too sensitive.
- Uterine contractions with orgasm may become painful.

Older women also need to know the importance of practicing "safe sex" and protecting themselves against STDs, especially when having intercourse with a new partner.

Patient Recommendations

Certain aspects of sexual health are likely to change in the natural process of aging. Methods for adapting to these changes include the following:

- Communication: Time needs to be spent in talking intimately as partners. Thoughts about lovemaking should be shared so that there is openness about what each partner is experiencing physically and emotionally.
- Ways to be intimate: Foreplay is important, and this may begin as early as a romantic dinner. Touch, massage, and words of intimacy can be a valuable component of sex.
- Safe sex: People of all ages, not just the young, need to practice safe sex. A condom should always be used when having sex with a new or different partner.

- Changes with aging: Women experience a number of naturally occurring changes in body shape and size as they age. This may result in a decrease in libido, orgasm capability, or feelings of sexual desirability.
- Medical conditions: Illnesses that involve the cardiovascular system, such as high blood pressure, diabetes, depression, or anxiety, and the treatments for them can pose problems with being sexually active. Surgical procedures that affect the pelvis or central nervous system can also influence the sexual response.
- Medications: Certain medications can inhibit the body's ability to become aroused or have an orgasm.
- Desire for sex: Differences in libido are common. Solutions needs to be discussed rather than accepting a pattern where one person initiates contact while the other avoids it.
- Illness: Pain, discomfort, medications, or worry can eclipse sexual desire in either partner. This gives the opportunity to discover other ways to be intimate.

CLINICAL PEARL

For some older individuals, advancing age is a time of freedom to explore sexual expression in ways never before realized.

CLINICAL PEARL

Of persons living with HIV/AIDS in the United States, 1 in 4 is 50 or older.

Disability and Mental Illness

Management of the health-care needs of individuals with disabilities and mental illness has shifted away from institutional care and toward less restrictive and community-based settings. Multiple comorbidities, polypharmacy, communication challenges, and developmental complexities are some of the considerations that predispose to vulnerability.

Special considerations for this population identified by health-care practitioners include the following:

- Situations may be encountered that they feel ill-equipped to manage.
- Identifying the most appropriate services can be challenging.
- The individual's ability to consent to care may be unclear.
- Identifying the effects and side effects of multiple medications is necessary.
- Collaboration with family is often essential.
- Communication is essential, as is learning to tune in to nonconventional communication signals.
- Components of care include advocacy, health promotion, assessment, and case management.

Tips for Providers

- Set clear boundaries.
- Develop risk assessment skills.
- Be firm, consistent, and empathetic.
- Develop skills for managing challenging behaviors, such as aggression and self-injurious behavior.
- Focus on the factors that promote a state of positive well-being rather than on disease management.
- Be vigilant about monitoring for side effects from polypharmacy.
- Be prepared to assist with self-care activities.
- Elicit recovery as defined by the individual.
- Manage risk factors.
- Encourage a sense of empowerment by assisting patients to acknowledge their resources rather than focusing on their disabilities.
- Be prepared to work collaboratively with families, groups, and communities.
- Develop strategies to avoid frustration or aggravation while providing appropriate reassurance.

Lesbian, Gay, Bisexual, and Transgender Individuals

The LGBT population is at increased risk for a number of health threats compared with their heterosexual peers. Reasons for this disparity include differences in sexual behavior, social and structural inequities, stigma, and discrimination. The experiences of LGBT individuals are not uniform and are shaped by race, ethnicity, socioeconomic status, geographical location, and age. Health concerns for this population include the following:

- Breast cancer and other gynecological cancers—concentration of risk factors
- Depression/anxiety—chronic stress from homophobic discrimination and social isolation
- Cardiovascular disease—obesity, diet, lack of exercise in older adults, and marginalization
- Tobacco/alcohol/substance use and use of other mechanisms to combat stress
- Domestic violence
- Osteoporosis—as an unintended consequence of tobacco/alcohol/substance use, abusive dieting, or lack of weight-bearing exercise

Special considerations in providing care to LGBT populations include invisibility, access, and disclosure.

Invisibility

- As individuals and as a group, there is limited health-care dialogue/research available.
- Self-identification is absent from much of the research.

Access

- Less likely to have insurance
- Less likely to benefit from screening and health-promotion procedures
- Lack of providers who are knowledgeable about LGBT health needs

- Fear of discrimination in health-care settings
- Reluctance to seek medical care through a traditional provider–patient relationship
- Support systems
  - LGBT elders are less likely to have children and more likely to rely on friends and others as caregivers rather than biological family members.
- Costs
  - Health care related to transgender issues may not be covered by insurance.

Disclosure

- Although many lesbians would prefer to "come out" to their health providers, many don't because of fear of negative reactions.
- Important health history components may be withheld from providers.

Tips for Providers

- Reassure patients that all information is confidential.
- Obtain permission to document sexual orientation and gender in the permanent record.
- Ask questions such as the following to elicit specific information:
  - Are you sexually active?
  - Are you sexually involved with a male or female?
  - Is there a need for birth control?
- Elicit history of all sexual contacts.
- Recommend routine Pap smears and breast health screening for lesbian patients.

CLINICAL PEARL

Unique risks for transgender women arise from cross-gender hormones. Estrogens increase the risk of blood clots, high blood pressure, elevated blood sugar, and water retention. Anti-androgens such as spironolactone may increase risks for dehydration, low blood pressure, and electrolyte disturbances.

> **CLINICAL PEARL**
>
> Some transgender women who desire physical feminization but do not want to wait for the effects of estrogen choose to use injectable silicone for instant curves. The mechanism of administration, often at "pumping parties" by nonmedical persons, may increase risks for hepatitis, migration, and subsequent disfigurement.

> **CLINICAL PEARL**
>
> LGBT youth are at increased risk for attempted suicide and depression, and they have higher rates of substance use than their heterosexual counterparts.

Immigrants/Non-English-Speaking Individuals

Providing patient-centered care empowers patients to be active participants in their health care and has been linked to improved recovery rates, fewer symptoms, and improved emotional health. When patients perceive that they have found common ground with their providers, their overall health status improves.

Special considerations in providing health care to immigrants and non-English speakers are discussed in the following subsections.

Communication Styles

- Tone of voice, volume of conversation, eye contact, and firm or limp handshake are examples of communication styles that vary by culture.

Views on Time

- Individuals from more tropical climates may perceive time conceptually, whereas those from more Nordic environments perceive time literally.
- Scheduling of appointments may warrant clarification and accommodation.

Paperwork

- The intake forms used in most health-care facilities may prove to be significantly challenging to new immigrants and non-English speakers.
- The level of detail may be unexpected and unanticipated.
- Concepts as seemingly benign as a birth date may be challenging for patients who are from cultures where birth is placed not by date but within the context of other significant events.
- New immigrants who are aware of significant adverse consequences from improperly completed immigration forms may experience undue anxiety at the need to complete health-care forms that are equally complex.

Explanatory Models of Care

- Explanatory models for disease etiology may differ; the patient's perception of what has caused disease (e.g., bad energy or the evil eye) may conflict with the biomedical model.
- The concept of disease without illness may be foreign to new immigrants, causing a refusal to participate in preventative health-care measures, which could place them at increased risk for significant health complications.

New Diseases Versus Old

Diseases such as tuberculosis and polio, which are considered to be eradicated in the United States, Western Europe, and the industrialized nations around the world, remain in parts of the developing world, including Asia, Africa, and Latin America, and may present in health-care settings.

Language Barriers

The U.S. Department of Health and Human Services Office of Minority Health (2013) recommends the following:

- Offer language assistance to individuals who have limited English proficiency or other communication needs, at no cost to them, to facilitate timely access to all health care and services.

- Inform all individuals of the availability of language assistance services clearly and in their preferred language, verbally and in writing.
- Ensure the competence of individuals providing language assistance, recognizing that the use of untrained individuals and/or minors as interpreters should be avoided.
- Provide easy-to-understand print and multimedia materials and signage in the languages commonly used by the populations in the service area.

Females Who Are Subject to Female Genital Cutting (Female Circumcision, Female Genital Mutilation)

According to the World Health Organization (WHO, 2017) female genital cutting (FGC) or female genital mutilation (FGM) comprises all procedures that involve partial or total removal of the external female genitalia or other injury to the female genital organs for nonmedical reasons.

Table 19-1 describes the types of FGM.

Etiology

- Cultural ideals of femininity and modesty
- Cultural and societal norms to conform and to be accepted

Epidemiology

- FGM is mostly carried out on young girls between infancy and age 15.
- The practice is most common in Asia, Africa, and the Middle East.
- Prevalence ranges between and within countries; for example, among women aged 15 to 49, prevalence estimates are 1% for Cameroon and 90% for Somalia.

Table 19-1 Classification of the Types of FGM

Type 1 Clitoridectomy	• Partial or total removal of the clitoris
Type 2 Excision	• Partial or total removal of the clitoris and the labia minora
Type 3 Infibulation	• Narrowing of the vaginal opening through the creation of a covering seal. The seal is formed by cutting and repositioning the labia minora or labia majora, or through stitching, with or without removal of the clitoris.
Type 4	• All other harmful procedures to the female genitalia for nonmedical purposes, such as pricking, piercing, incising, scraping, and cauterizing the genital area.

Data from World Health Organization. (2016). *Female genital mutilation*. Retrieved from http://www.who.int /mediacentre/factsheets/fs241/en/

CLINICAL PEARL

Deinfibulation refers to the practice of cutting open the sealed vaginal opening in a woman who has been infibulated. This is often necessary for improving health and well-being, to allow intercourse, or to facilitate childbirth.

Modified from World Health Organization. (2017). *Female genital mutilation*. Retrieved from http://www.who.int/mediacentre/factsheets/fs241/en/

Complications

Immediate

- Severe pain
- Excessive bleeding
- Genital tissue swelling
- Fever
- Infections
- Urinary problems
- Impaired wound healing
- Shock
- Death

Long Term

- Pain—tissue damage and scarring that may result in trapped or unprotected nerve endings
- Infections
  - Chronic genital infections
  - Chronic reproductive tract infections which may cause chronic back and pelvic pain.
- Painful urination caused by obstruction of the urethra and recurrent urinary tract infections (UTIs)
- Menstrual difficulties—dysmenorrhea, oligomenorrhea, and difficulty in passing menstrual blood
- Keloids—excessive scar tissue formation at the site of the cutting
- HIV
- Sexual health challenges—loss or decrease of libido, dyspareunia
- Obstetric complications
  - Increased risk of caesarean section
  - Postpartum hemorrhage
  - Recourse to episiotomy
  - Difficult/prolonged labor
  - Obstetric tears/lacerations
  - Obstetric fistula
    - There is a direct association between FGM and obstetric fistula.
- Perinatal risks
  - Obstetric complications can result in a higher incidence of infant resuscitation at delivery, intrapartum stillbirth, and neonatal death.
- Psychological consequences—posttraumatic stress disorder (PTSD), anxiety disorders, and depression

Tips for Providers

The following recommendations are summarized from Perron et al. (2013).

Communication

- Avoid verbal and nonverbal reactions to women with FGC that may make the women feel stigmatized.

- Be mindful of terminology, confidentiality, and privacy.
  - Women who have undergone the practice of FGC may not see themselves as different or mutilated, and many may be offended by the use of the term *female genital mutilation*. The term *female circumcision* is frequently used by practicing communities and may be the terminology of choice. Determine how the woman refers to the practice of FGM and use her terminology.
- Identify and document the woman's FGC status. Sample screening questions include the following:
  - Many women from your country have been circumcised or "closed" as children. If you do not mind telling me, were you circumcised or closed as a child?
  - Do you have any problems passing your urine? Does it take you a long time to urinate? (Note that women with obstruction may take several minutes to pass urine.)
  - Do you have any pain with menstruation? Does your menstrual blood get stuck?
  - Do you have any itching, burning, or discharge from your pelvic area?
  - If sexually active: Do you have any pain or difficulty when having sexual relations?
- Explore and assess the decision-making process of the woman and her family, and be sure to solicit the woman's views and wishes.

Sexual Health

- Sexual function may be normal in women with FGC even in the absence of the clitoris and/or labia.
- Currently accepted treatment for sexual dysfunction should be considered for women with FGC.

Adolescent Care

- The physical complications and management of FGC in adolescents are the same as those in adult women.

- Young women often have no recollection of FGC performed at an early age.
- Discussion about healthy sexual choices, contraception, and avoidance of STDs is always important, as is attention to any self-destructive behaviors (sexual promiscuity, substance abuse, eating disorders, suicidality).
- Well-woman examinations should be discussed.

Working with Families with At-Risk Daughters

- All health professionals providing care to families from communities that practice FGC should educate the parents about the illegality of the practice in the Western world.
- Health-care professionals have legal responsibilities to protect children, and thus to report FGC practices involving children.
- Health-care professionals should lend their voices to community-based initiatives seeking to promote the elimination of FGC.

TECHNICAL NOTE

Considerations for practitioners performing pelvic exams include the following:
- Well-woman examinations and cervical screenings need to be fully explained so that the woman understands the need for the tests.
- Women experiencing distressing symptoms related to vaginal obstruction or mass effect and those considering intercourse or pregnancy can be offered surgery, deinfibulation, or excision.
- Vaginal dilators may be appropriate for some women.
- A wide variety of small, narrow specula should be available to perform the exam with the least amount of discomfort.
- The use of a lubricant is encouraged.
- Requests for reinfibulation should be declined on medical grounds because repetitive cutting and suturing of the vulva is likely to increase scar tissue, thus causing or perpetuating dyspareunia or voiding difficulties.
- Gentle self-dilatation after deinfibulation may be required while the edges heal in the postpartum period.

Appendix

Websites
Websites with a Focus on Women's Health

HealthyWomen
http://www.healthywomen.org
MedlinePlus: Women's Health
http://www.nlm.nih.gov/medlineplus/womenshealth.html
National Institutes of Health: Women's Health
http://health.nih.gov/category/WomensHealth
Women's Health Resources—Women's Health Research from
the National Institutes of Health
http://www.womenshealthresources.nlm.nih.gov/index.html
Our Bodies, Ourselves
www.ourbodiesourselves.org/
Society for Women's Health Research
http://www.womenshealthresearch.org/
U.S. Department of Health and Human Services, Office of
Women's Health: womenshealth.gov
http://womenshealth.gov/

Breast and Cervical Cancer Screening Resources for the Uninsured and Underinsured

National Breast and Cervical Cancer Early Detection Program
(NBCCEDP)
Provides low-income, uninsured, and underserved women
access to timely breast and cervical cancer screening and
diagnostic tests.
https://www.cdc.gov/cancer/nbccedp/
Sage Clinics
Provide screening and early detection of breast, cervical, and
colorectal cancers free of charge to people who qualify.

http://www.health.state.mn.us/divs/healthimprovement/working
-together/who-we-are/sage.html

National Cancer Institute (NCI) Breast Cancer Risk Assessment
Tool (BCRAT)

Provides an estimated risk for women based on factors such as
age of menarche, race, and family history of cancer.

http://www.cancer.gov/bcrisktool/

Medical Education

https://www.cdc.gov/cancer/breast/young_women/bringyourbrave
/health_care_provider_education/resource.htm

Statistics

https://www.cancer.org/cancer/breast-cancer/understanding-a
-breast-cancer-diagnosis/breast-cancer-survival-rates.html

Support Groups

http://ww5.komen.org/Connect-with-Susan-G-Komen.aspx?utm
_source=komen.org&utm_medium=JoinOurCommunity&utm
_campaign=MoreThanPink

Drug, Herb, and Vitamin Resources

Pharmaceuticals—Dosages, Contraindications, and Side Effects

Drugs.com

https://www.drugs.com/professionals.html

Monthly Prescribing Reference

http://www.empr.com/browseby/brand/

RxList—The Internet Drug Index

http://www.rxlist.com/script/main/hp.asp

http://med.emory.edu/pa/about_us/mobile_medicine/free
_drug_reference_apps.html

American Association of Poison Control Centers

http://www.aapcc.org

Nutraceuticals—Dosages, Contraindications, Interactions, and Side Effects

American Botanical Council

http://abc.herbalgram.org/site/PageServer

Linus Pauling Institute Micronutrient Information Center
http://lpi.oregonstate.edu/mic
MedlinePlus
https://medlineplus.gov/druginfo/herb_All.html

Commonly Used Medications in Labor and Delivery and Their Side Effects

American College of Obstetricians and Gynecologists
http://www.acog.org/Patients/FAQs/Medications-for-Pain
-Relief-During-Labor-and-Delivery
Mayo Clinic
http://www.mayoclinic.org/healthy-lifestyle/labor-and-delivery
/in-depth/labor-and-delivery/art-20049326
American Pregnancy Association
http://americanpregnancy.org/labor-and-birth/narcotics/
RxList—The Internet Drug Index
http://www.rxlist.com/script/main/hp.asp

Postpartum Depression

National Women's Health Information Center
http://www.4women.gov
Postpartum Support International
http://www.chss.iup.edu/postpartum
Depression After Delivery
http://www.depressionafterdelivery.com

Birth Plan Template

http://www.marchofdimes.org/materials/birth-plan.pdf

DetoxPlans: Sample

https://www.standardprocess.com/Products/Literature/Patient
-Purification-Program-Guide

Resources for Abuse Situations

Department of Justice, Office of Justice Programs, Washington, DC
National Coalition Against Domestic Violence, Denver, CO

National Domestic Violence Hotline 1-800-799-7233 (1-800-799-SAFE)

National Resource Center on Domestic Violence, Harrisburg, PA

Online Resources for Health Literacy

Agency for Health Care Research and Quality—Health Literacy Measuring Tools

http://www.ahrq.gov/professionals/quality-patient-safety/quality-resources/tools/literacy/index.html#rapid

Centers for Disease Control and Prevention—Evaluate Skills & Programs

http://www.cdc.gov/healthliteracy/ResearchEvaluate/index.html

Health.gov—Literacy

http://health.gov/communication/literacy/

Health.gov—Quick Guide to Health Literacy Fact Sheet

http://health.gov/communication/literacy/quickguide/factsliteracy.htm

Online Resources for Disabilities

Americans with Disabilities Act

https://www.ada.gov/

Social Security Administration—Disability: Frequently Asked Questions

https://faq.ssa.gov/link/portal/34011/34019/

Disability Benefits Help—How to Apply for Social Security Disability

http://www.disability-benefits-help.org/content/how-apply

Chapter 1

Common Blood Tests and Normal Ranges

Blood Substance	Normal	If Low Count	If High Count
Hemoglobin (HgB)	Male (M): 13.8–17.2 g/dl Female (F): 12.1–15.1 g/dl	Bone marrow damage; leukemia; lymphoma; shortage of iron, vitamin B_{12}, or folate; blood loss; some types of chemotherapy and radiation; red cell lysis	Lung diseases, dehydration, congestive heart failure, renal disease
Hematocrit (HCT)	M: 40.7–50.3% F: 36.1–46.3%	Bone marrow damage; leukemia; lymphoma; shortage of iron, vitamin B_{12}, or folate; blood loss; some types of chemotherapy and radiation; red cell lysis	Lung diseases, dehydration, congestive heart failure, renal disease
Mean corpuscular volume (MCV)	80–95 fl	Iron deficiency	B_{12} or folate deficiency
Mean corpuscular hemoglobin (MCH)	23–31 pg	Iron deficiency	B_{12} or folate deficiency
Platelet count	150–400 thousand/mcl	Bone marrow failure, chemotherapy, radiation, viral infections, certain blood cancers	Myeloproliferative disease inflammatory conditions, certain blood cancers

Blood Substance	Normal	If Low Count	If High Count
White cell count (WBC)	4,500–10,000 cells/mcl	Bone marrow failure, chemotherapy, autoimmune diseases, immunosuppression	Infection, leukemia inflammation, corticosteroids, stress, extreme exercise
Lymphocytes (LY)	800–5,000 cells/mcl	Bone marrow failure, chemotherapy, HIV/AIDS, immunosuppression	Viral infections, lymphoma leukemia
Monocytes (MC)	400–1,000 cells/mcl	Bone marrow failure, chemotherapy, immunosuppression	Infection (chronic), leukemia, autoimmune diseases
Granulocytes (GR)	1,800–8,300 cells/mcl	Bone marrow failure, chemotherapy, immunosuppression	Inflammation, infection, leukemia, corticosteroids, extreme exercise, prolonged stress
Neutrophils (NE)	1,800–8,300 cells/mcl	Bone marrow failure, chemotherapy, immunosuppression	Inflammation, infections, corticosteroids, extreme exercise, prolonged stress
Eosinophils (EOS)	0–800 cells/mcl	No concern	Parasitic infection
Basophiles (BAS)	0–100 cells/mcl	No concern	Active allergic response

Red blood cell count (RBC)	M: 4.7–6.1 million/mcl F: 4.2–5.4 million/mcl	Bone marrow damage; leukemia; lymphoma; shortage of iron, vitamin B_{12}, or folate; blood loss; red cell lysis; types of chemotherapy and radiation	Lung diseases, dehydration, congestive heart failure, renal disease
Thyroid-stimulating hormone (TSH)	0.4–4.2 microunits per milliliter (mcU/mL)	Overactive thyroid (Graves), multinodular or toxic goiter, damage to pituitary gland secondary to taking too much thyroid medicine in first trimester of pregnancy.	Underactive thyroid, (Hashimoto's disease), not taking enough thyroid hormone medicine
Liver function tests ALT (SGPT) and AST (SGOT)	ALT: 7–55 units per liter (U/L) AST: 8–48 U/L	Rare but with other low liver enzymes may suggest liver cirrhosis	Liver disease or injury to liver
Kidney function tests Glomerular filtration rate (GFR) and blood urea nitrogen (BUN)	GFR: M: 1.4 W: 1.2 BUN: 7–20	Rare if low	Kidney damage; disease; with high BUN, certain drugs or supplements

Chapter 2
Additional Estrogen and Progesterone Concepts

Estrogens work by crossing the cell membrane into the cell and activating estrogen receptors in the nucleus of the cell. Each type of estrogen has a different receptor affinity and nuclear retention time—the stronger the receptor affinity and the longer the nuclear retention time, the more potent the physiological action of the estrogen. Estrogen receptors are proteins coded as alpha and beta. One of the functions of the estrogen receptor is to bind to DNA and regulate the activity of other genes. Alpha and beta receptors are not evenly distributed throughout the body.

Catechol Estrogens—Fast Facts

- Liver metabolites formed from estradiol and estrone
- Chemical structure of part estrogen and part catecholamine
- May decrease the growth of some existing cancers
- Inhibit abnormal growth of cardiac fibroblasts, thereby decreasing the risk of hypertension and myocardial infarction (MI)
- Inhibit the action of leukotrienes, thereby decreasing inflammation, arthrosclerosis, and osteoporosis
- Have antioxidant properties
- Types of catechol estrogens: 2-hydroxextradiol, 4-hydroxestradiol, 2-hydroxyestrone, and 4-hydroxyestrone

Progesterone

- Progesterone has different effects on target tissues and on the different cell types within each tissue.
- Progesterone has a different effect on normal versus diseased tissue. For example, progesterone is an antagonist to estrogen-driven growth in the endometrium and an agonist to estrogen-driven growth in the breast.
- Progesterone promotes proliferation of breast cancer cells and uterine fibroid growth and concurrently protects from endometrial cancer.

- Progesterone receptor (PR) expression within cells is substrate specific. For example, within the breast, PR is expressed in the mammary gland; within the endometrium, PR is expressed by both epithelial and stromal cells.
- Progesterone expression is mediated locally both by estrogen and progesterone; the presence of estrogen increases progesterone expression, and the presence of progesterone decreases further progesterone expression.
- Progesterone influences many metabolic pathways, including glycogenesis, nucleotide metabolism, and protein synthesis.
- In pregnancy, progesterone hinders myometrial contractility, in part by inhibiting local prostaglandin synthesis and decreasing intracellular calcium.

The use of progesterone as a treatment strategy can result in a net decrease in progesterone expression. Progesterone treatment can also oppose the effect of estrogen on PRs, resulting in a net decrease of progesterone expression. Researchers have found that despite the presence of high circulating progesterone and the absence of estrogen receptor in the late luteal phase, PR is barely detectable in glandular uterine tissue but strongly expressed in stromal and myometrial uterine tissue during this phase. Conversely, PR remains consistent in the breast throughout the follicular and luteal phases. Progesterone has the capacity both to stimulate and hinder uterine cell proliferation.

Chapter 3

Staging in Breast Cancer

https://cancerstaging.org/references-tools/quickreferences/ Documents/BreastSmall.pdf

Chapters 5 and 7

Note: All techniques should be performed by health-care practitioners certified in the technique.

Hiatal Hernia Maneuver

The patient is lying supine. The health-care provider stands or sits facing the patient, locates the sternum, and places two fingers (index and middle) just below the sternum. The area of greatest tension (commonly on the patient's left) is located just left of the midsternal line. The provider reinforces with the fingers on the other hand. The patient inhales; as the patient inhales, tissue slack is removed. Repeat, and as the patient exhales, gently but firmly traction the finger inferior and lateral (in pulses) to release the fascia. Repeat two to three times.

Concurrently assess for a chronic cough, sympathetic dominance, or internalized stress, and manage or refer as warranted.

Spinal Touch Technique[1]

The spinal touch treatment as described by Dr. W. La Mar Rosquist is as follows:

The patient is in a clinic gown that opens to the back and is placed in a plumb-line position with the eyes closed. The practitioner observes the following:

a. Position of the bottom of the neck in relation to the string
b. Tilt of head—forward, back, or straight up
c. Turn of head and angle, whether straight or cocked
d. Level of shoulders, whether one is low or high or more forward
e. Level of hips, high or low, or rotated
f. Line between buttocks in relation to string and line between the thighs
g. Line between thighs in relation to string and line between buttocks
h. Anterior (more forward) knee
i. Anterior (more forward) glut (the contact point is on this side, just below the gluteal crease)
j. Spine curvature (hyperlordosis or hypolordosis)
k. Spine curvature (such as "C" or "S" type of curve)

Determine the point of contact as indicated by the anterior (more forward) glut and the relation of the line between the gluts and thighs to the string, using contact point charts for exact contact.

Mark contact points on anterior (most forward) thigh just below the gluteal crease.

Kneel behind the patient and, using index finger, apply light pressure to the contact point, slightly upward (in the direction of appropriate contact point and back toward yourself) and note the subject's drift or movement back to the center of the plumb line. (This is the test to be certain the contact point is correct.)

After testing the contact point and making sure it's correct, place the patient face down on the treatment table. Raise the patient's ankles and hips with pillows, and be certain patient is comfortable and can relax.

Locate (and mark, if desired) all tender areas of the gluts, back, shoulders, neck, and abdominal areas.

Place thumb on contact point in proper attitude and direction and proceed to touch (and rub out) each of the muscle touch zones.

To work out tender and painful areas, hold the zones for a longer period of time

Do not overdo the treatment by keeping the patient at the plumb line for more than 30 seconds or on the table for more than 15 minutes.

Return the patient to the plumb line and note any/all changes.

[1]Adapted from German Therapology Inc., Salt Lake City, Utah.

Chapter 6

Food Allergy and Anaphylaxis Emergency Care Plan from Food Allergy Research and Education

http://www.foodallergy.org/file/emergency-care-plan.pdf

https://schoolnursenet.nasn.org/communities/community-home/librarydocuments/viewdocument?DocumentKey=c9aac2b4-bde9-4e95-8500-c14fe836dbc6

Chapter 7

Cross Crawl Exercises

Standing

March in place, ensuring that opposing limbs are moving simultaneously (right leg, left arm; left leg, right arm). Start slowly, with emphasis on increasing the range of motion of the arm and the leg with each march. Slowly build up speed, working up to 100 to 200 marches daily.

Raise the left arm to horizontal while simultaneously raising the right leg to horizontal. Raise the right arm to horizontal while simultaneously raising the left leg to horizontal. Work first on stability and then on speed. Work up to 50 repetitions daily.

Reach the right arm behind the body to touch the left foot. Reach the left hand behind the body to touch the right foot. Repeat.

Sitting

Raise the right knee to meet the left elbow or hand, then raise the left knee to meet the right elbow or hand. Repeat 50 times.

Crawling

Crawl on the floor ensuring that opposing limbs are moving simultaneously.

Swimming

Any kind of swimming is good.

In Utero Constraint (Webster Technique)

The patient lies prone on the examining table. The health-care provider flexes both of the patient's knees to bring the heels to the buttocks. If both knees are symmetric, the procedure is discontinued. If one side is restricted, the sacrum on the restricted side is adjusted for posterior rotation. The patient then is instructed to lie supine. The provider evaluates for a trigger-point-like nodule in the round ligament on the side of posterior rotation of the sacrum. To locate this point, a diagonal line is drawn from the anterior superior iliac spine (ASIS) toward the symphysis pubis and from the navel toward the anterior inferior iliac spine. The point of intersection of these two lines is the approximate location of this nodule. The nodule is massaged until it releases. No further treatment is given. The patient may need to have the procedure repeated on subsequent visits. The Webster technique should be performed by a health-care provider certified in the technique. For information on certification, see the website http://www.icpa4kids.com.

Buckled Sacrum Maneuver[2]

The buckled sacrum maneuver, as described by Dr. C. J. Phillips for relief of symptoms associated with increased pressure on the cervix, is as follows:

The mother stands several feet from a wall, facing the wall. Her feet are shoulder-width apart. She rests her hands against the wall.

The helper stands perpendicular to the mother with one hand just above the pubic region and the other hand on the lumbosacral spine, fingers pointed toward the floor. The hand on the back applies slight pressure and slides down the lumbo sacral and sacroiliac area. If the palm of the hand feels any resistance to the downward motion, downward pressure against the sacrum is maintained for several minutes or until the buckled sacral segments smooth out and the hand slides down without resistance. The hormones of pregnancy combined with pressure against the segments will allow the pliable sacrum to mold to the contour of the band. This is an extremely gentle maneuver. No pressure is applied toward the baby by either hand.

When the sacral segments realign, balance is restored to the uterine ligaments, and the uterus no longer applies pressure against the structures located in the front of the abdomen, resulting in resolution of the premature contractions and thigh pain.

Some patients are able to correct the buckled sacrum themselves by lying on the floor with a small rolled towel about 2 inches high and 4 inches wide slipped under the lower back. They slide the towel downward until the buckled segment of the sacrum restricts it; the weight of the mother's body resting on the towel works to help the sacrum realign itself.

[2]Reproduced from Phillips, C. J. (2001). *Hands of love, seven steps to the miracle of birth* (1st ed). St. Paul, MN: New Dawn Publishing.

Pelvic-Floor (Kegel) Exercises

To identify the correct muscles, the patient places a clean finger in the vagina, squeezes the finger, and identifies the muscles that contract around the finger. Next, the patient attempts to stop the flow of urine using just the pelvic-floor muscles while urinating and identifies the muscles used for this maneuver. (*In addition, the patient can attempt to stop a bowel movement and identify the muscles used for this maneuver*). These are the core muscle groups used in the pelvic-floor exercises (see Figure 1).

Once the muscles have been identified, the exercises are performed a minimum of three times daily. The patient contracts the muscles and sustains the contraction for 10 seconds followed by 10 seconds of rest. The cycle is repeated 10 times.

Additional guidelines:

- The exercise is best performed seated or standing, not supine.
- The exercise should be performed with an empty bladder.
- It is important to use only the pelvic-floor muscles and to avoid recruiting the quadriceps, gluteus muscles, and abdominals.
- The exercise should not cause strain. The patient should be relaxed during the exercise and breathe freely.

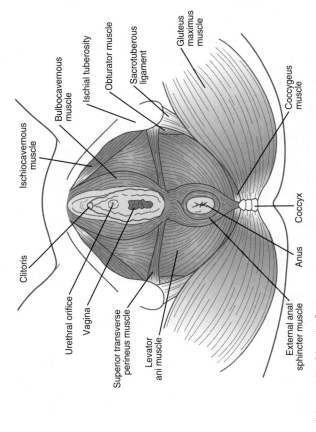

Figure 1 Core muscles of the pelvic floor

- Once the muscles have been identified, the exercise should not be performed while urinating because this can result in weaker muscles, incomplete emptying of the bladder, and bladder infections.
- Vaginal cones may be used to enhance the exercise.

Back Labor—The Side-Lying Maneuver
Four Steps to Reduce Back Labor [3]

The mother lies on her side at the edge of a table with the bottom leg straight and the head resting on a pillow. The examiner stands with his or her legs straddling the mother's belly.

The mother's hips and shoulders should be straight and perfectly perpendicular to the spine.

The mother drops the top leg off the table and allows it to hang downward for a few minutes. The provider hooks his or her thumbs into the anterior superior iliac spine (ASIS) while applying downward pressure to the ilia.

The resultant separation of the sacroiliac (SI) joint frees the sacrum and decreases the tone of the pelvic-floor muscles, which may free the baby's head, allowing it to turn from the pubic bone.

After a few minutes, the mother rolls over to her other side, and the procedure is repeated.

At home, the mother may be able to kneel on a step with her forearms on the floor and the hips above the head. The water floats toward the lungs, and the baby's head dislodges enough from the pelvic outlet to be able to rotate the face away from the pubic bone.

This technique does not work in the following situations:

The cord is wrapped tightly around the body, thereby restricting movements.

The extremities are trapped in a distorted position.

The infant is induced before the cranium has molded.

[3]Reproduced from Phillips, C. J. (2001). *Hands of love, seven steps to the miracle of birth* (1st ed). St. Paul, MN: New Dawn Publishing.

Dyad Bonding

Position	Description	Advantages	Illustration
Cradle or Madonna position	The infant is side-lying, facing the mother, with the side of the head and body resting on the mother's forearm of the arm next to the breast to be used.	This is the most commonly used nursing position and tends to feel most natural for the mother. However, it offers the least amount of control over the infant's head.	
Cross-cradle posture	The infant is side-lying, facing the mother, with the side resting on the mother's forearm of the arm on the opposite side of the breast being used.	This posture is considered especially useful for the mother of a newborn or preterm infant. It offers greater control over the infant's head	
Football or clutch	A sitting position in which the infant lies on her or his back, curled between the side of the mother's chest and her arm. The infant's upper body is supported by the mother's forearm. The mother's hand supports the infant's neck and shoulders. The infant's hips are flexed up along the chair back or other surface that the mother is leaning against.	This position is helpful for women post cesarean section and those who have large pendulous breasts or are nursing multiple infants.	

Figure 2 Common body positions for breastfeeding

565

Semi-reclining	The mother leans back and the infant lies against her body, in chest-to-chest contact, usually prone.	This is the most comfortable position for women recovering from a cesarean section, those who have large pendulous breasts, and those who choose to co-sleep with their infants.
Side-lying	The mother lies on her side. The infant is side-lying, chest to chest with the mother. The mother's arm closest to the mattress supports the infant's back.	This position is helpful for women who have had a cesarean section or have large or pendulous breasts.
Australian	The mother is "down-under," lying on her back, with the infant supported on her chest.	This posture allows the infant to be in maximal control of the feeding and is especially valuable when the milk flow is faster than the infant can handle.

Modified from International Lactation Consultant Association; Mannel, R., Martens, P. J., Walker, M. (Eds.). (2013). Core curriculum for lactation consultant practice (3rd ed.). Burlington, MA: Jones & Bartlett Learning.

Figure 2 (*Continued*)

Depression—Assessment Scales

Edinburgh Postnatal Depression Scale[4] (EPDS)

https://www.ncbi.nlm.nih.gov/pubmed/12668422

Postpartum depression is the most common complication of childbearing.[5] The 10-question EPDS is a valuable and efficient way of identifying patients at risk for "perinatal" depression. The EPDS is easy to administer and has proven to be an effective screening tool.

Mothers who score above 13 are likely to be suffering from a depressive illness of varying severity. The EPDS score should not override clinical judgment. A careful clinical assessment should be carried out to confirm the diagnosis. The scale indicates how the mother has felt *during the previous week*. In doubtful cases, it may be useful to repeat the tool after 2 weeks. The scale will not detect mothers with anxiety neuroses, phobias, or personality disorders.

[4]Source: Cox, J. L., Holden, J. M.,& Sagovsky, R. (1987.) Detection of postnatal depression: Development of the 10-item Edinburgh Postnatal Depression Scale. *British Journal of Psychiatry, 150,* 782–786.
[5]Source: Wisner, K. L., Parry, B. L., & Piontek, C. M. (2002). Postpartum depression. *New England Journal of Medicine, 347*(3), 194–199.

Center for Epidemiologic Studies Depression Scale (CES-D Scale)

The CESD screens for depression and depressive disorder using symptoms defined by the DSM-V as associated with a depressive episode. The screen may be accessed at http://cesd-r.com

Chapter 8

Pelvic Inflammatory Disease— Conventional Medications

Centers for Disease Control and Prevention (CDC) Guidelines
https://www.cdc.gov/std/tg2015/pid.htm

Chapter 9
Premenstrual Dysphoric Disorder (PMDD)

Validated rating scales over a 31 day cycle include the following:

• Felt depressed	• Had cravings for specific foods
• Felt hopeless	• Slept more, found it hard to get up when intended
• Felt worthless	
• Felt anxious	• Had trouble getting to sleep or staying asleep
• Experienced mood swings	
• Was more sensitive	• Felt overwhelmed
• Felt irritable	• Felt out of control
• Had less interest in usual activities	• Had breast tenderness
	• Experienced bloating or weight gain
• Had difficulty concentrating	
• Felt lethargic	• Had headache
• Experienced increased appetite	• Had joint or muscle pain

At work, school, home, or in daily routine, at least one of the problems noted above caused reduced productivity or inefficiency

At least one of the problems noted above interfered with hobbies or social activities

At least one of the problems noted above interfered with relationships with others

Figure 3 PMDD scale

Premenstrual Mood Symptoms

Visual analogue scales include the following:

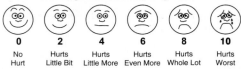

Wong-Baker FACES® Pain Rating Scale

0	2	4	6	8	10
No Hurt	Hurts Little Bit	Hurts Little More	Hurts Even More	Hurts Whole Lot	Hurts Worst

©1983 Wong-Baker FACES® Foundation. www.WongBakerFACES.org
Used with permission. Originally published in *Whaley & Wong's Nursing Care of Infants and Children.* ©Elsevier Inc.

Figure 4 Wong–Baker FACES scale

0	1	2	3	4	5	6	7	8	9	10
No Pain					Moderate Pain					Worst Pain

Figure 5 Visual analog scale

Symptoms Check all that apply

Month	1	2	3	4	5	6	7	8	9	10	12	13	14	15	16	17	18	19	20	22	23	24	25	26	27	28	29	30	31
Menstrual Bleeding																													
Increased appetite																													
Craving Salt																													
Craving Sugar																													
Breast Tenderness																													
Depression																													
Headache																													
Backache																													
Fatigue																													
Abdominal bloating																													
Anxiety																													
Nervous tension/Restlessness																													
Mood Swings																													
Irritability																													
Insomnia																													
Dizzy spells																													
Fatigue																													
Fainting																													
Weight Gain/Swelling																													
Forgetfulness																													
Other Symptoms																													

Figure 6 Premenstrual tension syndrome rating scale

Chapter 13
Sacral Nerve Stimulation

Sacral nerve stimulation is a surgical procedure used to treat incontinence that is not responsive to other treatments. It is specifically used to treat urge incontinence and urinary frequency, and it is not recommended for people with stress incontinence or men with overflow incontinence. A small electrical device is used to transmit electrical impulses to the sacral nerve to decrease urgency. The system is surgically placed under the skin once efficacy has been established.

Chapter 19
Assessment for Dementia/Wandering and Cognitive Function

MINI-COG
http://mini-cog.com
http://mini-cog.com/mini-cog-instrument/administering-the-mini-cog/
http://mini-cog.com/mini-cog-instrument/scoring-the-mini-cog/

Falls/Mobility Risk Assessment

Centers for Disease Control and Prevention (CDC) Algorithm
https://www.cdc.gov/steadi/pdf/algorithm_2015-04-a.pdf

Medications/Polypharmacy

Beers Criteria
http://www.americangeriatrics.org/files/documents/beers/201
    2AGSBeersCriteriaCitations.pdf

Chart of Body Mass Index

Body Mass Index Table

BMI	19	20	21	22	23	24	25	26	27	28	29	30	31	32	33	34	35	36	37	38	39	40	41	42	43	44	45	46	47	48	49	50	51	52	53	54
	Normal						Overweight					Obese										Extreme Obesity														
Height (inches)												Body Weight (pounds)																								
58	91	96	100	105	110	115	119	124	129	134	138	143	148	153	158	162	167	172	177	181	186	191	196	201	205	210	215	220	224	229	234	239	244	248	253	258
59	94	99	104	109	114	119	124	128	133	138	143	148	153	158	163	168	173	178	183	188	193	198	203	208	212	217	222	227	232	237	242	247	252	257	262	267
60	97	102	107	112	118	123	128	133	138	143	148	153	158	163	168	174	179	184	189	194	199	204	209	215	220	225	230	235	240	245	250	255	261	266	271	276
61	100	106	111	116	122	127	132	137	143	148	153	158	164	169	174	180	185	190	195	201	206	211	217	222	227	232	238	243	248	254	259	264	269	275	280	285
62	104	109	115	120	126	131	136	142	147	153	158	164	169	175	180	186	191	196	202	207	213	218	224	229	235	240	246	251	256	262	267	273	278	284	289	295
63	107	113	118	124	130	135	141	146	152	158	163	169	175	180	186	191	197	203	208	214	220	225	231	237	242	248	254	259	265	270	278	282	287	293	299	304
64	110	116	122	128	134	140	145	151	157	163	169	174	180	186	192	197	204	209	215	221	227	232	238	244	250	256	262	267	273	279	285	291	296	302	308	314
65	114	120	126	132	138	144	150	156	162	168	174	180	186	192	198	204	210	216	222	228	234	240	246	252	258	264	270	276	282	288	294	300	306	312	318	324
66	118	124	130	136	142	148	155	161	167	173	179	186	192	198	204	210	216	223	229	235	241	247	253	260	266	272	278	284	291	297	303	309	315	322	328	334
67	121	127	134	140	146	153	159	166	172	178	185	191	198	204	211	217	223	230	236	242	249	255	261	268	274	280	287	293	299	306	312	319	325	331	338	344
68	125	131	138	144	151	158	164	171	177	184	190	197	203	210	216	223	230	236	243	249	256	262	269	276	282	289	295	302	308	315	322	328	335	341	348	354
69	128	135	142	149	155	162	169	176	182	189	196	203	209	216	223	230	236	243	250	257	263	270	277	284	291	297	304	311	318	324	331	338	345	351	358	365
70	132	139	146	153	160	167	174	181	188	195	202	209	216	222	229	236	243	250	257	264	271	278	285	292	299	306	313	320	327	334	341	348	355	362	369	376
71	136	143	150	157	165	172	179	186	193	200	208	215	222	229	236	243	250	257	265	272	279	286	293	301	308	315	322	329	338	343	351	358	365	372	379	386
72	140	147	154	162	169	177	184	191	199	206	213	221	228	235	242	250	258	265	272	279	287	294	302	309	316	324	331	338	346	353	361	368	375	383	390	397
73	144	151	159	166	174	182	189	197	204	212	219	227	235	242	250	257	265	272	280	288	295	302	310	318	325	333	340	348	355	363	371	378	386	393	401	408
74	148	155	163	171	179	186	194	202	210	218	225	233	241	249	256	264	272	280	287	295	303	311	319	326	334	342	350	358	365	373	381	389	396	404	412	420
75	152	160	168	176	184	192	200	208	216	224	232	240	248	256	264	272	279	287	295	303	311	319	327	335	343	351	359	367	375	383	391	399	407	415	423	431
76	156	164	172	180	189	197	205	213	221	230	238	246	254	263	271	279	287	295	304	312	320	328	336	344	353	361	369	377	385	394	402	410	418	426	435	443

Source: Adapted from Clinical Guidelines on the Identification, Evaluation, and Treatment of Overweight and Obesity in Adults: The Evidence Report

Figure 7 BMI chart

Reproduced from National Heart, Lung, and Blood Institute. (n.d.). Body Mass Index table 1. Retrieved from https://www.nhlbi.nih.gov/health/educational/lose_wt/BMI/bmi_tbl.htm

Screening Tests for Women

Annual screening tests include the following:

- Dental Health Assessment
- Mental Health Assessment
- Nutritional Assessment
- Spinal Health assessment

See Table 1 for additional screening guidelines by age

Table 1 Screening Tests for Women

Screening Tests	Ages 18–39	Ages 40–49	Ages 50–64	Ages 65 and Older
Blood pressure test	Get tested at least every 2 years if you have normal blood pressure (lower than 120/80). Get tested once a year if you have blood pressure between 120/80 and 139/89. Discuss treatment with your doctor or nurse if you have blood pressure 140/90 or higher.	Get tested at least every 2 years if you have normal blood pressure (lower than 120/80). Get tested once a year if you have blood pressure between 120/80 and 139/89. Discuss treatment with your doctor or nurse if you have blood pressure 140/90 or higher.	Get tested at least every 2 years if you have normal blood pressure (lower than 120/80). Get tested once a year if you have blood pressure between 120/80 and 139/89. Discuss treatment with your doctor or nurse if you have blood pressure 140/90 or higher.	Get tested at least every 2 years if you have normal blood pressure (lower than 120/80). Get tested once a year if you have blood pressure between 120/80 and 139/89. Discuss treatment with your doctor or nurse if you have blood pressure 140/90 or higher.
Bone mineral density test (osteoporosis screening)			Discuss with your doctor or nurse if you are at risk of osteoporosis.	Get this test at least once at age 65 or older. Talk to your doctor or nurse about repeat testing.

(continues)

Table 1 Screening Tests for Women

Screening Tests	Ages 18–39	Ages 40–49	Ages 50–64	Ages 65 and Older
Breast cancer screening (mammogram)		Discuss with your doctor or nurse.	Starting at age 50, get screened every 2 years.	Get screened every 2 years through age 74. Age 75 and older, ask your doctor or nurse if you need to be screened.
Cervical cancer screening (Pap test)	Get a Pap test every 3 years if you are 21 or older and have a cervix. If you are 30 or older, you can get a Pap test and HPV test together every 5 years.	Get a Pap test and HPV test together every 5 years if you have a cervix.	Get a Pap test and HPV test together every 5 years if you have a cervix.	Ask your doctor or nurse if you need to get a Pap test.
Chlamydia test	Get tested for chlamydia yearly through age 24 if you are sexually active or pregnant. Age 25 and older, get tested for chlamydia if you are at increased risk, pregnant or not pregnant.	Get tested for chlamydia if you are sexually active and at increased risk, pregnant or not pregnant.	Get tested for chlamydia if you are sexually active and at increased risk.	Get tested for chlamydia if you are sexually active and at increased risk.

Cholesterol test	Starting at age 20, get a cholesterol test regularly if you are at increased risk for heart disease. Ask your doctor or nurse how often you need your cholesterol tested.	Get a cholesterol test regularly if you are at increased risk for heart disease. Ask your doctor or nurse how often you need your cholesterol tested.	Get a cholesterol test regularly if you are at increased risk for heart disease. Ask your doctor or nurse how often you need your cholesterol tested.	Get a cholesterol test regularly if you are at increased risk for heart disease. Ask your doctor or nurse how often you need your cholesterol tested.
Colorectal cancer screening (using fecal occult blood testing, sigmoidoscopy, or colonoscopy)			Starting at age 50, get screened for colorectal cancer. Talk to your doctor or nurse about which screening test is best for you and how often you need it.	Get screened for colorectal cancer through age 75. Talk to your doctor or nurse about which screening test is best for you and how often you need it.
Diabetes screening	Get screened for diabetes if your blood pressure is higher than 135/80 or if you take medicine for high blood pressure.	Get screened for diabetes if your blood pressure is higher than 135/80 or if you take medicine for high blood pressure.	Get screened for diabetes if your blood pressure is higher than 135/80 or if you take medicine for high blood pressure.	Get screened for diabetes if your blood pressure is higher than 135/80 or if you take medicine for high blood pressure.

(*continues*)

Table 1 Screening Tests for Women

Screening Tests	Ages 18–39	Ages 40–49	Ages 50–64	Ages 65 and Older
Gonorrhea test	Get tested for gonorrhea if you are sexually active and at increased risk, pregnant or not pregnant.	Get tested for gonorrhea if you are sexually active and at increased risk, pregnant or not pregnant.	Get tested for gonorrhea if you are sexually active and at increased risk.	Get tested for gonorrhea if you are sexually active and at increased risk.
HIV test	Get tested for HIV at least once. Discuss your risk with your doctor or nurse because you may need more frequent tests. All pregnant women need to be tested for HIV.	Get tested for HIV at least once. Discuss your risk with your doctor or nurse because you may need more frequent tests. All pregnant women need to be tested for HIV.	Get tested for HIV at least once. Discuss your risk with your doctor or nurse because you may need more frequent tests.	Get tested for HIV at least once if you are age 65 and have never been tested. Get tested if you are at increased risk for HIV. Discuss your risk with your doctor or nurse.
Syphilis test	Get tested for syphilis if you are at increased risk or pregnant.	Get tested for syphilis if you are at increased risk or pregnant.	Get tested for syphilis if you are at increased risk.	Get tested for syphilis if you are at increased risk.

Reproduced from Office on Womens Health. (2013). Screening Tests for women. Retrieved from https://www.womenshealth.gov/screening-tests-and-vaccines/screening-tests-for-women/

References

Chapter 2

Prather, H., Dugan, S., Fitzgerald, C., Hunt, D. (2009). Review of anatomy, evaluation, and treatment of musculoskeletal pelvic floor pain in women. *PM&R, 1*(4), 346–358.

Chapter 3

American Cancer Society. (2016). Breast cancer survival rates, by stage. Retrieved from http://www.cancer.org/cancer/breastcancer/detailedguide/breast-cancer-survival-by-stage

American Cancer Society. (2017). *Breast cancer treatment*. Retrieved from https://www.cancer.org/cancer/breast-cancer/treatment.html

Marriott, M., Masino, K., & Casella, G. (2014). *Breast cancer care gets personal*. Retrieved from http://www.americannursetoday.com/breast-cancer-care-gets-personal/

National Cancer Institute. (2012). *Breast cancer risk in American women*. Retrieved from http://www.cancer.gov/cancertopics/types/breast/risk-fact-sheet

Song, N., Choi, J-Y., Sung, H., Jeon, S., Chung, S., Park, S. K., . . . Kang, D. (2015). Prediction of breast cancer survival using clinical and genetic markers by tumor subtypes. *PLoS ONE, 10*(4): e0122413. doi:10.1371/journal.pone.0122413

World Health Organization. (2014). *Breast cancer burden*. Retrieved from http://www.who.int/cancer/detection/breastcancer/en/index1.html

Chapter 4

American Cancer Society. (2016). *Key statistics for lung cancer*. Retrieved from http://www.cancer.org/cancer/non-small-cell-lung-cancer/about/key-statistics.html

American College of Obstetricians and Gynecologists. (2013). *OB-GYNs issue task force report on hypertension in pregnancy*. Retrieved from http://www.acog.org/About-ACOG/News-Room/News-Releases/2013/Ob-Gyns-Issue-Task-Force-Report-on-Hypertension-in-Pregnancy

Centers for Disease Control. (2012). Venous thromboembolism in adult hospitalizations, United States, 2007–2009. *Morbidity and Mortality Weekly Report, 61*(22). Retrieved from https://www.cdc.gov/mmwr/pdf/wk/mm6122.pdf

Hathcock, J. N., Azzi, A., Blumberg, J., Bray, T., Dickinson, A., Frei, B., . . . Traber, M. G. (2005). Vitamins E and C are safe across a broad range of intakes. *American Journal of Clinical Nutrition, 81*(4), 736–745.

National Health Service. (2012). *Lung cancer rates in women*. Retrieved from http://www.nhs.uk/news/2012/11November/Pages/Lung-cancer-rates-in-women-to-soar-by-2040.aspx

National Institutes of Health. (2015). *Systolic Blood Pressure Intervention Trial (SPRINT) overview*. Retrieved from https://www.nhlbi.nih.gov/news/spotlight/fact-sheet/systolic-blood-pressure-intervention-trial-sprint-overview

National Institutes of Health. (2016). *Varicose veins overview*. Retrieved from https://www.ncbi.nlm.nih.gov/pubmedhealth/PMH0072431/

References

National Stroke Association. (2011). *Stroke facts*. Retrieved from https://www.google
.com/?client=safari&channel=mac_bm#channel=mac_bm&q=National+Stroke
+Association:+•%09%3CBL%3ETen+percent+of+stroke+survivors+recover+almost
+completely.+•%09Twenty-five+percent+recover+with+

World Health Organization. (2016). *Burden of COPD*. Retrieved from http://www.who
.int/respiratory/copd/burden/en/

Chapter 5

World Health Organization. (2013). *Diarrhoeal diseases*. Retrieved from http://www.who
.int/mediacentre/factsheets/fs330/en/

Chapter 6

Amsel, R., Totten, P. A., Spiegel, C. A., Chen, K., Eschenbach, D., & Holmes, K. K.
(1983). Nonspecific vaginitis: Diagnostic criteria and microbial and epidemiologic
associations. *American Journal of Medicine, 74*(1), 14–22.

Centers for Disease Control and Prevention. (2010). *Seroprevalence of herpes simplex virus
type 2*. Retrieved from https://www.cdc.gov/mmwr/preview/mmwrhtml/mm5915a3.htm

Centers for Disease Control and Prevention. (2015a). *Cervical cancer screening for
average-risk women*. Retrieved from https://www.cdc.gov/cancer/cervical/pdf/guidelines
.pdf

Centers for Disease Control and Prevention. (2015b). *Food allergy in schools*. Retrieved
from https://www.cdc.gov/healthyschools/foodallergies/index.htm

Centers for Disease Control and Prevention. (2016a). *Bacterial vaginosis treatment and
care*. Retrieved from https://www.cdc.gov/std/bv/treatment.htm

Centers for Disease Control and Prevention. (2016b). *CDC recommends only two HPV
shots for younger adolescents*. Retrieved January 17, 2017 from https://www.cdc.gov
/media/releases/2016/p1020-hpv-shots.html

Centers for Disease Control and Prevention. (2016c). *Chlamydia*. Retrieved from https://
www.cdc.gov/std/chlamydia/

Centers for Disease Control and Prevention. (2016d). *Facts about stillbirth*. Retrieved
from https://www.cdc.gov/ncbddd/stillbirth/facts.html

Centers for Disease Control and Prevention. (2016e). *Hepatitis C. FAQ for health professionals*. Retrieved from https://www.cdc.gov/hepatitis/hcv/hcvfaq.htm

Centers for Disease Control and Prevention. (2016f). *HIV fact sheets*. Retrieved from
https://www.cdc.gov/hiv/library/factsheets/

Centers for Disease Control and Prevention. (2016g). *Statistics (HIV)*. Retrieved from
https://www.cdc.gov/hiv/statistics/overview/

Centers for Disease Control and Prevention. (2016h). *STD—Gonorrhea fact sheet*.
Retrieved from https://www.cdc.gov/std/gonorrhea/stdfact-gonorrhea.htm

Centers for Disease Control and Prevention. (2016i). *Trends in food allergy*. Retrieved from
https://www.cdc.gov/nchs/products/databriefs/db10.htm

Centers for Disease Control and Prevention. (2016j). *Vulvovaginal candidiasis*. Retrieved
from https://www.cdc.gov/std/tg2015/candidiasis.htm

Masese, L., Baeten, J. M., Richardson, B. A., Bukusi, E., John-Stewart, G., Jaoko, W., . . .
McClelland, R. S. (2014). Incident herpes simplex virus type 2 infection increases
the risk of subsequent episodes of bacterial vaginosis. *Journal of Infectious Diseases,
209*(7), 1023–1027. doi:10.1093/infdis/jit634

References

Mohammadzadeh, F., Dolatian, M., Jorjani, M., & Majd, H. A. (2015). Diagnostic value of Amsel's clinical criteria for diagnosis of bacterial vaginosis. *Global Journal of Health Science, 7*(3), 8–14. doi:10.5539/gjhs.v7n3p8

National Asthma Education and Prevention Program, Third Expert Panel on the Diagnosis and Management of Asthma, & National Heart, Lung, and Blood Institute. (2007). *Guidelines for the diagnosis and management of asthma* (NIH Publication No. 08-5846). Bethesda, MD: NHLBI.

National Cancer Institute. (2010). *Guidelines: Urge exercise for cancer patients, survivors.* Retrieved from https://www.cancer.gov/about-cancer/treatment/research/exercise-before-after-treatment

National Center for Complementary and Integrative Health. (2015). *Yoga for health.* Retrieved from https://nccih.nih.gov/health/providers/digest/yoga

Osborne, C. (2012). *Pre- and perinatal massage therapy: A comprehensive guide to prenatal, labor, and postpartum practice.* Philadelphia, PA: Wolters Kluwer Health/Lippincott Williams & Wilkins.

Petri, M., Orbai, A. M., Alarcón, G. S., Gordon, C., Merrill, J. T., Fortin, P. R., & Magder, L. S. (2012). Derivation and validation of the Systemic Lupus International Collaborating Clinics classification criteria for systemic lupus erythematosus. *Arthritis and Rheumatology, 64*(8), 2677.

Pollart, S. M., & Elward, K. S. (2009). Overview of changes to asthma guidelines: Diagnosis and screening. *American Family Physician, 79*(9), 761–767.

Planned Parenthood. (2017). *Public lice (crabs).* Retrieved from https://www.plannedparenthood.org/learn/stds-hiv-safer-sex/pubic-lice

Straface, G., Selmin, A., Zanardo, V., De Santis, M., Ercoli, A., Scambia, G. (2012). Herpes simplex virus infection in pregnancy. *Infectious Diseases in Obstetrics and Gynecology, 2012,* 385697. doi:10.1155/2012/385697

U.S. Preventive Services Task Force. (2012). *Cervical cancer screening.* Retrieved from https://www.uspreventiveservicestaskforce.org/Page/Document/RecommendationStatementFinal/cervical-cancer-screening

Chapter 7

American College of Obstetricians and Gynecologists. (2013). *Hypertension in pregnancy.* Washington, DC: Author.

American College of Obstetricians and Gynecologists. (2014). *Frequently asked questions. Gynecological problems. FAQ022: Contraception.* Retrieved from http://www.acog.org/-/media/For-Patients/faq022.pdf?dmc=1&ts=20150721T1436130143

American College of Obstetricians and Gynecologists (2015). Physical activity and exercise during pregnancy and the postpartum period. Committee Opinion No. 650. *Obstetrics and Gynecology, 126,* e135–e142.

American College of Obstetricians and Gynecologists. (n.d.). *Preeclampsia and Hypertension in Pregnancy: Resource Overview.* Retrieved from http://www.acog.org/Womens-Health/Preeclampsia-and-Hypertension-in-Pregnancy

American Diabetes Association. (2016). Management of diabetes in pregnancy. *Diabetes Care, 39*(Suppl. 1), S94–S98.

American Psychiatric Association. (2013). *Diagnostic and statistical manual of mental disorders* (5th ed.). Arlington, VA: American Psychiatric Publishing.

Bedsider.org. (2016). *Birth control methods.* Retrieved from https://providers.bedsider.org

Grant, M. D., Marbella, A., Wang, A. T., Pines, E., Hoag, J., Bonnell, C., . . . Aronson, N. (2015). *Menopausal symptoms: Comparative effectiveness of therapies* (Report

No. 15-EHC005-EF). Rockville, MD: Agency for Healthcare Research and Quality. Retrieved from https://www.ncbi.nlm.nih.gov/books/NBK285463/

Grimes, D. A., Gallo, M. F., Grigorieva, V., Nanda, K., Schulz, K. F. (2004). Fertility awareness-based methods for contraception. *Cochrane Database of Systematic Reviews*, (4), CD004860.

Henshaw, S. (2008). Induced abortion. *Global Library of Women's Medicine*. Retrieved from http://www.glowm.com/section_view/heading/Induced%20Abortion:%20 Epidemiologic%20Aspects/item/436. doi:10.3843/GLOWM.10437

Nelson, R. (2015). *The pill has prevented 400,000 cases of endometrial cancer*. Retrieved from http://www.medscape.com/viewarticle/849065.

Shih, G. (2015). Does being overweight affect your birth control? *Bedsider.org*. Retrieved from http://bedsider.org/features/164-does-being-overweight-affect-your-birth-control

US. Food and Drug Administration. (2015). *Ella (ulipristal acetate)*. Retrieved from https:// www.accessdata.fda.gov/drugsatfda_docs/label/2015/022474s007lbl.pdf

Chapter 8

American Psychiatric Association. (2013). *Diagnostic and statistical manual of mental disorders* (5th ed.). Arlington, VA: American Psychiatric Publishing.

Bertone-Johnson, E. R., Hankinson, S. E., Bendich, A., Johnson, S. R., Willett, W. C., & Manson, J. E. (2005). Calcium and vitamin D intake and risk of incident premenstrual syndrome. *Archives of Internal Medicine*, 165(11), 1246–1252.

Centers for Disease Control. (2016). *PID fact sheet*. Retrieved from https://www.cdc.gov /std/pid/stdfact-pid.htm

Dadkhah, H., Ebrahimi, E., & Fathizadeh, N. (2016). Evaluating the effects of vitamin D and vitamin E supplement on premenstrual syndrome: A randomized, double-blind, controlled trial. *Iranian Journal of Nursing and Midwifery Research*, 21(2), 159–164. doi:10.4103/1735-9066.178237

Hollins-Martin, C., van den Akker, O., Martin, S., & Preedy, V. R. (Eds.). (2014). *Handbook of diet and nutrition in the menstrual cycle, periconception and fertility*. Human Health Handbooks No. 7. Wageningen, Netherlands: Wageningen Academic Publishers.

Koninckx, P. R., Ussia, A., Keckstein, J., Wattiez, A., & Adamyan, L. (2016). Epidemiology of subtle, typical, cystic, and deep endometriosis: A systematic review. *Gynaecological Surgery, 13*, 457–467.

Męczekalski, B., & Czyżyk, A. (2015). *Vitex agnus castus* in the treatment of hyperprolactinemia and menstrual disorders—A case report. *Polski Merkuriusz Lekarski, 39*(229), 43–46.

Shaw, K., Turner, J., & Del Mar, C. (2002). Tryptophan and 5-hydroxytryptophan for depression. *Cochrane Database of Systematic Reviews, 1*, CD003198.

Stefansson, H., Geirsson, R., Steinthorsdottir, V., Jonsson, H., Manolescu, A., Kong, A., . . . Stefansson, K. (2002). Genetic factors contribute to the risk of developing endometriosis. *Human Reproduction, 17*(3), 555–559. doi:10.1093/humrep/17.3.555

Steinthorsdottir, V., Steinthorsdottir, V., Thorleifsson, G., Aradottir, K., Feenstra, B., Sigurdsson, A., . . . Thorsteinsdottir, U. (2016). Common variants upstream of KDR encoding VEGFR2 and in TTC39B associate with endometriosis. *Nature Communications, 7*, 12350. doi:10.1038/ncomms12350

Tartagni, M., Cicinelli, M. V., Tartagni, M. V., Alrasheed, H., Matteo, M., Baldini, D., . . . Montagnani, M. (2016). Vitamin D supplementation for premenstrual syndromerelated mood disorders in adolescents with severe hypovitaminosis D. *Journal of Pediatric and Adolescent Gynecology, 29*(4), 357–361.

References

Van Die, M. D., Burger, H. G., Teede, H. J., & Bone, K. M. (2013). *Vitex agnus-castus* extracts for female reproductive disorders: a systematic review of clinical trials. *Planta Medica, 79*(7), 562–575.

Won, H. R., & Abbott, J. (2010). Optimal management of chronic cyclical pelvic pain: An evidence-based and pragmatic approach. *International Journal of Women's Health, 2,* 263–277. doi:10.2147/IJWH.S7991

Chapter 9

Dunn, T. M., Bratman, S. (2016). On orthorexia nervosa: A review of the literature and proposed diagnostic criteria. *Eating Behaviors, 21,*11–17.

Kratina, K. (2016). *Orthorexia nervosa.* Retrieved from https://www.nationaleatingdisorders .org/orthorexia-nervosa

National Institutes of Health (2016a). *Anxiety disorders.* Retrieved from https://www.nimh .nih.gov/health/topics/anxiety-disorders/index.shtml

National Institutes of Health. (2016b). *Major depression among adults.* Retrieved from https:// www.nimh.nih.gov/health/statistics/prevalence/major-depression-among-adults.shtml

QPR Institute. (2016). *Question, persuade and refer.* Retrieved from https://www .qprinstitute.com/about-qpr

Chapter 10

Hahner, S., Loeffler, M., Bleicken, B., Drechsler, C., Milovanovic, D., Fassnacht, M., . . . Allolio, B. (2010). Epidemiology of adrenal crisis in chronic adrenal insufficiency: The need for new prevention strategies. *European Journal of Endocrinology, 62*(3), 597–602.

Chapter 11

Ablin, J., Fitzcharles, M.-A., Buskila, D., Shir, Y., Sommer, C., & Häuser, W. (2013). Treatment of fibromyalgia syndrome: Recommendations of recent evidence-based interdisciplinary guidelines with special emphasis on complementary and alternative therapies. *Evidence-Based Complementary and Alternative Medicine,* 485272. doi:10.1155/2013/485272

Centers for Disease Control. (2010). *Prevalence of doctor-diagnosed arthritis and arthritis-attributable activity limitation—United States, 2007–2009.* Retrieved from https://www .cdc.gov/mmwr/preview/mmwrhtml/mm5939a1.htm

Centers for Disease Control. (2016). *Arthritis-related statistics.* Retrieved from https:// www.cdc.gov/arthritis/data_statistics/arthritis-related-stats.htm

Menzies, V. (2016). Fibromyalgia syndrome: Current considerations in symptom management. *American Journal of Nursing, 116*(1), 24–32.

North American Menopause Society. (2010). Position statement: Management of osteoporosis in postmenopausal women: 2010 position statement of the North American Menopause Society. *Menopause, 17*(1), 25–54.

Speroff, L., & Fritz, M. A. (2005). *Clinical gynecologic endocrinology and infertility* (7th ed.). Philadelphia, PA: Lippincott Williams & Wilkins.

Wolfe, F., Clauw, D. J., Fitzcharles, M. A., Goldenberg, D. L., Katz, R. S., Mease, P., . . . Yunus, M. B. (2010). The American College of Rheumatology preliminary diagnostic criteria for fibromyalgia and measurement of symptom severity. *Arthritis Care and Research, 62*(5), 600–610.

Wolfe, F., Fitzcharles, M. A., Goldenberg, D. L., Häuser, W., Katz, R. L., Mease, P. J., . . . Walitt, B. (2016). Comparison of physician-based and patient-based criteria for the diagnosis of fibromyalgia. *Arthritis Care and Research*, 68(5), 652–659.

Zavanelli-Morgan, B. A. (2007, October). *Amenorrhea*. Presentation at Institute of Women's Health and Integrative Medicine, Portland, OR.

Chapter 13

National Institute of Diabetes and Digestive and Kidney Diseases. (2016). *Treatment for interstitial cystitis*. Retrieved from https://www.niddk.nih.gov/health-information /urologic-diseases/interstitial-cystitis-painful-bladder-syndrome/treatment

Qaseem, A., Dallas, P., Forciea, M. A., Starkey, M., Denberg, T. D., & Shekelle, P. (2014). Nonsurgical management of urinary incontinence in women: A clinical practice guideline from the American College of Physicians. *Annals of Internal Medicine, 161*(6), 429–440.

Chapter 14

Betancourt, J. R., Green, A. R., & Carrillo, J. E. (2002). *Cultural competence in health care: Emerging frameworks and practical approaches* (Vol. 576). New York, NY: Commonwealth Fund, Quality of Care for Underserved Populations.

Boscardin, C. K., Grbic, D., Grumbach, K., & O'Sullivan, P. (2014). Educational and individual factors associated with positive change in and reaffirmation of medical students' intention to practice in underserved areas. *Academic Medicine, 89*(11), 1490–1496.

Dauvrin, M., & Lorant, V. (2015). Leadership and cultural competence of healthcare professionals: A social network analysis. *Nursing Research, 64*(3), 200–210. doi:10.1097 /NNR.0000000000000092

Donald, F., Martin-Misener, R., Carter, N., Donald, E. E., Kaasalainen, S., Wickson-Griffiths, A., . . . DiCenso, A. (2013). A systematic review of the effectiveness of advanced practice nurses in long-term care. *Journal of Advanced Nursing, 69*(10), 2148–2161.

Hayman, B., & Wilkes, L. (2016). Older lesbian women's health and healthcare: A narrative review of the literature. *Journal of Clinical Nursing, 25*(23–24), 3454–3468.

Institute of Medicine. (2014). *The health of lesbian, gay, bisexual, and transgender people: Building a foundation for better understanding*. Washington, DC: The National Academies Press; 2011. Retrieved from http://www.nap.edu/catalog.php?record_id=13128

National Center for Cultural Competence. (2016). *Conceptual frameworks/models, guiding values and principles*. Retrieved from https://nccc.georgetown.edu/foundations /frameworks.html#ccdefinition

Núñez, A. E. (2000). Transforming cultural competence into cross-cultural efficacy in women's health education. *Academic Medicine, 75*(11), 1071–1080.

Understanding Prejudice. (2017). *Exercises: Implicit Association Test*. Retrieved from http:// www.understandingprejudice.org/iat/noflash.htm

U.S. Department of Health and Human Services, Office of Minority Health. (2016). *The national CLAS standards*. Retrieved from https://minorityhealth.hhs.gov/omh/browse. aspx?lvl=2&lvlid=53

Chapter 15

Bureau of Justice Statistics. (2016). *Publications and products: Intimate partner violence*. Retrieved from https://www.bjs.gov/index.cfm?ty=pbse&sid=78

Chapter 16

Agency for Health Care Research and Quality. (2016). *Health literacy measuring tools.* Retrieved from http://www.ahrq.gov/professionals/quality-patient-safety/quality-resources/tools/literacy/index.html#rapid

Hartzler, A., & Pratt, W. (2011). Managing the personal side of health: How patient expertise differs from the expertise of clinicians. *Journal of Medical Internet Research, 13*(3), e62. doi:10.2196/jmir.1728

Hersh, L., Salzman, B., Snyderman, D. (2015). Health literacy in primary care practice. *American Family Physician, 92*(2), 118–124.

Robinson, T., White, G., & Houchins, J. (2006). Improving communication with older patients: Tips from the literature. *Family Practice Management, 13*(8), 73–78.

U.S. Department of Health and Human Services. (2008). *Literacy.* Retrieved from http://health.gov/communication/literacy/

U.S. Department of Health and Human Services. (2015a). *Health Literacy fact sheet.* Retrieved from https://health.gov/communication/literacy/quickguide/factsbasic.htm

U.S. Department of Health and Human Services. (2015b) *Quick guide to health literacy.* Retrieved January 30, 2017 from https://health.gov/communication/literacy/quickguide/services.htm

U.S. Department of Health and Human Services. (n.d.). *Quick guide to health literacy fact sheet.* Retrieved from http://health.gov/communication/literacy/quickguide/factsliteracy.htm

Chapter 17

Centers for Disease Control and Prevention. (2016). *Defining adult overweight and obesity.* Retrieved from https://www.cdc.gov/obesity/adult/defining.html

National Center for Health Statistics. (2016). *Health E-Stats.* Retrieved from https://www.cdc.gov/nchs/products/hestats.htm

Institute of Medicine. (2009). *Weight gain during pregnancy: Reexamining the guidelines.* Washington, DC: National Academies Press.

Chapter 19

Fryar, C. D., & Ogden, C. L. (2012). *Prevalence of underweight among adults aged 20 years and over.* Retrieved from https://www.cdc.gov/nchs/data/hestat/underweight_adult_07_10/underweight_adult_07_10.htm

Institute of Medicine. (2012). *The mental health and substance use workforce for older adults: In whose hands?* Washington, DC: National Academies Press. Retrieved from https://www.nap.edu/catalog/13400/the-mental-health-and-substance-use-workforce-for-older-adults

Perron, L., Senikas, V., Burnett, M., Davis, V., & Society of Obstetricians and Gynaecologists of Canada. (2013). Clinical practice guidelines: Female genital cutting. *Journal of Obstetrics and Gynaecology Canada, 35*(11), e1–e18.

U.S. Department of Health and Human Services, Office of Minority Health. (2013). *National standards for culturally and linguistically appropriate services in health care.* Retrieved from https://www.thinkculturalhealth.hhs.gov/pdfs/EnhancedCLASSStandardsBlueprint.pdf

World Health Organization. (2017). *Female genital mutilation.* Retrieved from http://www.who.int/mediacentre/factsheets/fs241/en/

Bibliography

Health Fundamentals

American Physiological Society. (2016, January 12). Not the weaker sex: Estrogen protects women against the flu, study finds: Study in human cells supports why the flu may hit men harder than women. *ScienceDaily*. Retrieved from http://www.sciencedaily.com /releases/2016/01/160112093424.htm

Arslan, A. A., Koenig, K. L., & Lenner, P., et al. (2014). Circulating estrogen metabolites and risk of breast cancer in postmenopausal women. *Cancer Epidemiology, Biomarkers, and Prevention, 23*(7), 1290–1297. doi:10.1158/1055-9965.EPI-14-0009

Colborn, T., Dumanoski, D., & Myers, J. P. (1997). *Our stolen future*. New York, NY: Penguin.

Dallal, C., & Taioli, E. (2010). Urinary 2/16 estrogen metabolite ratio levels in healthy women: A review of the literature. *Mutation Research, 705*(2), 154–162. doi:10.1016/j. mrrev.2010.06.004

Hodges, R. E., & Minich, D. M. (2015). Modulation of metabolic detoxification pathways using foods and food-derived components: A scientific review with clinical application. *Journal of Nutrition and Metabolism, 760689*. doi:10.1155/2015/760689

Jindal, S., Gao, D., Bell, P., Albrektsen, G., Edgerton, S. M., Ambrosone, C. B., . . . Schedin, P. (2014). Postpartum breast involution reveals regression of secretory lobules mediated by tissue-remodeling. *Breast Cancer Research, 16*(2), R31. doi:10.1186 /bcr3633

Obi, N., Vrieling, A., Heinz, J., & Chang-Claude, J. (2011). Estrogen metabolite ratio: Is the 2-hydroxyestrone to 16α-hydroxyestrone ratio predictive for breast cancer? *International Journal of Women's Health, 3*, 37–51. doi:10.2147/IJWH.S7595

Pollycove, R., Naftolin, F., & Simon, J. A. (2011). The evolutionary origin and significance of Menopause. *Menopause, 18*(3), 336–342. doi:10.1097/gme.0b013e3181ed957a

Radisky, D. C., & Hartmann, L. C. (2009). Mammary involution and breast cancer risk: Transgenic models and clinical studies. *Journal of Mammary Gland Biology and Neoplasia, 14*(2), 181–191. doi:10.1007/s10911-009-9123-y

Ruan, X., Seeger, H., Wallwiener, D., Huober, J., & Mueck, A. O. (2015). The ratio of the estradiol metabolites 2-hydroxyestrone (2-OHE1) and 16α-hydroxyestrone (16-OHE1) may predict breast cancer risk in postmenopausal but not in premenopausal women: Two case-control studies. *Archives of Gynecology and Obstetrics, 291*(5), 1141–1146.

Samavat, H., & Kurzer, M. S. (2015). Estrogen metabolism and breast cancer. *Cancer Letters, 356*(2 Pt. A), 231–243.

Seetharam, P., & Rodrigues, G. (2015). Benign breast disorders: An insight with a detailed literature review. *Breast, 6*(1), WMC004806. doi:10.9754/journal.wmc.2015.004806

Menstrual Cycle

Campeau, S., Liberzon, I., Morilak, D., & Ressler, K. (2011). Stress modulation of cognitive and affective processes. *Stress, 14*(5), 503–519. doi:10.3109/10253890.2011. 596864

Bibliography

Clarke-Pearson, D. L., & Dawood, M. Y. (1990). *Green's gynecology: Essentials of clinical practice* (4th ed.). Boston, MA: Little, Brown & Co.

Dasharathy, S. S., Mumford, S. L., Pollack, A. Z., Perkins, N. J., Mattison, D. R., Wactawski-Wende, J., & Schisterman, E. F. (2012). Menstrual bleeding patterns among regularly menstruating women. *American Journal of Epidemiology, 175*(6), 536–545. doi:10.1093/aje/kwr356

Gordon, J. L., & Girdler, S. S. (2014). Mechanisms underlying hemodynamic and neuroendocrine stress reactivity at different phases of the menstrual cycle. *Psychophysiology, 51*(4), 309–318. doi:10.1111/psyp.12177

Ling, F. W., & Duff, P. (2001). *Obstetrics and gynecology principles for practice.* New York, NY: McGraw-Hill.

Santos, I. S., Minten, G. C., Valle, N. C., Giovana, C. T., Alessandra, B. S., Guilherme, A. R. P., & Joaquim, F. C. (2011). Menstrual bleeding patterns: A community-based cross-sectional study among women aged 18–45 years in southern Brazil. *BMC Women's Health, 11*, 26. doi:10.1186/1472-6874-11-26

Shechter, A., & Boivin, D. B. (2010). Sleep, hormones, and circadian rhythms throughout the menstrual cycle in healthy women and women with premenstrual dysphoric disorder. *International Journal of Endocrinology, 259345.* doi:10.1155/2010/259345

Shephard, B. D., & Shephard, C. A. (1990). *The complete guide to women's health* (2nd ed.). New York, NY: Plume.

Sundström Poromaa, I., & Gingnell, M. (2014). Menstrual cycle influence on cognitive function and emotion processing—From a reproductive perspective. *Frontiers in Neuroscience, 8*, 380. doi:10.3389/fnins.2014.00380

Vollman, R. F. (1977). The Menstrual Cycle. In E. Friedman (Ed.), *Major problems of obstetrics and gynecology* (pp. 11–193). Philadelphia, PA: W.B. Saunders.

White, C. P., Hitchcock, C. L., Vigna, Y. M., & Prior, J. C. (2011). Fluid retention over the menstrual cycle: 1-year data from the prospective ovulation cohort. *Obstetrics and Gynecology International, 138451.* doi:10.1155/2011/138451

Progesterone Concepts

Blanks, A. M., & Brosens, J. J. (2012). Progesterone action in the myometrium and decidua in preterm birth. *Facts, Views, and Visions in ObGyn, 4*(3), 33–43.

Conneely, O. M., Lydon, J. P., De Mayo, F., & O'malley, B. W. (2000). Reproductive functions of the progesterone receptor. *Journal of the Society for Gynecologic Investigation, 7*(Suppl. 1), S25–S32.

Diep, C. H., Daniel, A. R., Mauro, L. J., Knutson, T. P., & Lange, C. A. (2015). Progesterone action in breast, uterine, and ovarian cancers. *Journal of Molecular Endocrinology, 54*(2), R31–R53. doi:10.1530/JME-14-0252

Graham, J. D., & Clarke, C. L. (2011). Physiological action of progesterone in target tissues. *Endocrine Reviews, 18*(4), 502–519.

Jacobsen, B. M., & Horwitz, K. B. (2012). Progesterone receptors, their isoforms and progesterone regulated transcription. *Molecular and Cellular Endocrinology, 357*(1–2), 18–29. doi:10.1016/j.mce.2011.09.016

Kim, C. H. (2015). A functional relay from progesterone to vitamin D in the immune system. *DNA and Cell Biology, 34*(6), 379–382.

Kim, J. J., Kurita, T., & Bulun, S. E. (2013). Progesterone action in endometrial cancer, endometriosis, uterine fibroids, and breast cancer. *Endocrine Reviews, 34*(1), 130–162. doi:10.1210/er.2012-1043

Bibliography

Li, X., Feng, Y., Lin, J-F., Billig, H., & Shao, R. (2014). Endometrial progesterone resistance and PCOS. *Journal of Biomedical Science, 21*(1), 2. doi:10.1186/1423-0127-21-2

Mesiano, S., Wang, Y., & Norwitz, E. R. (2011). Progesterone receptors in the human pregnancy uterus: Do they hold the key to birth timing? *Reproductive Sciences, 18*(1), 6–19.

Obr, A., & Edwards, D. P. (2012). The biology of progesterone receptor in the normal mammary gland and in breast cancer. *Molecular and Cellular Endocrinology, 357*(1–2), 4–17. doi:10.1016/j.mce.2011.10.030

Scarpin, K. M., Graham, J. D., Mote, P. A., & Clarke, C. L. (2009). Progesterone action in human tissues: regulation by progesterone receptor (PR) isoform expression, nuclear positioning and coregulator expression. *Nuclear Receptor Signaling, 7*, e009. doi:10.1621/nrs.07009

Reproductive Anatomy

Clarke-Pearson, D. L., & Dawood, M. Y. (1990). *Green's gynecology: Essentials of clinical practice* (4th ed.). Boston, MA: Little, Brown & Co.

Marshall, J. C., Dalkin, A. C., Haisenleder, D. J., Paul, S. J., Ortolano, G. A., & Kelch, R. P. (1991). Gonadotropin-releasing hormone pulses: Regulators of gonadotropin synthesis and ovulatory cycles. *Recent Progress in Hormone Research, 47*, 155–189.

Oyelowo, T. (2007). *Mosby's guide to women's health: A handbook for health professionals.* St. Louis, MO: Elsevier.

Scott, J. R., Gibbs, R. S., Karlan, B. Y., & Haney, A. F. (2003). Danforth's obstetrics and gynecology (9th ed.). Philadelphia, PA: Lippincott Williams and Wilkins.

Shephard, B. D., & Shephard, C. A. (1990). *The complete guide to women's health* (2nd ed.). New York, NY: Plume.

Speroff, L., & Fritz, M. A. (2005). *Clinical gynecologic endocrinology and infertility* (7th ed.). Philadelphia, PA: Lippincott Williams and Wilkins.

Youngkin, E. Q., & Davis, M. S. (1998). *Women's health: A primary care clinical guide* (2nd ed.). Stamford, CT: Appleton and Lange.

Pregnancy

Bowe, S., Adams, J., Lui, C. W., & Sibbritt, D. (2015). A longitudinal analysis of self-prescribed complementary and alternative medicine use by a nationally representative sample of 19,783 Australian women, 2006–2010. *Complementary Therapies in Medicine, 23*(5), 699–704.

Feijen-de Jong, E. I., Jansen, D. E., Baarveld, F., Spelten, E., Schellevis, F., & Reijneveld, S. A. (2015). Determinants of use of care provided by complementary and alternative health care practitioners to pregnant women in primary midwifery care: A prospective cohort study. *BMC Pregnancy and Childbirth, 15*, 140. doi:10.1186/s12884-015-0555-7

Frawley, J., Adams, J., Sibbritt, D., Steel, A., Broom, A., & Gallois, C. (2013). Prevalence and determinants of complementary and alternative medicine use during pregnancy: Results from a nationally representative sample of Australian pregnant women. *Australian and New Zealand Journal of Obstetrics and Gynaecology, 53*(4), 347–352.

Hall, H. G., Griffiths, D. L., & McKenna, L. G. (2011). The use of complementary and alternative medicine by pregnant women: a literature review. *Midwifery, 27*(6), 817–824.

Holden, S. C., Gardiner, P., Birdee, G., Davis, R. B., & Yeh, G. Y. (2015). Complementary and alternative medicine use among women during pregnancy and childbearing years. *Birth, 42*(3), 261–269.

Peng, W., Adams, J., Hickman, L., & Sibbritt, D. W. (2015). Association between consultations with complementary/alternative medicine practitioners and menopause-related symptoms: A cross-sectional study. *Climacteric, 18*(4), 551–558.

U.S. Department of Health and Human Services. (2015). *Complementary, alternative, or integrative health: What's in a name.* Retrieved from https://nccih.nih.gov/health/integrative-health

Adrenal Function

Alghadir, A. H., & Gabr, S. A. (2015). Physical activity and environmental influences on adrenal fatigue of Saudi adults: Biochemical analysis and questionnaire survey. *Journal of Physical Therapy Science, 27*(7), 2045–2051. doi:10.1589/jpts.27.2045

Alijaniha, F., Naseri, M., Afsharypuor, S., Fallahi, F., Noorbala, A., Mosaddegh, M., . . . Sadrai, S. (2015). Heart palpitation relief with *Melissa officinalis* leaf extract: Double blind, randomized, placebo controlled trial of efficacy and safety. *Journal of Ethnopharmacology, 164,* 378–384.

Allolio, B., Arlt, W., & Hahner, S. (2007). DHEA: Why, when, and how much—DHEA replacement in adrenal insufficiency. *Annales d'Endocrinologie, 68*(4), 268–273.

Cases, J., Ibarra, A., Feuillère, N., Roller, M., & Sukkar, S. G. (2011). Pilot trial of *Melissa officinalis* L. leaf extract in the treatment of volunteers suffering from mild-to-moderate anxiety disorders and sleep disturbances. *Mediterranean Journal of Nutrition and Metabolism, 4*(3), 211–218. doi:10.1007/s12349-010-0045-4

Dhatariya, K. K., Greenlund, L. J. S., Bigelow, M. L., Thapa, P., Oberg, A. L., Ford, G. C., . . . Nair, K. S. (2008). Dehydroepiandrosterone replacement therapy in hypoadrenal women: Protein anabolism and skeletal muscle function. *Mayo Clinic Proceedings, 83*(11), 1218–1225.

Farahani, M. S., Bahramsoltani, R., Farzaei, M. H., Abdollahi, M., & Rahimi, R. (2015). Plant-derived natural medicines for the management of depression: An overview of mechanisms of action. *Reviews in Neuroscience, 26*(3), 305–321.

Gurnell, E. M., Hunt, P. J., Curran, S. E., Conway, C. L., Pullenayegum, E. M., Huppert, F. A., . . . Chatterjee, V. K. K. (2008). Long-term DHEA replacement in primary adrenal insufficiency: A randomized, controlled trial. *Journal of Clinical Endocrinology and Metabolism, 93*(2), 400–409. doi:10.1210/jc.2007-1134

Head, K. A., & Kelly, G. S. (2009). Nutrients and botanicals for treatment of stress: Adrenal fatigue, neurotransmitter imbalance, anxiety, and restless sleep. *Alternative Medicine Review, 14*(2), 114–140.

Kalani, A., Bahtiyar, G., & Sacerdote, A. (2012). *Ashwagandha* root in the treatment of non-classical adrenal hyperplasia. *BMJ Case Reports,* bcr2012006989. doi:10.1136/bcr-2012-006989

Neary, N., & Nieman, L. (2010). Adrenal insufficiency—Etiology, diagnosis and treatment. *Current Opinion in Endocrinology, Diabetes, and Obesity, 17*(3), 217–223. doi:10.1097/MED.0b013e328338f608

Amenorrhea

Bousfiha, N., Errarhay, S., Saadi, H., Ouldim, K., Bouchikhi, C., & Banani, A. (2010). Gonadal dysgenesis 46, XX associated with Mayer-Rokitansky-Kuster-Hauser syndrome: One case report. *Obstetrics and Gynecology International,* 847370. doi:10.1155/2010/847370

Deligeoroglou, E., Athanasopoulos, N., Tsimaris, P., Dimopoulos, K. D., Vrachnis, N., & Creatsas, G. (2010). Evaluation and management of adolescent amenorrhea. *Annals of the New York Academy of Sciences, 1205*, 23–32.

Fourman, L. T., & Fazeli, P. K. (2015). Neuroendocrine causes of amenorrhea—An update. *Journal of Clinical Endocrinology and Metabolism, 100*(3), 812–824.

Klein, D. A., & Poth, M. A. (2013). Amenorrhea: An approach to diagnosis and management. *American Family Physician, 87*(11), 781–788.

Kumar, S., & Kaur, G. (2013). Intermittent fasting dietary restriction regimen negatively influences reproduction in young rats: A study of hypothalamo-hypophysial-gonadal axis. *PLoS ONE, 8*(1), e52416. doi:10.1371/journal.pone.0052416

Kwon, S-K., Chae, H-D., Lee K-H., Kim S-H., Kim C-H., & Kang B-M. (2014). Causes of amenorrhea in Korea: Experience of a single large center. *Clinical and Experimental Reproductive Medicine, 41*(1), 29–32. doi:10.5653/cerm.2014.41.1.29

Narita, K., Nagao, K., Bannai, M., Ichimaru, T., Nakano, S., Murata, T., . . . Takahashi, M. (2011). Dietary deficiency of essential amino acids rapidly induces cessation of the rat estrous cycle. *PLoS ONE, 6*(11), e28136. doi:10.1371/journal.pone.0028136

Bladder Syndromes

American College of Obstetricians and Gynecologists. (2011). *Gynecological problems: Urinary incontinence.* Retrieved from http://www.acog.org/~/media/for patients/faq081.pdf?dmc=1&ts=20121218t1703471630

American College of Obstetricians and Gynecologists. (2014). *Surgery for stress urinary incontinence.* Retrieved from http://www.acog.org/~/media/forpatients/faq166.pdf?dmc=1&ts=20130102t2043435319

Berry, S. H., Elliott, M. N., Suttorp, M., Bogart, L. M., Stoto, M. A., Eggers, P., . . . Clemens, J. Q. (2011). Prevalence of symptoms of bladder pain syndrome/interstitial cystitis among adult females in the United States. *Journal of Urology, 186*, 540–544.

Dowling-Castronovo, A., & Bradway, C. *Nursing standard of practice protocol: Urinary incontinence (UI) in older adults admitted to acute care.* Retrieved from https://consultgeri.org/geriatric-topics/urinary-incontinence

Dowling-Castronovo, A., & Specht, J. K. (2012). How to try this. *American Journal of Nursing, 11*(1), 62–71. Retrieved from http://consultgerirn.org/uploads/file/trythis/try_this_11_1.pdf

Lian, A., Zhang, W., & Wang, S. (2015). Mild and moderate female stress urinary incontinence treated with transcutaneous acupoint electrical stimulation: A randomized controlled trial. *Zhongguo Zhen Jiu, 35*(4), 327–329.

National Institute of Diabetes and Digestive and Kidney Diseases. (2011). Interstitial cystitis/painful bladder syndrome. Retrieved from http://www.niddk.nih.gov/health-information/health-topics/urologic-disease/interstitial-cystitis-painful-bladder-syndrome/pages/facts.aspx

Qaseem, A., Dallas, P., Forciea, M. A., Starkey, M., Denberg, T. D., & Shekelle, P. (2014, September 16). Clinical Guidelines Committee of the American College of Physicians. Nonsurgical management of urinary incontinence in women: A clinical practice guideline from the American College of Physicians. *Annals of Internal Medicine, 161*(6), 429–440.

Breast Conditions

Akseev, N. P., Vladimir, I. I., & Nadezhda, T. E. (2015). Pathological postpartum breast engorgement: Prediction, prevention, and resolution. *Breastfeeding Medicine, 10*(4), 203–208. doi:10.1089/bfm.2014.0047

Bibliography

Arslan, A. A., Koenig, K. L., Lenner, P., Afanasyeva, Y., Shore, R. E., Chen, Y., . . . Zeleniuch-Jacquotte, A. (2014). Circulating estrogen metabolites and risk of breast cancer in postmenopausal women. *Cancer Epidemiology, Biomarkers, and Prevention, 23*(7), 1290–1297. doi:10.1158/1055-9965.EPI-14-0009

Bjelakovic, G., Gluud, L. L., Nikolova, D., Whitfield, K., Krstic, G., Wetterslev, J., & Gluud, C. (2014). Vitamin D supplementation for prevention of cancer in adults. *Cochrane Database of Systematic Reviews, 6,* CD007469.

Cadeau, C., Fournier, A., Mesrine, S., Clavel-Chapelon, F., Fagherazzi, G., & Boutron-Ruault, M. C. (2015). Interaction between current vitamin D supplementation and menopausal hormone therapy use on breast cancer risk: Evidence from the E3N cohort. *American Journal of Clinical Nutrition, 102*(4), 966–973.

Centers for Disease Control and Prevention. (2015). *United States Cancer Statistics (USCS) 1999–2012.* Retrieved from https://nccd.cdc.gov/uscs/

Chen, J-H., Liu, H., Baek, H-M., Nalcioglu, O., & Su, M-Y. (2008). MR imaging features of fibrocystic change of the breast. *Magnetic Resonance Imaging, 26*(9), 1207–1214. doi:10.1016/j.mri.2008.02.004

Colonese, F., Laganà, A. S., Colonese, E., Sofo, V., Salmeri, F. M., Granese, R., & Triolo, O. (2015). The pleiotropic effects of vitamin D in gynaecological and obstetric diseases: An overview on a hot topic. *BioMed Research International,* 986281. doi:10.1155/2015/986281

Cui, Y., Shikany, J. M., Liu, S., Shagufta, Y., & Rohan, T. E. (2008). Selected antioxidants and risk of hormone receptor-defined invasive breast cancers among postmenopausal women in the Women's Health Initiative Observational Study. *American Journal of Clinical Nutrition, 87*(4), 1009–1018.

Denlinger, C. S., Ligibel, J. A., Are, M., Baker, K. S., Demark-Wahnefried, W., Dizon, D., . . . National Comprehensive Cancer Network. (2014). Survivorship: Nutrition and weight management, version 2.2014: Clinical practice guidelines in oncology. *Journal of the National Comprehensive Cancer Network, 12*(10), 1396–1406.

Diep, C. H., Daniel, A. R., Mauro, L. J., Knutson, T. P., & Lange, C. A. (2015). Progesterone action in breast, uterine, and ovarian cancers. *Journal of Molecular Endocrinology, 54*(2), R31–R53. doi:10.1530/JME-14-0252

Duthie, S. J. (2011). Folate and cancer: How DNA damage, repair and methylation impact on colon carcinogenesis. *Journal of Inherited Metabolic Disease, 34,* 101–109.

Fabian, C. J., Kimler, B. F., & Hursting, S. D. (2015). Omega-3 fatty acids for breast cancer prevention and survivorship. *Breast Cancer Research, 17*(1), 62. doi:10.1186/s13058-015-0571-6

Falconer, I. R. (2006). Are endocrine disrupting compounds a health risk in drinking water? *International Journal of Environmental Research and Public Health, 3*(2), 180–184.

Garrido-Maraver, J., Cordero, M. D., Oropesa-Ávila, M., Vega, A. F., de la Mata, M., Pavón, A. D., . . . Sánchez-Alcázar, J. A. (2014). Coenzyme q10 therapy. *Molecular Syndromology, 5*(3–4), 187–197. doi:10.1159/000360101

Harris, H. R., Orsini, N., & Wolk, A. (2014). Vitamin C and survival among women with breast cancer: A Meta-analysis. *European Journal of Cancer, 50*(7), 1223–1231. doi:10.1016/j.ejca.2014.02.013

Hutchinson, J., Burley, V. J., Greenwood, D. C., Thomas, J. D., & Cade, J. E. (2010). High-dose vitamin C supplement use is associated with self-reported histories of breast cancer and other illnesses in the UK Women's Cohort Study. *Public Health Nutrition, 14*(5), 768–777. doi:10.1017/S1368980010002739

Iyengar, N. M., Hudis, C. A., & Gucalp, A. (2013). Omega-3 fatty acids for the prevention of breast cancer: An update and state of the science. *Current Breast Cancer Reports, 5*(3), 247–254. doi:10.1007/s12609-013-0112-1

Kim, J. J., Kurita, T., & Bulun, S. E. (2013). Progesterone Action in endometrial cancer, endometriosis, uterine fibroids, and breast cancer. *Endocrine Reviews, 34*(1), 130–162. doi:10.1210/er.2012-1043

Kim, J., Lim, S-Y., Shin, A., Sung, M. K., Ro, J., Kang, H. S., . . . Lee, E. S. (2009). Fatty fish and fish omega-3 fatty acid intakes decrease the breast cancer risk: A case-control study. *BMC Cancer, 9,* 216. doi:10.1186/1471-2407-9-216

Lesser, G. J., Case, D., Stark, N., Williford, S., Giguere, J., Garino, L. A., . . . Wake Forest University Community Clinical Oncology Program Research Base. (2013). A randomized, double-blind, placebo-controlled study of oral coenzyme Q10 to relieve self-reported treatment-related fatigue in newly diagnosed patients with breast cancer. *Journal of Supportive Oncology, 11*(1), 31–42.

Lockwood, K., Moesgaard, S., Hanioka, T., & Folkers, K. (1994). Apparent partial remission of breast cancer in "high risk" patients supplemented with nutritional antioxidants, essential fatty acids and coenzyme Q10. *Molecular Aspects of Medicine,* 15(Suppl.), 231–240.

Mangesi, L., & Dowswell, T. (2010). Treatments for breast engorgement during lactation. *Cochrane Database of Systematic Reviews, 9,* CD006946. doi:10.1002/14651858. CD006946.pub2

Mannion, C., Page, S., Bell, L. H., & Verhoef, M. (2011). Components of an anticancer diet: Dietary recommendations, restrictions and supplements of the Bill Henderson protocol. *Nutrients, 3*(1), 1–26. doi:10.3390/nu3010001

Marriott, M., Masino, K., & Casella, G. (2014). *Breast cancer care gets personal.* Retrieved from http://www.americannursetoday.com/breast-cancer-care-gets-personal

Mason, J. K., Chen, J., & Thompson, L. U. (2010). Flaxseed oil-trastuzumab interaction in breast cancer. *Food and Chemical Toxicology, 48,* 2223–2226.

Michels, K. B., & Willett, W. C. (2009). The Women's Health Initiative Randomized Controlled Dietary Modification Trial: A post-mortem. *Breast Cancer Research and Treatment, 114,* 1–6.

Misotti, A. M., & Gnagnarella, P. (2013). Vitamin supplement consumption and breast cancer risk: A review. *Ecancermedicalscience, 7,* 365. doi:10.3332/ecancer.2013.365

Narvaez, C. J., Matthews, D., LaPorta, E., Simmons, K. M., Beaudin, S., & Welsh, J. (2014). The impact of vitamin D in breast cancer: Genomics, pathways, metabolism. *Frontiers in Physiology, 5,* 213. doi:10.3389/fphys.2014.00213

National Cancer Institute. (2014). *Coenzyme Q10.* Retrieved from http://www.cancer.gov /about-cancer/treatment/cam/patient/coenzyme-q10-pdq/#link/_24

National Cancer Institute. (2015). *High-dose vitamin C.* Retrieved from http://www.cancer .gov/about-cancer/treatment/cam/hp/vitamin-c-pdq#section/_14

Pan, S. Y., Zhou, J., Gibbons, L., Morrison, H., & Wen, S. W. (2011). Antioxidants and breast cancer risk—A population-based case-control study in Canada. *BMC Cancer, 11,* 372. doi:10.1186/1471-2407-11-372

Papandreou, C. N., Doxani, C., Zdoukopoulos, N., Vlachostergios, P. J., Hatzidaki, E., Bakalos, G., . . . Zintzaras, E. (2012). Evidence of association between methylene-tetrahydrofolate reductase gene and susceptibility to breast cancer: A candidate-gene association study in a South-eastern European population. *DNA and Cell Biology, 31,* 193–198.

Pooja, S., Carlus, J., Sekhar, D., Francis, A., Gupta, N., Konwar, R., . . . Rajender, S. (2015). MTHFR 677C>T polymorphism and the risk of breast cancer: Evidence from an original study and pooled data for 28031 cases and 31880 controls. *PLoS ONE, 10*(3), e0120654. doi:10.1371/journal.pone.0120654

Rai, V. (2014). Methylenetetrahydrofolate reductase A1298C polymorphism and breast cancer risk: A meta-analysis of 33 studies. *Annals of Medical and Health Sciences Research, 4*(6), 841–851. doi:10.4103/2141-9248.144873

Rehm, J. (2015). Light or moderate drinking is linked to alcohol related cancers, including breast cancer. *British Medical Journal, 351.* doi:10.1136/bmj.h4400

Ruan, X., Seeger, H., Wallwiener, D., Huober, J., & Mueck, A. O. (2015). The ratio of the estradiol metabolites 2-hydroxyestrone (2-OHE1) and 16α-hydroxyestrone (16-OHE1) may predict breast cancer risk in postmenopausal but not in premenopausal women: Two case-control studies. *Archives of Gynecology and Obstetrics, 291*(5), 1141–1146.

Saggar, J. K., Chen, J., Corey, P., & Thompson, L. U. (2010). Dietary flaxseed lignan or oil combined with tamoxifen treatment affects MCF-7 tumor growth through estrogen receptor- and growth factor-signaling pathways. *Molecular Nutrition and Food Research, 54,* 415–425.

Saini, P., & Saini, R. (2014). Cabbage leaves and breast engorgement. *Indian Journal of Public Health, 58,* 291–292. Retrieved from http://www.ijph.in/text .asp?2014/58/4/291/146309

Samavat, H., & Kurzer, M. S. (2015). Estrogen metabolism and breast cancer. *Cancer Letters, 356*(2 Pt. A), 231–243.

Seo, B. R., Bhardwaj, P., Choi, S., Gonzalez, J., Andresen Eguiluz, R. C., Wang, K., . . . Fischbach, C. (2015). Obesity-dependent changes in interstitial ECM mechanics promote breast tumorigenesis. *Science Translational Medicine, 7,* 301–301. doi:10.1126/scitranslmed.3010467

Silva, C. P., Otero, M., & Esteves, V. (2012). Processes for the elimination of estrogenic steroid hormones from water: A review. *Environmental Pollution, 165,* 38–58.

Sun, Y., Huang, H., Sun, Y., Wang, C., Shi, X., Hu, H., . . . Fujie, K. (2013). Ecological risk of estrogenic endocrine disrupting chemicals in sewage plant effluent and reclaimed water. *Environmental Pollution, 180,* 339–344.

Suzuki, T., Matsuo, K., Hirose, K., Hiraki, A., Kawase, T., Watanabe, M., . . . Tajima, K. (2008). One-carbon metabolism-related gene polymorphisms and risk of breast cancer. *Carcinogenesis, 29,* 356–362.

Tagliabue, E., Raimondi, S., & Gandini, S. (2015). Meta-analysis of vitamin D-binding protein and cancer risk. *Cancer Epidemiology, Biomarkers, and Prevention, 24*(11), 1758–1765.

Wang, D., Vélez de-la-paz, O. I., Zhai, J. X., & Liu, D. W. (2013). Serum 25-hydroxyvitamin D and breast cancer risk: A meta-analysis of prospective studies. *Tumor Biology, 34*(6), 3509–3517.

Weng, J-R., Tsai, C-H., Kulp, S. K., & Chen, C-S. (2008). Indole-3-carbinol as a chemopreventive and anti-cancer agent. *Cancer Letters, 262*(2), 153. doi:10.1016/j .canlet.2008.01.033

Weylandt, K. H., Serini, S., Chen, Y. Q., Su, H., Lim, K., Cittadini, A., & Calviello, G. (2015). Omega-3 polyunsaturated fatty acids: The way forward in times of mixed evidence. *BioMed Research International, 2015,* 143109. doi:10.1155/2015/143109

Yan, B., Stantic, M., Zobalova, R., Bezawork-Geleta, A., Stapelberg, M., Stursa, J., Prokopova, K., . . . Neuzil, J. (2015). Mitochondrially targeted vitamin E succinate efficiently kills breast tumour-initiating cells in a complex II-dependent manner. *BMC Cancer, 15,* 401–401. doi:10.1186/s12885-015-1394-7

Bibliography

Cardiovascular Disease

Astrup, A. (2014). Yogurt and dairy product consumption to prevent cardiometabolic diseases: epidemiologic and experimental studies. *American Journal of Clinical Nutrition, 99*(Suppl. 5), 1235S–1242S.

Bakris, G., Dickholtz, M., Meyer, P. M., Kravitz, G., Avery, E., Miller, M., . . . Bell, B. (2007). Atlas vertebra realignment and achievement of arterial pressure goal in hypertensive patients: A pilot study. *Journal of Human Hypertension, 21*(5), 347–352.

Bonci, E., Chiesa, C., Versacci, P., Anania, C., Silvestri, L., & Pacifico, L. (2015). Association of nonalcoholic fatty liver disease with subclinical cardiovascular changes: A systematic review and meta-analysis. *BioMed Research International,* 213737. doi:10.1155/2015/213737

Chronic Heart Failure: National Clinical Guideline for Diagnosis and Management in Primary and Secondary Care: Partial Update. *National Clinical Guideline Centre:* 34–47. Aug 2010. PMID 22741186.

Dantas AP, Jimenez-Altayo F, Vila E (August 2012). "Vascular aging: facts and factors". *Frontiers in Vascular Physiology* 3 (325): 1–2.

Eikenberg, J. D., & Davy, B. M. (2013). Prediabetes: A prevalent and treatable, but often unrecognized clinical condition. *Journal of the Academy of Nutrition and Dietetics, 113*(2), 213–218.

Hauner, H., Bechthold, A., Boeing, H., Brönstrup, A., Buyken, A., Leschik-Bonnet, E., . . . German Nutrition Society. (2012). Evidence-based guideline of the German Nutrition Society: carbohydrate intake and prevention of nutrition-related diseases. *Annals of Nutrition and Metabolism, 60*(Suppl. 1), 1–58.

Holmes, L., Hossain, J., Ward, D., & Opara, F. (2012). Racial/ethnic variability in hypertension prevalence and risk factors in National Health Interview Survey. *ISRN Hypertension,* 1–8. doi:10.5402/2013/257842

Kratz, M., Baars, T., & Guyenet, S. (2013). The relationship between high-fat dairy consumption and obesity, cardiovascular, and metabolic disease. *European Journal of Nutrition, 52*(1), 1–24.

Kuipers, R. S., De graaf, D. J., Luxwolda, M. F., Muskiet, M. H., Dijck-Brouwer, D. A., & Muskiet, F. A. (2011). Saturated fat, carbohydrates and cardiovascular disease. *Netherlands Journal of Medicine, 69*(9), 372–378.

Liao, I-C., Chen, S-L., Wang, M-Y., & Tsai, P-S. (2014). Effects of massage on blood pressure in patients with hypertension and prehypertension. *Journal of Cardiovascular Nursing, 31*(1), 73–83.

Mangum, K., Partna, L., & Vavrek, D. (2012). Spinal manipulation for the treatment of hypertension: A systematic qualitative literature review. *Journal of Manipulative and Physiological Therapeutics, 35*(3), 235–243. doi:10.1016/j.jmpt.2012.01.005

Mayo Clinic Heart attack. (2014). Retrieval from http://www.mayoclinic.org /diseases-conditions/heart-attack/basics/definition/con-20019520

Mendis, S., Puska, P., & Norrving, B. (2011). *Global atlas on cardiovascular disease prevention and control.* Geneva: World Health Organization, World Heart Federation, and World Stroke Organization.

Ried, K., Frank, O. R., & Stocks, N. P. (2012). Aged garlic extract reduces blood pressure in hypertensives: a dose–response trial. *European Journal of Clinical Nutrition, 67*(1), 64–70. doi:10.1038/ejcn.2012.178

Siri-Tarino, P. W., Sun, Q., Hu, F. B., & Krauss, R. M. (2010). Saturated fat, carbohydrate, and cardiovascular disease. *American Journal of Clinical Nutrition, 91*(3), 502–509. doi:10.3945/ajcn.2008.26285

Strange, R. C., Shipman, K. E., & Ramachandran, S. (2015). Metabolic syndrome: A review of the role of vitamin D in mediating susceptibility and outcome. *World Journal of Diabetes, 6*(7), 896–911. doi:10.4239/wjd.v6.i7.896

WHO Regional Office for South East Asia. (2011). *Hypertension fact sheet.* Retrieved from http://www.searo.who.int/entity/noncommunicable_diseases/media/non _communicable_diseases_hypertension_fs.pdf

Coccydynia

Hodges, S. D., Eck, J. C., & Humphreys, S. C. (2004). A treatment and outcomes analysis of patients with coccydynia. *Spine Journal, 4*(2), 138–140.

Howard, P. D., Dolan, A. N., Falco, A. N., Holland, B. M., Wilkinson, C. F., & Zink, A. M. (2013). A comparison of conservative interventions and their effectiveness for coccydynia: a systematic review. *Journal of Manual and Manipulative Therapy, 21*(4), 213–219. doi:10.1179/2042618613Y.0000000040

Kwon, H. D., Schrot, R. J., Kerr, E. E., & Kim, K. D. (2012). Coccygodynia and coccygectomy. *Korean Journal of Spine, 9*(4), 326–333. doi:10.14245/kjs.2012.9.4.326

Maigne, J. Y., Lagauche, D., & Doursounian, L. (2000). Instability of the coccyx in coccydynia. *Journal of Bone and Joint Surgery, 82*(7), 1038–1041.

Maigne, J. Y., Doursounian, L., & Chatellier, G. (2000). Causes and mechanisms of common coccydynia: Role of body mass index and coccygeal trauma. *Spine, 25*(23), 3072–3079.

Maigne, J. Y., & Chatellier, G. (2001). Comparison of three manual coccydynia treatments: A pilot study. *Spine, 26*(20), E479–E483.

Maigne, J. Y., Chatellier, G., Faou, M. L., & Archambeau, M. (2006). The treatment of chronic coccydynia with intrarectal manipulation: A randomized controlled study. *Spine, 31*(18), E621–E627.

Maigne, J. Y., Pigeau, I., Aguer, N., Doursounian, L., & Chatellier, G. (2011). Chronic coccydynia in adolescents. A series of 53 patients. *European Journal of Physical and Rehabilitation Medicine, 47*(2), 245–251.

Maigne, J. Y., Rusakiewicz, F., & Diouf, M. (2012). Postpartum coccydynia: A case series study of 57 women. *European Journal of Physical and Rehabilitation Medicine, 48*(3), 387–392.

Nathan, S. T., Fisher, B. E., & Roberts, C. S. (2010). Coccydynia: A review of pathoanatomy, aetiology, treatment and outcome. *Journal of Bone and Joint Surgery, 92*(12), 1622–1627.

Polkinghorn, B. S, & Colloca, C. J. (1999, July 22). Chiropractic treatment of coccygodynia via instrumental adjusting procedures using activator methods chiropractic technique. *Journal of Manipulative and Physiological Therapeutics, 6,* 411–416.

Ramieri, A., Domenicucci, M., Cellocco, P., Miscusi, M., & Costanzo, G. (2013). Acute traumatic instability of the coccyx: Results in 28 consecutive coccygectomies. *European Spine Journal, 22*(Suppl. 6), 939–944. doi:10.1007/s00586-013-3010-3

Ryder, I., & Alexander, J. (2000, June). Coccydynia: A woman's tail. *Midwifery, 16*(2), 155–160.

Diabetes

Abeywardena, M. Y., & Patten, G. S. (2011). Role of ω3 long-chain polyunsaturated fatty acids in reducing cardio-metabolic risk factors. *Endocrine, Metabolic, and Immune Disorders—Drug Targets, 11*(3), 232–246.

Bibliography

Alaei Shahmiri, F., Soares, M. J., Zhao, Y., & Sherriff, J. (2013). High-dose thiamine supplementation improves glucose tolerance in hyperglycemic individuals: A random-ized, double-blind cross-over trial. *European Journal of Nutrition, 52*(7), 1821–1824.

Ali, A., Ma, Y., Reynolds, J., Wise, J. P., Inzucchi, S. E., & Katz, D. L. (2011). Chromium effects on glucose tolerance and insulin sesitivity in persons at risk for diabetes mellitus. *Endocrine Practice, 17*(1), 16–25. doi:10.4158/EP10131.OR

Evert, A. B., & Boucher, J. L. (2014). New diabetes nutrition therapy recommenda-tions: What you need to know. *Diabetes Spectrum, 27*(2), 121–130. doi:10.2337/diaspect.27.2.121

Evert, A. B., Boucher, J. L., Cypress, M., Dunbar, S. A., Franz, M. J., Mayer-Davis, E. J., . . . American Diabetes Association. (2013). Nutrition therapy recommendations for the management of adults with diabetes. *Diabetes Care, 36*(11), 3821–3842. doi:10.2337/dc13-2042

Franz, M. J., Boucher, J. L., & Evert, A. B. (2014). Evidence-based diabetes nutrition therapy recommendations are effective: the key is individualization. *Diabetes, Metabolic Syndrome, and Obesity: Targets and Therapy, 7*, 65–72. doi:10.2147/DMSO.S45140

Franz, M. J., Boucher, J. L., Rutten-Ramos, S., & Vanwormer, J. J. (2015). Lifestyle weight-loss intervention outcomes in overweight and obese adults with type 2 diabetes: A systematic review and meta-analysis of randomized clinical trials. *Journal of the Academy of Nutrition and Dietetics, 115*(9), 1447–1463.

Franz, M. J., Powers, M. A., Leontos, C., Holzmeister, L. A., Kulkarni, K., Monk, A., . . . Gradwell, E. (2010). The evidence for medical nutrition therapy for type 1 and type 2 diabetes in adults. *Journal of the American Dietetic Association, 110*(12), 1852–1889.

George, P. S., Pearson, E. R., & Witham, M. D. (2012). Effect of vitamin D supplemen-tation on glycaemic control and insulin resistance: A systematic review and meta-analysis. *Diabetes Medicine, 29*(8), e142–e150.

Jahnke, R., Larkey, L., Rogers, C., Etnier, J., & Lin, F. (2010). A Comprehensive review of health benefits of qigong and tai chi. *American Journal of Health Promotion, 24*(6), e1–e25. doi:10.4278/ajhp.081013-LIT-248

Kuhnt, K., Fuhrmann, C., Köhler, M., Kiehntopf, M., & Jahreis, G. (2014). Dietary echium oil increases long-chain n–3 PUFAs, including docosapentaenoic acid, in blood fractions and alters biochemical markers for cardiovascular disease independently of age, sex, and metabolic syndrome. *Journal of Nutrition, 144*(4), 447–460. doi:10.3945/jn.113.180802

Landman, G. W., Bilo, H. J., Houweling, S. T., & Kleefstra, N. (2014). Chromium does not belong in the diabetes treatment arsenal: Current evidence and future perspectives. *World Journal of Diabetes, 5*(2), 160–164. doi:10.4239/wjd.v5.i2.160

Lee, T. C., Ivester, P., Hester, A. G., Sergeant, S., Case, L. D., Morgan, T., . . . Chilton, F. H. (2014). The impact of polyunsaturated fatty acid-based dietary supplements on disease biomarkers in a metabolic syndrome/diabetes population. *Lipids in Health and Disease, 13*, 196. doi:10.1186/1476-511X-13-196

Ogbera, A. O., Ezeobi, E., Unachukwu, C., & Oshinaike, O. (2014). Treatment of diabe-tes mellitus-associated neuropathy with vitamin E and Eve primrose. *Indian Journal of Endocrinology and Metabolism, 18*(6), 846–849. doi:10.4103/2230-8210.140270

Ramalingum, N., & Mahomoodally, M. F. (2014). The therapeutic potential of medici-nal foods. *Advances in Pharmacological Sciences, 354264*. doi:10.1155/2014/354264

Strange, R. C., Shipman, K. E., & Ramachandran, S. (2015). Metabolic syndrome: A review of the role of vitamin D in mediating susceptibility and outcome. *World Journal of Diabetes, 6*(7), 896–911. doi:10.4239/wjd.v6.i7.896

U.S. Department of Health and Human Services & U.S. Department of Agriculture. (2010). *Dietary guidelines for Americans, 2010.* Retrieved from http://www.health.gov /dietaryguidelines

Dysmenorrhea

Benjamin-Pratt, A. R., & Howard, F. M. (2013). Management of chronic pelvic pain. *Minerva Ginecologica, 62*(5), 447–465.

Chiarioni, G., Asteria, C., & Whitehead, W. E. (2011). Chronic proctalgia and chronic pelvic pain syndromes: New etiologic insights and treatment options. *World Journal of Gastroenterology, 17*(40), 4447–4455. doi:10.3748/wjg.v17.i40.4447

Chiarioni, G. (2011). Treatment of levator ani syndrome: Update and future developments. *Recenti Progressi in Medicina, 102*(5), 196–201.

Cho, S. H., & Hwang, E. W. (2010). Acupuncture for primary dysmenorrhoea: A systematic review. *BJOG, 117*(5), 509–521.

Daily, J. W., Zhang, X., Kim, D. S., & Park, S. (2015). Efficacy of ginger for alleviating the symptoms of primary dysmenorrhea: A systematic review and meta-analysis of randomized clinical trials. *Pain Medicine, 16*(12), 2243–2255.

Doggweiler, R., & Stewart, A. F. (2011). Pelvic floor therapies in chronic pelvic pain syndrome. *Current Urology Reports, 12*(4), 304–311.

Fenton, B., Brobeck, L., Witten, E., & Gruenigen, V. V. (2012). Chronic pelvic pain syndrome-related diagnoses in an outpatient office setting. *Gynecologic and Obstetric Investigation, 74*(1), 64–67. doi:10.1159/000336768

Habibi N., Huang, M. S., Gan, W. Y., Zulida, R., & Safavi, S. M. (2015). Prevalence of primary dysmenorrhea and factors associated with its intensity among undergraduate students: A cross-sectional study. *Pain Management Nursing, 16*(6), 855–881.

Iorno, V., Burani, R., Bianchini, B., Minelli, E., Martinelli, F., & Ciatto, S. (2008). Acupuncture treatment of dysmenorrhea resistant to conventional medical treatment. *Evidence-Based Complementary and Alternative Medicine, 5*(2), 227–230. doi:10.1093 /ecam/nem020

Johantgen, M., Fountain, L., Zangaro, G., Newhouse, R., Stanik-Hutt, J., & White, K. (2011). Comparison of labor and delivery care provided by certified nurse-midwives and physicians: A systematic review, 1990 to 2008. *Women's Health Issues, 22*(1), 73–81. doi:10.1016/j.whi.2011.06.005

Lacovides, S., Avidon, I., & Baker, F. C. (2015). What we know about primary dysmenorrhea today: A critical review. *Human Reproduction, 21*(6), 762–778.

McFarlin, B. L., Gibson, M. H., O'Rear, J., & Harman, P. (1999). A national survey of herbal preparation use by nurse-midwives for labor stimulation. Review of the literature and recommendations for practice. *Journal of Nurse-Midwifery, 44*(3), 205–216.

Mirabi, P., Dolatian, M., Mojab, F., & Majd, H. A. (2011). Effects of valerian on the severity and systemic manifestations of dysmenorrhea. *International Journal of Gynecology and Obstetrics, 115*(3), 285–288.

Powell, J. (2014). The approach to chronic pelvic pain in the adolescent. *Obstetrics and Gynecology Clinics of North America, 41*(3), 343–355. doi:10.1016/j.ogc.2014.06.001

Proctor M., & Farquhar, C. (2006). Diagnosis and management of dysmenorrhoea. *British Medical Journal, 332*(7550), 1134–1138.

Rahnama, P., Montazeri, A., Huseini, H. F., Kianbakht, S., & Naseri, M. (2012). Effect of *Zingiber officinale R. rhizomes* (ginger) on pain relief in primary dysmenorrhea: A placebo randomized trial. *BMC Complementary and Alternative Medicine, 12*, 92. doi:10.1186/1472-6882-12-92

Shin, J. H., & Howard, F. M. (2011). Management of chronic pelvic pain. *Current Pain and Headache Reports, 15*(5), 377–385.

Smith, C. A., Crowther, C. A., Petrucco, O., Beilby, J., & Dent, H. (2011). Acupuncture to treat primary dysmenorrhea in women: A randomized controlled trial. *Evidence-Based Complementary and Alternative Medicine*, 1–11. doi:10.1093/ecam/nep239

Smith, C. A., Zhu, X., He, L., & Song, J. (2011). Acupuncture for primary dysmenorrhoea. *Cochrane Database of Systematic Reviews, 1*, CD007854.

Sriprasert, I., Suerungruang, S., Athilarp, P., Matanasarawoot, A., & Teekachunhatean, S. (2015). Efficacy of acupuncture versus combined oral contraceptive pill in treatment of moderate-to-severe dysmenorrhea: A randomized controlled trial. *Evidence-Based Complementary and Alternative Medicine*, 735690. doi:10.1155/2015/735690

Stein, S. L. (2013). Chronic pelvic pain. *Gastroenterology Clinics of North America, 42*(4), 785–800. doi:10.1016/j.gtc.2013.08.005

Valiani, M., Babae, E., Heshmat, R., & Zare, Z. (2010). Comparing the effects of reflexology methods and Ibuprofen administration on dysmenorrhea in female students of Isfahan University of Medical Sciences. *Iranian Journal of Nursery and Midwifery Research, 15*(1), 371–378.

Won, H. R., & Abbott, J. (2010). Optimal management of chronic cyclical pelvic pain: An evidence-based and pragmatic approach. *International Journal of Women's Health, 2*, 263–277. doi:10.2147/IJWH.S7991

Dyspareunia

Benjamin-Pratt, A. R., & Howard, F. M. (2013). Management of chronic pelvic pain. *Minerva Ginecologica, 62*(5), 447–465.

Chervenak, J. L. (2010). Reproductive aging, sexuality and symptoms. *Seminars in Reproductive Medicine, 28*(5), 380–387.

Davis, S. R., & Jane, F. (2011). Sex and perimenopause. *Australian Family Physician, 40*(5), 274–278.

Fenton, B., Brobeck, L., Witten, E., Gruenigen, V. V. (2012). Chronic pelvic pain syndrome-related diagnoses in an outpatient office setting. *Gynecologic and Obstetric Investigation, 74*(1), 64–67. doi:10.1159/000336768

Graziottin, A., Gambini, D., & Bertolasi, L. (2015). Genital and sexual pain in women. In D. B. Vodusek & F. Boller (Eds.), *Handbook of Clinical Neurology* (pp. 395–412). Amsterdam, Netherlands: Elsevier.

Huang, A. J., Moore, E. E., Boyko, E. J., Scholes, D., Lin, F., Vittinghoff, E., & Fihn, S. D. (2010). Vaginal symptoms in postmenopausal women: Self-reported severity, natural history, and risk factors. *Menopause, 17*(1), 121–126. doi:10.1097/gme.0b013e3181acb9ed

Hutchinson-colas, J., & Segal, S. (2015). Genitourinary syndrome of menopause and the use of laser therapy. *Maturitas*. doi:10.1016/j.maturitas.2015.08.001

Jobling, P., O'Hara, K., & Hua, S. (2014). Female reproductive tract pain: Targets, challenges, and outcomes. *Frontiers in Pharmacology, 5*, 17. doi:10.3389/fphar.2014.00017

Kao, A., Binik, Y. M., Kapuscinski, A., & Khalifé, S. (2008). Dyspareunia in postmenopausal women: A critical review. *Pain Research and Management, 13*(3), 243–254.

Lahaie, M. A., Amsel, R., Khalifé, S., Boyer, S., Faaborg-Andersen, M., & Binik, Y. M. (2015). Can fear, pain, and muscle tension discriminate vaginismus from dyspareunia/provoked vestibulodynia? Implications for the new *DSM-5* diagnosis of genito-pelvic pain/penetration disorder. *Archives of Sexual Behavior, 44*(6), 1537–1550.

Portman, D. J., & Gass, M. L. (2014). Genitourinary syndrome of menopause: New terminology for vulvovaginal atrophy from the International Society for the Study of Women's Sexual Health and the North American Menopause Society. *Climacteric, 17*(5), 557–563.

Rao, T. S. S., & Nagaraj, A. K. M. (2015). Female sexuality. *Indian Journal of Psychiatry, 57*(Suppl. 2), S296–S302. doi:10.4103/0019-5545.161496

Rocker, I. (1990). *Pelvic pain in women: Diagnosis and management.* London, England: Springer-Verlag.

Santoro, N., Epperson, C. N., & Mathews, S. B. (2015). Menopausal symptoms and their management. *Endocrinology and Metabolism Clinics of North America, 44*(3), 497–515.

Seehusen, D. A., Baird, D. C., & Bode, D. V. (2014). Dyspareunia in women. *American Family Physician, 90*(7), 465–470.

Travel, J., & Simons, D. (2015). *The trigger point manual.* Baltimore, MD: William & Wilkins.

Endometriosis

Acién, P., & Velasco, I. (2013). Endometriosis: A disease that remains enigmatic. *ISRN Obstetrics and Gynecology,* 242149. doi:10.1155/2013/242149

Brosens, I., Gordts, S., & Benagiano, G. (2013). Endometriosis in adolescents is a hidden, progressive and severe disease that deserves attention, not just compassion. *Human Reproduction, 28*(8), 2026–2031. doi:10.1093/humrep/det243

Chen, Y., Pei, H., Chang, Y., Chen, M., Wang, H., Xie, H., & Yao, S. (2014). The impact of endometrioma and laparoscopic cystectomy on ovarian reserve and the exploration of related factors assessed by serum anti-Mullerian hormone: A prospective cohort study. *Journal of Ovarian Research, 7,* 108. doi:10.1186/s13048-014-0108-0

Cochrane, S., Smith, C. A., Possamai-Inesedy, A., & Bensoussan, A. (2014). Acupuncture and women's health: an overview of the role of acupuncture and its clinical management in women's reproductive health. *International Journal of Women's Health, 6,* 313–325. doi:10.2147/IJWH.S38969

Giri, A., Sturgeon, S. R., Luisi, N., Bertone-Johnson, E., Balasubramanian, R., & Reeves, K. W. (2011). Caffeinated coffee, decaffeinated coffee and endometrial cancer risk: A prospective cohort study among US postmenopausal women. *Nutrients, 3*(11), 937–950. doi:10.3390/nu3110937

Gordts, S., Puttemans, P., Gordts, S., & Brosens, I. (2015). Ovarian endometrioma in the adolescent: A plea for early-stage diagnosis and full surgical treatment. *Gynecological Surgery, 12*(1), 21–30. doi:10.1007/s10397-014-0877-x

Harris, H. R., Chavarro, J. E., Malspeis, S., Willett, W. C., & Missmer, S. A. (2013). Dairy-FOOD, calcium, magnesium, and vitamin D intake and endometriosis: A prospective cohort study. *American Journal of Epidemiology, 177*(5), 420–430. doi:10.1093/aje/kws247

Havens, C. S., & Sullivan, N. D. (2002). *Manual of outpatient gynecology.* Philadelphia, PA: Lippincott Williams & Wilkins.

Jamieson, D. J., Terrell, M. L., Aguocha, N. N., Small, C. M., Cameron, L. L., & Marcus, M. (2011). Dietary exposure to brominated flame retardants and abnormal pap test results. *Journal of Women's Health, 20*(9), 1269–1278. doi:10.1089/jwh.2010.2275

Kim, J. J., Kurita, T., & Bulun, S. E. (2013). Progesterone action in endometrial cancer, endometriosis, uterine fibroids, and breast cancer. *Endocrine Reviews, 34*(1), 130–162. doi:10.1210/er.2012-1043

Kresch, J. A. (1993). Clinical assessment. In D. C. Martin (Ed.), *An atlas of endometriosis* (pp. 3.1–3.8). New York, NY: Grower Medical Publishing.

Lee, J. R., Hanley, J., & Hopkins, V. (1999). *What your doctor may not tell you about pre-menopause*. New York, NY: Warner Books.

Lieke, T., Steinberg, C. E. W, Ju, J., & Saul, N. (2015). Natural marine and synthetic xenobiotics get on nematode's nerves: Neuro-stimulating and neurotoxic findings in *Caenorhabditis elegans*. *Marine Drugs, 13*(5), 2785–2812. doi:10.3390/md13052785

Raffi, F., Metwally, M., & Amer, S. (2012). The impact of excision of ovarian endometrioma on ovarian reserve: a systematic review and meta-analysis. *Journal of Clinical Endocrinology and Metabolism,* 97(9), 3146–3154.

Rahmioglu, N., Missmer, S. A., Montgomery, G. W., & Zondervan, K. T. (2012). Insights into assessing the genetics of endometriosis. *Current Obstetrics and Gynecology Reports, 1*(3), 124–137.

Shaw, S. D., Blum, A., Weber, R., Kannan, K., Rich, D., Lucas, D., . . . Birnbaum, L. S. (2010). Halogenated flame retardants: Do the fire safety benefits justify the risks? *Reviews on Environmental Health,* 25(4), 261–305.

Trabert, B., Peters, U., De Roos, A. J., Scholes, D., & Holt, V. L. (2011). Diet and risk of endometriosis in a population-based case-control study. *British Journal of Nutrition, 105*(3), 459–467. doi:10.1017/S0007114510003661

Fecal Incontinence

Alavi, K., Chan, S., Wise, P., Kaise, A., Sudan, R., & Bordeianou, L. (2015). Fecal incontinence: Etiology, diagnosis and management. *Journal of Gastrointestinal Surgery, 19*(10), 1910–1921.

Bliss, D. Z., Savik, K., Jung, H. J., Whitebird, R., Lowry, A., & Sheng, X. (2014). Dietary fiber supplementation for fecal incontinence: A randomized clinical trial. *Research in Nursing and Health,* 37(5), 367–378.

Kegel, A. M. (1951). Physiologic therapy for urinary stress incontinence. *JAMA, 146*, 915–917.

Norton, C., & Cody, J. D. (2012). Biofeedback and/or sphincter exercises for the treatment of faecal incontinence in adults. *Cochrane Database of Systematic Reviews,* 7, CD002111.

Nygaard, I. E., & Shaw, J. M. (2015). Physical activity and the pelvic floor. *American Journal of Obstetrics and Gynecology,* 214(2), 164–171.

Patel, A. S., Saratzis, A., Arasaradnam, R., & Harmston, C. (2015). Use of antegrade continence enema for the treatment of fecal incontinence and functional constipation in adults: A systematic review. *Diseases of the Colon and Rectum,* 58(10), 999–1013.

Rosenblatt, P. (2015). New developments in therapies for fecal incontinence. *Current Opinion in Obstetrics and Gynecology,* 27(5), 353–358.

Shamliyan, T., Wyman, J., Bliss, D. Z., Kane, R. L., & Wilt, T. J. (2007). Prevention of urinary and fecal incontinence in adults. *Evidence Report/Technology Assessment, 161*, 1–379.

Female Athlete Triad

Ackerman, K. E., & Misra, M. (2011). Bone health in adolescent athletes with a focus on female athlete triad. *The Physician and Sportsmedicine,* 39(1), 131–141. doi:10.3810/psm.2011.02.1871.

Bonci, C. M., Bonci, L. J., Granger, L. R., Johnson, C. L., Malina, R. M., Milne, L. W., . . . Vanderbunt, E. M. (2008). National athletic trainers' association position statement: Preventing, detecting, and managing disordered eating in athletes. *Journal of Athletic Training,* 43(1), 80–108.

Chen, Y.-T., Tenforde, A. S., & Fredericson, M. (2013). Update on stress fractures in female athletes: Epidemiology, treatment, and prevention. *Current Reviews in Musculoskeletal Medicine, 6*(2), 173–181. doi:10.1007/s12178-013-9167-x

Coelho, G. M. O., Gomes A. I. S, Ribeiro, B. G., & Soares, E. A. (2014). Prevention of eating disorders in female athletes. *Open Access Journal of Sports Medicine, 5*, 105–113. doi:10.2147/OAJSM.S36528

Laframboise, M. A., Borody, C., & Stern, P. (2013). The female athlete triad: A case series and narrative overview. *Journal of the Canadian Chiropractic Association, 57*(4), 316–326.

Mallinson, R. J., & De Souza, M. J. (2014). Current perspectives on the etiology and manifestation of the "silent" component of the female athlete triad. *International Journal of Women's Health, 6*, 451–467. doi:10.2147/IJWH.S38603

Nazem, T. G., & Ackerman, K. E. (2012). The female athlete triad. *Sports Health, 4*(4), 302–311. doi:10.1177/1941738112439685

Fibroids/Uterine Leiomyoma

Baird, D. D., Hill, M. C., Schectman, J. M., & Hollis, B. W. (2013). Vitamin D and the risk of uterine fibroids. *Epidemiology, 24*(3), 447–453.

Brunengraber, L. N., Jayes, F. L., & Leppert, P. C. (2014). Injectable *Clostridium histolyticum* collagenase as a potential treatment for uterine fibroids. *Reproductive Sciences, 21*(12), 1452–1459.

Commandeur, A. E., Styer, A. K., & Teixeira, J. M. (2015). Epidemiological and genetic clues for molecular mechanisms involved in uterine leiomyoma development and growth. *Human Reproduction, 21*(5), 593–615.

Eltoukhi, H. M., Modi, M. N., Weston, M., Armstrong, A. Y., & Stewart, E. A. (2014). The health disparities of uterine fibroids for African American women: A public health issue. *American Journal of Obstetrics and Gynecology, 210*(3), 194–199. doi:10.1016/j.ajog.2013.08.008

Formoso, G., Perrone, E., Maltoni, S., Balduzzi, S., D'Amico, R., Bassi, C., . . . Maestri, E. (2012). Short and long term effects of tibolone in postmenopausal women. *Cochrane Database of Systematic Reviews, 2*, CD008536.

Guadarrama-López, A. L., Valdés-Ramos, R., & Martínez-Carrillo, B. E. (2014). Type 2 diabetes, PUFAs, and vitamin D: Their relation to inflammation. *Journal of Immunology Research*, 1–13.

Hart, R. (2003, September). Unexplained infertility, endometriosis, and fibroids. *British Medical Journal, 327*, 721–724.

Islam, M. S., Akhtar, M. M., Ciavattini, A., Giannubilo, S. R., Protic, O., Janjusevic, M., . . . Ciarmela, P. (2014). Use of dietary phytochemicals to target inflammation, fibrosis, proliferation, and angiogenesis in uterine tissues: Promising options for prevention and treatment of uterine fibroids? *Molecular Nutrition and Food Research, 58*(8), 1667–1684. doi:10.1002/mnfr.201400134

Islam, M. S., Protic, O., Stortoni, P., Grechi, G., Lamanna, P., Petraglia, F., . . . Ciarmela, P. (2013). Complex networks of multiple factors in the pathogenesis of uterine leiomyoma. *Fertility and Sterility, 100*(1), 178–193.

Jacoby, V. L., Jacoby, A., Learman, L. A., Schembri, M., Gregorich, S. E., Jackson, R., & Kuppermann, M. (2014). Use of medical, surgical and complementary treatments among women with fibroids. *European Journal of Obstetrics and Gynecology and Reproductive Biology, 182*, 220–225.

Bibliography

Jensen, A. M., Bewketu, B., & Sanford, D. (2011). Intermittent low back pain referred from a uterine adenomyosis: A case report. *Journal of Chiropractic Medicine, 10*(1), 64–69. doi:10.1016/j.jcm.2010.08.004

Kim, J. J., Kurita, T., & Bulun, S. E. (2013). Progesterone action in endometrial cancer, endometriosis, uterine fibroids, and breast cancer. *Endocrine Reviews, 34*(1), 130–162. doi:10.1210/er.2012-1043

Kim, J. J., & Sefton, E. C. (2012). The role of progesterone signaling in the pathogenesis of uterine leiomyoma. *Molecular and Cellular Endocrinology, 358*(2), 223–231. doi:10.1016/j.mce.2011.05.044

Latthe, P., Mignini, L., Gray, R., Hills, R., & Khan, K. (2006). Factors predisposing women to chronic pelvic pain: Systematic review. *British Medical Journal, 332*(7544), 749–755.

Lattimer, J. M., & Haub, M. D. (2010). Effects of dietary fiber and its components on metabolic health. *Nutrients, 2*(12), 1266–1289.

Malik, M., Mendoza, M., Payson, M., & Catherino, W. H. (2009). Curcumin, a nutritional supplement with antineoplastic activity, enhances leiomyoma cell apoptosis and decreases fibronectin expression. *Fertility and Sterility, 91*(Suppl. 5), 2177–2184.

Moorman, P. G., Leppert, P., Myers, E. R., & Wang, F. (2013). Comparison of characteristics of fibroids in African American and white women undergoing pre-menopausal hysterectomy. *Fertility and Sterility, 99*(3), 768–776. doi:10.1016/j.fertnstert.2012.10.039

Ouldamer, L., & Marret, H. (2011). Therapeutic alternatives of uterine fibroids except medicinal treatment and embolization. *Journal de Gynécologie Obstétrique et Biologie de la Reproduction, 40*(8), 928–936.

Peddada, S. D., Laughlin, S. K., Miner, K., Guyon, J. P., Haneke, K., Vahdat, H. L., . . . Baird, D. D. (2008). Growth of uterine leiomyomata among premenopausal black and white women. *Proceedings of the National Academy of Sciences of the United States of America, 105*(50), 19887–19892. doi:10.1073/pnas.0808188105

Plewka, D., Marczyński, J., Morek, M., Bogunia, E., & Plewka, A. (2014). Receptors of hypothalamic-pituitary-ovarian-axis hormone in uterine myomas. *BioMed Research International,* 521313. doi:10.1155/2014/52131

Roshdy, E., Rajaratnam, V., Maitra, S., Sabry, M., Allah, A. S. A., & Al-Hendy, A. (2013). Treatment of symptomatic uterine fibroids with green tea extract: A pilot randomized controlled clinical study. *International Journal of Women's Health, 5,* 477–486. doi:10.2147/IJWH.S41021

Ross, S. M. (2014). Efficacy of a standardized isopropanolic black cohosh (*Actaea racemosa*) extract in treatment of uterine fibroids in comparison with tibolone among patients with menopausal symptoms. *Holistic Nursing Practice, 28*(6), 386–391.

Sabry, M., & Al-Hendy, A. (2012). Medical treatment of uterine leiomyoma. *Reproductive Sciences, 19*(4), 339–353. doi:10.1177/1933719111432867

Santulli, P., Borghese, B., Lemaréchal, H., Leconte, M., Millischer, A., Batteux, F., . . . Borderie, D. (2013). Increased serum oxidative stress markers in women with uterine leiomyoma. *PLoS ONE, 8*(8), e72069. doi:10.1371/journal.pone.0072069

Taylor, D. K., Holthouser, K., Segars, J. H., & Leppert, P. C. (2015). Recent scientific advances in leiomyoma (uterine fibroids) research facilitates better understanding and management. *F1000Research, 4*(F1000 Faculty Rev.), 183. doi:10.12688/f1000research.6189.

Trefoux Bourdet, A., Luton, D., & Koskas, M. (2015). Clinical utility of ulipristal acetate for the treatment of uterine fibroids: Current evidence. *International Journal of Women's Health, 7,* 321–330. doi:10.2147/IJWH.S50016

Vilos, G. A., Allaire, C., Laberge, P. Y., Leyland, N., Special Contributors, Vilos, A. G., . . . Chen, I. (2015). The management of uterine leiomyomas. *Journal of Obstetrics and Gynaecology Canada, 37*(2), 157–181.

Wise, L., Palmer, J. R., Harlow, B. L., Spiegelman, D. B., Stewart, E. A., Adams Campbell, L. L., & Rosenberg, L. (2004). Risk of uterine leiomyomata in relation to tobacco, alcohol and caffeine consumption in the Black Women's Health Study. *Human Reproduction (Oxford, England), 19*(8), 1746–1754. http://doi.org/10.1093/humrep/deh309

Xi, S., Liske, E., Wang, S., Liu, J., Zhang, Z., Geng, L., . . . Bai, W. (2014). Effect of Isopropanolic *Cimicifuga racemosa* extract on uterine fibroids in comparison with tibolone among patients of a recent randomized, double blind, parallel-controlled study in Chinese women with menopausal symptoms. *Evidence-based Complementary and Alternative Medicine,* 717686. doi:10.1155/2014/717686

Fibromyalgia

Arnold, L. M., Clauw, D. J., McCarberg, B. H., for the FibroCollaborative. (2011). Improving the Recognition and Diagnosis of Fibromyalgia. *Mayo Clinic Proceedings, 86*(5), 457–464. doi:10.4065/mcp.2010.0738.

Arnold, L. M., Clauw, D. J., Dunegan, L. J., Turk, D. C., FibroCollaborative. (2012). A framework for fibromyalgia management for primary care providers. *Mayo Clinic Proceedings, 87*(5), 488–496. doi:10.1016/j.mayocp.2012.02.010

Baron, R., Perrot, S., Guillemin, I., Alegre, C., Dias-Barbosa, C., Choy, E., . . . Arnould, B. (2014). Improving the primary care physicians' decision making for fibromyalgia in clinical practice: Development and validation of the fibromyalgia detection (FibroDetect®) screening tool. *Health and Quality of Life Outcomes, 12*, 128. doi:10.1186/s12955-014-0128-x

Bellato, E., Marini, E., Castoldi, F., Barbasetti, N., Mattei, L., Bonasia, D. E., & Blonna, D. (2012). Fibromyalgia syndrome: Etiology, pathogenesis, diagnosis, and treatment. *Pain Research and Treatment,* 426130. doi:10.1155/2012/426130.

Dadabhoy, D., Crofford, L. J., Spaeth, M., Russell, I. J., & Clauw, D. J. (2008). Biology and therapy of fibromyalgia. Evidence-based biomarkers for fibromyalgia syndrome. *Arthritis Research and Therapy, 10*(4), 211. doi:10.1186/ar2443

Dawczynski, C., Hackermeier, U., Viehweger, M., Stange, R., Springer, M., & Jahreis, G. (2011). Incorporation of n-3 PUFA and γ-linolenic acid in blood lipids and red blood cell lipids together with their influence on disease activity in patients with chronic inflammatory arthritis—A randomized controlled human intervention trial. *Lipids in Health and Disease, 10*(130), 130.

Dussias, P., Kalali, A. H., & Staud, R. M. (2010). Treatment of fibromyalgia. *Psychiatry, 7*(5), 15–18.

Fitzcharles, M-A., Ste-Marie, P. A., Goldenberg, D. L., Pereira, J. X., Abbey, S., Choinière, M., . . . National Fibromyalgia Guideline Advisory Panel. (2012). Canadian guidelines for the diagnosis and management of fibromyalgia syndrome: Executive summary. *Pain Research and Management, 18*(3), 119–126.

Hadianfard, M. J., & Hosseinzadeh-Parizi, M. (2012). A randomized clinical trial of fibromyalgia treatment with acupuncture compared with fluoxetine. *Iranian Red Crescent Medical Journal, 14*(10), 631–640.

Häuser, W., Walitt, B., Fitzcharles, M-A., & Sommer, C. (2014). Review of pharmacological therapies in fibromyalgia syndrome. *Arthritis Research and Therapy, 16*(1), 201. doi:10.1186/ar4441

Häuser, W., Klose, P., Langhorst, J., Moradi, B., Steinbach, M., Schiltenwolf, M., & Busch, A. (2010). Efficacy of different types of aerobic exercise in fibromyalgia syndrome: A systematic review and meta-analysis of randomized controlled trials. *Arthritis Research and Therapy, 12*(3), R79. doi:10.1186/ar3002

Häuser, W., Arnold, B., Eich, W., Felde, E., Flügge, C., Henningsen, P., . . . Kopp, I. (2008). Management of fibromyalgia syndrome—An interdisciplinary evidence-based guideline. *German Medical Science, 6,* Doc. 14.

Khasar, S. G., Burkham, J., Dina, O. A., Brown, A. S., Bogen, O., Alessandri-Haber, N., . . . Levine, J. D. (2008). Stress induces a switch of intracellular signaling in sensory neurons in a model of generalized pain. *Journal of Neuroscience, 28*(22), 5721–5730.

Kim, D-H., Yoo, T-H., Lee, S. H., Kang, H. Y., Nam, B. Y., Kwak, S. J., . . . Kang, S. W. (2012). Gamma linolenic acid exerts anti-inflammatory and anti-fibrotic effects in diabetic nephropathy. *Yonsei Medical Journal, 53*(6), 1165–1165.

Malin, K., & Littlejohn, G. O. (2012). Personality and fibromyalgia syndrome. *The Open Rheumatology Journal, 6,* 273–285. doi:10.2174/1874312901206010273

McAllister, S. J., Vincent, A., Hassett, A. L., Whipple, M. O., Oh, T. H., Benzo, R. P., & Toussaint, L. L. (2013). Psychological resilience, affective mechanisms, and symptom burden in a tertiary care sample of patients with fibromyalgia. *Stress and Health.* doi:10.1002/smi.2555

Mist, S. D., Firestone, K. A., & Jones, K. D. (2013). Complementary and alternative exercise for fibromyalgia: A meta-analysis. *Journal of Pain Research, 6,* 247–260. doi:10.2147/JPR.S32297

Okifuji, A., & Hare, B. D. (2013). Management of fibromyalgia syndrome: Review of evidence. *Pain and Therapy, 2*(2), 87–104. doi:10.1007/s40122-013-0016-9

Wolfe, F., Clauw, D. J., Fitzcharles, M.-A., Goldenberg, D. L., Katz, R. S., Mease, P., . . . Yunus, M. B. (2010), The American College of Rheumatology preliminary diagnostic criteria for fibromyalgia and measurement of symptom severity. *Arthritis Care Research, 62,* 600–610. doi:10.1002/acr.20140

Menstrual Disorders

Alijaniha, F., Naseri, M., Afsharypuor, S., Fallahi, F., Noorbala, A., Mosaddegh, M., . . . Sadrai, S. (2015). Heart palpitation relief with *Melissa officinalis* leaf extract: Double blind, randomized, placebo controlled trial of efficacy and safety. *Journal of Ethnopharmacology, 164,* 378–384.

Alramadhan, E., Hanna, M. S., Hanna, M. S., Goldstein, T. A., Avila, S. M., &Weeks, B. S. (2012). Dietary and botanical anxiolytics. *Medical Science Monitor, 18*(4), RA40–RA48. doi:10.12659/MSM.882608

Amos, T., Stein, D. J., & Ipser, J. C. (2014). Pharmacological interventions for preventing post-traumatic stress disorder (PTSD). *Cochrane Database of Systematic Reviews, 7,* CD006239.

Barbee, J. G. (1998). Mixed symptoms and syndromes of anxiety and depression: Diagnostic, prognostic, and etiologic issues. *Annals of Clinical Psychiatry, 10,* 15–29.

Biggs, W. S., & Demuth, R. H. (2011). Premenstrual syndrome and premenstrual dysphoric disorder. *American Family Physician, 84*(8), 918–924.

Bubnov, R. V., Spivak, M. Y., Lazarenko, L. M., Bomba, A., & Boyko, N. V. (2015). Probiotics and immunity: Provisional role for personalized diets and disease prevention. *The EPMA Journal, 6*(1), 14. doi:10.1186/s13167-015-0036-0

Bunevicius, A., Leserman, J., & Girdler, S. (2012). Hypothalamic-pituitary-thyroid axis function in women with a menstrually related mood disorder: Association with histories of sexual abuse. *Psychosomatic Medicine, 74*(8), 810–816. doi:10.1097/PSY.0b013e31826c3397

Bunevicius, A., Rubinow, D. R., Calhoun, A., Leserman, J., Richardson, E., Rozanski, K., & Girdler, S. S. (2013). The association of migraine with menstrually related mood disorders and childhood sexual abuse. *Journal of Women's Health, 22*(10), 871–876. doi:10.1089/jwh.2013.4279

Bystritsky, A., Khalsa, S. S., Cameron, M. E., & Schiffman, J. (2013). Current diagnosis and treatment of anxiety disorders. *Pharmacy and Therapeutics, 38*(1), 30–57.

Cases, J., Ibarra, A., Feuillère, N., Roller, M., & Sukkar, S. G. (2011). Pilot trial of *Melissa officinalis* L. leaf extract in the treatment of volunteers suffering from mild-to-moderate anxiety disorders and sleep disturbances. *Mediterranean Journal of Nutrition and Metabolism, 4*(3), 211–218. doi:10.1007/s12349-010-0045-4

Cooley, K., Szczurko, O., Perri, D., Mills, E. J., Bernhardt, B., Zhou, Q., & Seely, D. (2009). Naturopathic care for anxiety: A randomized controlled trial ISRCTN78958974. *PLoS ONE, 4*(8), e6628. doi:10.1371/journal.pone.0006628

Dash, S., Clarke, G., Berk, M., & Jacka, F. N. (2015). The gut microbiome and diet in psychiatry: Focus on depression. *Current Opinions in Psychiatry, 28*(1), 1–6.

Delara, M., Ghofranipour, F., Azadfallah, P., Tavafian, S. S., Kazemnejad, A., & Montazeri, A. (2012). Health related quality of life among adolescents with premenstrual disorders: A cross-sectional study. *Health and Quality of Life Outcomes, 10*, 1. doi:10.1186/1477-7525-10-1

Demirci, K., Akgönül, M., Demirdaş, A., & Akpınar, A. (2015). Does *Melissa officinalis* cause withdrawal or dependence? *Medical Archives, 69*(1), 60–61. doi:10.5455/medarh.2015.69.60-61

Farahani, M. S., Bahramsoltani, R., Farzaei, M. H., Abdollahi, M., & Rahimi, R. (2015). Plant-derived natural medicines for the management of depression: An overview of mechanisms of action. *Reviews in Neuroscience, 26*(3), 305–321.

Fleischman, D. S., Bunevicius, A., Leserman, J., & Girdler, S. S. (2014). Menstrually related mood disorders and a history of abuse: Moderators of pain sensitivity. *Health Psychology, 33*(2), 147–154.

Foster, J. A., & McVey Neufeld, K. A. (2013). Gut-brain axis: How the microbiome influences anxiety and depression. *Trends in Neuroscience, 36*(5), 305–312.

Head, K. A., & Kelly, G. S. (2009). Nutrients and botanicals for treatment of stress: adrenal fatigue, neurotransmitter imbalance, anxiety, and restless sleep. *Alternative Medicine Review, 14*(2), 114–140.

Ipser, J. C., Wilson, D., Akindipe, T. O., Sager, C., & Stein, D. J. (2015). Pharmacotherapy for anxiety and comorbid alcohol use disorders. *Cochrane Database of Systematic Reviews, 1*, CD007505.

Kleinstäuber, M., Witthöft, M., Steffanowski, A., Van marwijk, H., Hiller, W., & Lambert, M. J. (2014). Pharmacological interventions for somatoform disorders in adults. *Cochrane Database of Systematic Reviews, 11*, CD010628.

Lakhan, S. E., & Vieira, K. F. (2010). Nutritional and herbal supplements for anxiety and anxiety-related disorders: Systematic review. *Nutrition Journal, 9*, 42. doi:10.1186/1475-2891-9-42

Moloney, R. D., Desbonnet, L., Clarke, G., Dinan, T. G., & Cryan, J. F. (2014). The microbiome: Stress, health and disease. *Mammalian Genome, 25*(1–2), 49–74.

National Institutes of Health and National Institute of Mental Health. (n.d.) *Anxiety disorders*. Retrieved from http://www.nimh.nih.gov/health/topics/anxiety-disorders/index.shtml

Pratte, M. A., Nanavati, K. B., Young, V., & Morley, C. P. (2014). An alternative treatment for anxiety: A systematic review of human trial results reported for the Ayurvedic herb Ashwagandha (*Withania somnifera*). *Journal of Alternative and Complementary Medicine, 20*(12), 901–908. doi:10.1089/acm.2014.0177

Puetz, T. W., Youngstedt, S. D., & Herring, M. P. (2015). Effects of pharmacotherapy on combat-related PTSD, anxiety, and depression: A systematic review and meta-regression analysis. *PLoS ONE, 10*(5), e0126529. doi:10.1371/journal.pone.0126529

Ross, S. M. (2014). Psychophytomedicine: An overview of clinical efficacy and phyto-pharmacology for treatment of depression, anxiety and insomnia. *Holistic Nursing Practice, 28*(4), 275–280.

Sarris, J., Laporte, E., & Schweitzer, I. (2011). Kava: A comprehensive review of efficacy, safety, and psychopharmacology. *Australian and New Zealand Journal of Psychiatry, 45*(1), 27–35.

Sarris, J., Stough, C., Bousman, C. A., Wahid, Z. T., Murray, G., Teschke, R., . . . Schweitzer, I. (2013). Kava in the treatment of generalized anxiety disorder: A double-blind, randomized, placebo-controlled study. *Journal of Clinical Psychopharmacology, 33*(5), 643–648.

Van dessel, N., Den boeft, M., Van der wooden, J. C., Kleinstäuber, M., Leone, S. S., Terluin, B., . . . van Marwijk, H. (2014). Non-pharmacological interventions for somatoform disorders and medically unexplained physical symptoms (MUPS) in adults. *Cochrane Database of Systematic Reviews, 11*, CD011142.

Osteoporosis

Adami, S., Idolazzi, L., Fracassi, E., Gatti, D., & Rossini, M. (2013). Osteoporosis treatment: When to discontinue and when to re-start. *Bone Research, 1*(4), 323–335. doi:10.4248/BR201304003

Agency for Healthcare Research and Quality. (2012). *Comparative effectiveness review summary guides for clinicians: Treatment to prevent osteoporotic fractures: An update.* Retrieved from http://www.ncbi.nlm.nih.gov/books/NBK107167/

Balvers, M. G. J., Brouwer-Brolsma, E. M., Endenburg, S., de Groot, L. C. P. G. M, Kok, F. J., & Gunnewiek, J. K. (2015). Recommended intakes of vitamin D to optimise health, associated circulating 25-hydroxyvitamin D concentrations, and dosing regimens to treat deficiency: Workshop report and overview of current literature. *Journal of Nutritional Science, 4*, e23. doi:10.1017/jns.2015.10

Bernabei, R., Martone, A. M., Ortolani, E., Landi, F., & Marzetti, E. (2014). Screening, diagnosis and treatment of osteoporosis: A brief review. *Clinical Cases in Mineral and Bone Metabolism, 11*(3), 201–207.

Cooper, C., Reginster, J. Y., Cortet, B., Diaz-Curiel, M., Lorenc, R. S., Kanis, J. A., & Rizzoli, R. (2012). Long-term treatment of osteoporosis in postmenopausal women: A review from the European Society for Clinical and Economic Aspects of Osteoporosis and Osteoarthritis (ESCEO) and the International Osteoporosis Foundation (IOF). *Current Medical Research and Opinion, 28*(3), 475–491.

Cranney, A., Horsley, T., O'Donnell, S., Weiler, H., Puil, L., Ooi, D., . . . Mamaladze, V. (2007). Effectiveness and safety of vitamin D in relation to bone health. *Evidence Report/Technology Assessment, 158*, 1–235.

Haworth, A. E., & Webb, J. (2012). Skeletal complications of bisphosphonate use: What the radiologist should know. *British Journal of Radiology, 85*(1018), 1333–1342. doi:10.1259/bjr/99102700

Bibliography

Hiligsmann, M., Bours, S. P. G., & Boonen, A. (2015). A review of patient preferences for osteoporosis drug treatment. *Current Rheumatology Reports, 17*(9), 61. doi:10.1007/s11926-015-0533-0

Jahnke, R., Larkey, L., Rogers, C., Etnier, J., & Lin, F. (2010). A comprehensive review of health benefits of qigong and tai chi. *American Journal of Health Promotion, 24*(6), e1–e25. doi:10.4278/ajhp.081013-LIT-248

Leung, P.-C., & Siu, W-S. (2013). Herbal treatment for osteoporosis: A current review. *Journal of Traditional and Complementary Medicine, 3*(2), 82–87. doi:10.4103/2225-4110.110407

Levis, S., & Theodore, G. (2012). Summary of AHRQ's comparative effectiveness review of treatment to prevent fractures in men and women with low bone density or osteoporosis: Update of the 2007 report. *Journal of Managed Care Pharmacy, 18*(4, Suppl. B), S1–S15.

Liu, R-H., Kang, X., Xu, L-P., Nian, H-L., Yang, X-W., Shi, H-T., & Wang, X-J. (2015). Effects of the combined extracts of *Herba epimedii* and *Fructus ligustri lucidi* on bone mineral content and bone turnover in osteoporotic rats. *BMC Complementary and Alternative Medicine, 15,* 112. doi:10.1186/s12906-015-0641-4

Reginster, J. Y. (2011). Antifracture efficacy of currently available therapies for postmenopausal osteoporosis. *Drugs, 71*(1), 65–78.

Rizzoli, R., Reginster, J-Y., Boonen, S., Bréart, G., Diez-Perez, A., Felsenberg, D., . . . Cooper, C. (2011). Adverse reactions and drug–drug interactions in the management of women with postmenopausal osteoporosis. *Calcified Tissue International, 89*(2), 91–104. doi:10.1007/s00223-011-9499-8

Saylor, P. J. (2014). Bone targeted therapies for the prevention of skeletal morbidity in men with prostate cancer. *Asian Journal of Andrology, 16*(3), 341–347. doi:10.4103/1008-682X.122591

Silverman, S., Calderon, A., Kaw, K., Childers, T. B., Stafford, B. A., Brynildsen, W., . . . Gold, D. T. (2013). Patient weighting of osteoporosis medication attributes across racial and ethnic groups: A study of osteoporosis medication preferences using conjoint analysis. *Osteoporosis International, 24*(7), 2067–2077.

Silverman, S., & Christiansen, C. (2012). Individualizing osteoporosis therapy. *Osteoporosis International, 23*(3), 797–809.

Stevenson, J. C. (2011). Prevention of osteoporosis: One step forward, two steps back. *Menopause International, 17*(4), 137–141.

Pelvic Inflammatory Disease

Braundmeier, A. G., Lenz, K. M., Inman, K. S., Chia, N., Jeraldo, P., Walther-António, M. R. S., . . . White, B. A. (2015). Individualized medicine and the microbiome in reproductive tract. *Frontiers in Physiology, 6,* 97. doi:10.3389/fphys.2015.00097

Dhasmana, D., Hathorn, E., McGrath, R., Tariq, A., & Ross, J. D. (2014). The effectiveness of nonsteroidal anti-inflammatory agents in the treatment of pelvic inflammatory disease: A systematic review. *Systematic Reviews, 3,* 79. doi:10.1186/2046-4053-3-79

Duarte, R., Fuhrich, D., & Ross, J. D. (2015). A review of antibiotic therapy for pelvic inflammatory disease. *International Journal of Antimicrobial Agents, 46*(3), 272–277.

Jaiyeoba, O., Lazenby, G., & Soper, D. E. (2011). Recommendations and rationale for the treatment of pelvic inflammatory disease. *Expert Review of Anti-infective Therapy, 9*(1), 61–70.

Rizzo, A., Fiorentino, M., Buommino, E., Donnarumma, G., Losacco, A., & Bevilacqua, N. (2015). *Lactobacillus crispatus* mediates anti-inflammatory cytokine interleukin-10 induction in response to *Chlamydia trachomatis* infection in vitro. *International Journal of Medical Microbiology, 305*(8), 815–827. doi:10.1016/j.ijmm.2015.07.005

Soper, D. E. (2010). Pelvic inflammatory disease. *Obstetrics and Gynecology, 116*(2 Pt. 1), 419–428.

Tepper, N. K., Steenland, M. W., Gaffield, M. E., Marchbanks, P. A., & Curtis, K. M. (2013). Retention of intrauterine devices in women who acquire pelvic inflammatory disease: A systematic review. *Contraception, 87*(5), 655–660.

Terzić, M., & Kocijancić, D. (2010). Pelvic inflammatory disease: Contemporary diagnostic and therapeutic approach, *Srpski arhiv za celokupno lekarstvo, 138*(9–10), 658–663.

Perimenopause

Chai, W., Novotny, R., Maskarinec, G., Le Marchand, L., Franke, A. A., & Cooney, R. V. (2014). Serum coenzyme Q10, α-tocopherol, γ-tocopherol, and C-reactive protein levels and body mass index in adolescent and premenopausal females. *Journal of the American College of Nutrition, 33*(3), 192–197. doi:10.1080/07315724.2013.862490

Clark, C., Rodgers, B., Caldwell, T., Power, C., & Stansfeld, S. (2007). Childhood and adulthood psychological ill health as predictors of midlife affective and anxiety disorders. *Archives of General Psychiatry, 64*(6), 668–678.

Demirci, K., Akgönül, M., Demirdaş, A., Akpınar, A. (2015). Does Melissa officinalis cause withdrawal or dependence? *Medical Archives, 69*(1), 60–61. doi:10.5455/medarh.2015.69.60-61

Doshi, S. B., & Agarwal, A. (2013). The role of oxidative stress in menopause. *Journal of Mid-Life Health, 4*(3), 140–146. doi:10.4103/0976-7800.118990

Drewe, J., Bucher, K. A., & Zahner, C. (2015). A systematic review of non-hormonal treatments of vasomotor symptoms in climacteric and cancer patients. *SpringerPlus, 4*, 65. doi:10.1186/s40064-015-0808-y

Luzia, A. L., Aldrighi, M. J., Damasceno, T. N., Sampaio, R. G., Soares, A. M. R., Silva, T. I., . . . Torres, F. S. E. (2015). Fish oil and vitamin E change lipid profiles and anti-LDL-antibodies in two different ethnic groups of women transitioning through menopause. *Nutricion Hospitalaria, 32*(1), 165–174.

Malik, S. (2013). Midlife disorders. *Journal of Mid-Life Health, 4*(3), 139. doi:10.4103/0976-7800.118989

Nastri, C. O., Lara, L. A., Ferriani, R. A., Rose-E-Silva, A. C., Figueiredo, J. B., & Martins, W. P. (2013). Hormone therapy for sexual function in perimenopausal and postmenopausal women. *Cochrane Database of Systematic Reviews, 6*, CD009672. doi:10.1002/14651858.CD009672.pub2

Parazzini, F. (2015). Resveratrol, tryptophanum, glycine and vitamin E: A nutraceutical approach to sleep disturbance and irritability in peri- and post-menopause. *Minerva Ginecologica, 67*(1), 1–5.

Prior, J. C. (2011). Progesterone for symptomatic perimenopause treatment—Progesterone politics, physiology and potential for perimenopause. *Facts, Views, and Vision in ObGyn, 3*(2), 109–120.

Ruiz, A. D., Daniels, K. R., Barner, J. C., Carson, J. J., & Frei, C. R. (2011). Effectiveness of compounded bioidentical hormone replacement therapy: An observational cohort study. *BMC Women's Health, 11*, 27. doi:10.1186/1472-6874-11-27

Saensak, S., Vutyavanich, T., Somboonporn, W., & Srisurapanont, M. (2014). Relaxation for perimenopausal and postmenopausal symptoms. *Cochrane Database of Systematic Reviews, 7*, CD008582. doi:10.1002/14651858.CD008582.pub2

Polycystic Ovarian Syndrome

American College of Obstetricians and Gynecologists. (2011). *Polycystic ovary syndrome.* Retrieved from http://www.acog.org/~/media/For%20Patients/faq121.pdf?dmc=1&ts =20120510T1116545699

Amini, L., Tehrani, N., Movahedin, M., Ramezani Tehrani, F., & Ziaee, S. (2015). Antioxidants and management of polycystic ovary syndrome in Iran: A systematic review of clinical trials. *Iranian Journal of Reproductive Medicine, 13*(1), 1–8.

Andrews, M. A., Schliep, K. C., Wactawski-Wende, J., Stanford, J. B., Zarek, S. M., Radin, R. G., . . . Mumford, S. L. (2015). Dietary factors and luteal phase deficiency in healthy eumenorrheic women. *Human Reproduction (Oxford, England), 30*(8), 1942–1951. http://doi.org/10.1093/humrep/dev133

Cappelli, V., Di Sabatino, A., Musacchio, M. C., & De leo, V. (2013). Evaluation of a new association between insulin-sensitizers and α-lipoic acid in obese women affected by PCOS. *Minerva Ginecologia, 65*(4), 425–433.

Cochrane, S., Smith, C., Possamai-Inesedy, A., & Bensoussan, A. (2014). Acupuncture and women's health: An overview of the role of acupuncture and its clinical management in women's reproductive health. *International Journal of Women's Health, 6,* 313–325. doi:10.2147/IJWH.S38969

Cui, W., Li, J., Sun, W., & Wen, J. (2011). Effect of electroacupuncture on oocyte quality and pregnancy of patients with PCOS undergoing in vitro fertilization and embryo transfer. *World Journal of Acupuncture—Moxibustion, 31*(8), 687–691.

De Leo, V., Tosti, C., Cappelli, V., Morgante, G., & Cianci, E. A. (2014). Combination inositol and glucomannan in PCOS patients. *Minerva Ginecologica, 66*(6), 527–533.

He, C., Lin, Z., Robb, S. W., & Ezeamama, A. E. (2015). Serum vitamin D levels and polycystic ovary syndrome: A systematic review and meta-analysis. *Nutrients, 7*(6), 4555–4577. doi:10.3390/nu7064555

Jakimiuk, A. J., & Szamatowicz, J. (2014). The role of inositol deficiency in the etiology of polycystic ovary syndrome disorders. *Ginekologia Polska, 85*(1), 54–57.

Johansson, J., & Stener-Victorin, E. (2013). Polycystic ovary syndrome: Effect and mechanisms of acupuncture for ovulation induction. *Evidence-Based Complementary and Alternative Medicine,* 762615. doi:10.1155/2013/762615

Krul-Poel, Y. H., Snackey, C., Louwers, Y., Lips, P., Lambalk, C., Laven, J., & Simsek, S. (2013). The role of vitamin D in metabolic disturbances in polycystic ovary syndrome: A systematic review. *European Journal of Endocrinology, 169*(6), 853–865.

Lim, S. S., Norman, R. J., Davies, M. J., & Moran, L. J. (2013). The effect of obesity on polycystic ovary syndrome: a systematic review and meta-analysis. *Obesity Reviews, 14*(2), 95–109.

Lin, A. W., & Lujan, M. E. (2014). Comparison of dietary intake and physical activity between women with and without polycystic ovary syndrome: A review. *Advances in Nutrition, 5*(5), 486–496. doi:10.3945/an.113.005561

Moran, L. J., Hutchison, S. K., Norman, R. J., & Teede, H. J. (2011). Lifestyle changes in women with polycystic ovary syndrome. *Cochrane Database of Systematic Reviews, 7,* CD007506.

Musacchio, M. C., Cappelli, V., Di Sabatino, A., Morgante, G., & De Leo, V. (2013). Evaluation of the myo-inositol-monacolin K association on hyperandrogenism and on the lipidic metabolism parameters in PCOS women. *Minerva Ginecologica, 65*(1), 89–97.

Nadjarzadeh, A., Dehghani Firouzabadi, R., Vaziri, N., Daneshbodi, H., Lotfi, M. H., & Mozaffari-Khosravi, H. (2013). The effect of omega-3 supplementation on androgen profile and menstrual status in women with polycystic ovary syndrome: A randomized clinical trial. *Iranian Journal of Reproductive Medicine, 11*(8), 665–672.

Sacchinelli, A., Venturella, R., Lico, D., Di Cello, A., Lucia, A., Rania, E., . . . Zullo, F. (2014). The efficacy of inositol and n-acetyl cysteine administration (Ovaric HP) in improving the ovarian function in infertile women with PCOS with or without insulin resistance. *Obstetrics and Gynecology International,* 141020. doi:10.1155/2014/141020.

Sahin, S., Eroglu, M., & Selcuk, S., Turkgeldi, L., Kozali, S., Davutoglu, S., & Muhcu, M. (2014). Intrinsic factors rather than vitamin D deficiency are related to insulin resistance in lean women with polycystic ovary syndrome. *European Review for Medical and Pharmacological Sciences, 18*(19), 2851–2856.

Shahnazi, V., Zaree, M., Nouri, M., Mehrzad-Sadaghiani, M., Fayezi, S., Darabi, M. . . . Darabi, M. (2015). Influence of ω-3 fatty acid eicosapentaenoic acid on IGF-1 and COX-2 gene expression in granulosa cells of PCOS women. *Iranian Journal of Reproductive Medicine, 13*(2), 71–78.

Unfer, V., Carlomagno, G., Dante, G., & Facchinetti, F. (2012). Effects of myo-inositol in women with PCOS: a systematic review of randomized controlled trials. *Gynecology and Endocrinology, 28*(7), 509–515.

Unfer, V., & Porcaro, G. (2014). Updates on the myo-inositol plus D-chiro-inositol combined therapy in polycystic ovary syndrome. *Expert Review of Clinical Pharmacology, 7*(5), 623–631.

United States Department of Health and Human Services. (n.d.). *Treatment of PCOS.* Retrieved from http://www.nichd.nih.gov/health/topics/PCOS/conditioninfo/Pages /relieve.aspx

Pregnancy

Adams, R., White, B., & Beckett, C. (2010). The effects of massage therapy on pain management in the acute care setting. *International Journal of Therapeutic Massage and Bodywork, 3*(1), 4–11.

Begley, C. M., Gyte, G. M., Murphy, D. J., Devane, D., Mcdonald, S. J., & Mcguire, W. (2010). Active versus expectant management for women in the third stage of labour. *Cochrane Database of Systematic Reviews, 7,* CD007412.

Bergström, C., Persson, M., & Mogren, I. (2014). Pregnancy-related low back pain and pelvic girdle pain approximately 14 months after pregnancy—Pain status, self-rated health and family situation. *BMC Pregnancy and Childbirth, 14,* 48. doi:10.1186/1471-2393-14-48

Copp, S. (2010a). Craniosacral therapy (1): From conception to birth. *Practicing Midwife, 13*(5), 20–22.

Copp, S. (2010b). Craniosacral therapy (2): Postnatal care for parents and babies. *Practicing Midwife, 13*(6), 31–32.

Dante, G., Bellei, G., Neri, I., & Facchinetti, F. (2014). Herbal therapies in pregnancy: What works? *Current Opinion in Obstetrics and Gynecology, 26*(2), 83–91.

Dean, S. V., Lassi, Z. S., Imam, A. M., & Bhutta, Z. A. (2014). Preconception care: Nutritional risks and interventions. *Reproductive Health, 11*(Suppl. 3), S3. doi:10.1186 /1742-4755-11-S3-S3

Djakovic, I., Djakovic, Z., Bilić, N., & Košec, V. (2015). Third stage of labor and acupuncture. *Medical Acupuncture, 27*(1), 10–13.

Drouillet-Pinard, P., Huel, G., Slama, R., Forhan, A., Sahuquillo, J., Goua, V., . . . Charles, M.-A. (2010). Prenatal mercury contamination: relationship with maternal seafood consumption during pregnancy and fetal growth in the "EDEN mother-child" cohort. *British Journal of Nutrition, 104*(8), 1096–1100. doi:10.1017 /S0007114510001947

Eberhard-gran, M., Slinning, K., & Rognerud, M. (2014). Screening for postnatal depression—A summary of current knowledge. *Tidsskr Nor Laegeforen, 134*(3), 297–301.

Elden, H., Östgaard, H. C., Glantz, A., Marciniak, P., Linnér, A. C., & Olsén, M. F. (2013). Effects of craniosacral therapy as adjunct to standard treatment for pelvic girdle pain in pregnant women: A multicenter, single blind, randomized controlled trial. *Acta Obstetricia et Gynecologica Scandinavica, 92*(7), 775–782.

Engel, S. M., & Wolff, M. S. (2013). Causal inference considerations for endocrine disruptor research in children's health. *Annual Review of Public Health, 34,* 139–158. doi:10.1146/annurev-publhealth-031811-124556

Epstein, J. B. (1980). The mouth: A window on systemic disease. *Canadian Family Physician, 26,* 953–957.

Gruber, C. W., & O'Brien, M. (2011). Uterotonic plants and their bioactive constituents. *Planta Medica, 77*(3), 207–220. doi:10.1055/s-0030-1250317

Gürsoy, M., Zeidán-Chuliá, F., Könönen, E., Moreira, J. C. F., Liukkonen, J., Sorsa, T., Gürsoy, U. K. (2014). Pregnancy-induced gingivitis and OMICS in dentistry: *In silico* modeling and in vivo prospective validation of estradiol-modulated inflammatory biomarkers. *OMICS, 18*(9), 582–590. doi:10.1089/omi.2014.0020

Gutke, A., Betten, C., Degerskär, K., Pousette, S., & Fagevik Olsén, M. (2015). Treatments for pregnancy-related lumbopelvic pain: A systematic review of physiotherapy modalities. *Acta Obstetricia et Gynecologica Scandinavica, 94*(11), 1156–1167. doi:10.1111/aogs.12681

Hall, H. G., Griffiths, D. L., & McKenna, L. G. (2011). The use of complementary and alternative medicine by pregnant women: A literature review. *Midwifery, 27*(6), 817–824.

Hines, E. P., Calafat, A. M., Silva, M. J., Mendola, P., & Fenton, S. E. (2009). Concentrations of phthalate metabolites in milk, urine, saliva, and serum of lactating North Carolina women. *Environmental Health Perspectives, 117*(1), 86–92. doi:10.1289 /ehp.11610

Hines, E. P., Mendola, P., Von Ehrenstein, O. S., Ye, X., Calafat, A. M., & Fenton, S. E. (2015). Concentrations of environmental phenols and parabens in milk, urine and serum of lactating North Carolina women. *Reproductive Toxicology, 54,* 120–128.

Holden, S. C., Gardiner, P., Birdee, G., Davis, R. B., & Yeh, G. Y. (2015). Complementary and alternative medicine use among women during pregnancy and childbearing years. *Birth, 42*(3), 261–269.

Kelley, K. E., Hernández-Díaz, S., Chaplin, E. L., Hauser, R., & Mitchell, A. A. (2012). Identification of phthalates in medications and dietary supplement formulations in the United States and Canada. *Environmental Health Perspectives, 120*(3), 379–384. doi:10.1289/ehp.1103998

Lassi, Z. S., Imam, A. M., Dean, S. V., & Bhutta, Z. A. (2014). Preconception care: Caffeine, smoking, alcohol, drugs and other environmental chemical/radiation exposure. *Reproductive Health, 11*(Suppl. 3), S6. doi:10.1186/1742-4755-11-S3-S6

Lassi, Z. S, Mansoor, T., Salam, R. A., Das, J. K., & Bhutta, Z. A. (2014). Essential prepregnancy and pregnancy interventions for improved maternal, newborn and child health. *Reproductive Health, 11*(Suppl. 1), S2. doi:10.1186/1742-4755-11-S1-S2

Lewis, S. J., Araya, R., Leary, S., Smith, G. D., & Ness, A. (2012). Folic acid supplementation during pregnancy may protect against depression 21 months after pregnancy, an effect modified by MTHFR C677T genotype. *European Journal of Clinical Nutrition, 66*(1), 97–103.

Bibliography

Lu, H-X., Xu, W., Wong, M. C. M., Wei, T-Y., & Feng, X-P. (2015). Impact of periodontal conditions on the quality of life of pregnant women: A cross-sectional study. *Health and Quality of Life Outcomes, 13*, 67. doi:10.1186/s12955-015-0267-8

Lyall, K., Munger, K. L., O'Reilly, É. J., Santangelo, S. L., & Ascherio, A. (2013). Maternal dietary fat intake in association with autism spectrum disorders. *American Journal of Epidemiology, 178*(2), 209–220. doi:10.1093/aje/kws433

Matthews, A., Dowswell, T., Haas, D. M., Doyle, M., & O'Mathúna, D. P. (2010). Interventions for nausea and vomiting in early pregnancy. *Cochrane Database of Systematic Reviews, 9,* CD007575. doi:10.1002/14651858.CD007575.pub2

Matthews, A., Haas, D. M., O'Mathúna, D. P., Dowswell, T., & Doyle, M. (2014). Interventions for nausea and vomiting in early pregnancy. *Cochrane Database of Systematic Reviews, 3,* CD007575.

Oladapo, O. T., Okusanya, B. O., & Abalos, E. (2012). Intramuscular versus intravenous prophylactic oxytocin for the third stage of labour. *Cochrane Database of Systematic Reviews, 2,* CD009332.

Peterson, C. K., Mühlemann, D., & Humphreys, B. K. (2014). Outcomes of pregnant patients with low back pain undergoing chiropractic treatment: A prospective cohort study with short term, medium term and 1 year follow-up. *Chiropractic and Manual Therapies, 22,* 15. doi:10.1186/2045-709X-22-15

Pistollato, F., Sumalla Cano, S., Elio, I., Masias Vergara, M., Giampieri, F., & Battino, M. (2015). Plant-based and plant-rich diet patterns during gestation: Beneficial effects and possible shortcomings. *Advances in Nutrition, 6*(5), 581–591.

Poomalar, G. K. (2015). Changing trends in management of gestational diabetes mellitus. *World Journal of Diabetes, 6*(2), 284–295. doi:10.4239/wjd.v6.i2.284

Rogozińska, E., Chamillard, M., Hitman, G. A., Khan, K. S., & Thangaratinam, S. (2015). Nutritional manipulation for the primary prevention of gestational diabetes mellitus: A meta-analysis of randomised studies. *PLoS ONE, 10*(2), e0115526. doi:10.1371/journal.pone.0115526

Sadr, S., Pourkiani-Allah-Abad, N., & Stuber, K. J. (2012). The treatment experience of patients with low back pain during pregnancy and their chiropractors: A qualitative study. *Chiropractic and Manual Therapies, 20,* 32. doi:10.1186/2045-709X-20-32

Segre, L. S., O'Hara, M. W., Arndt, S., & Beck, C. T. (2010). Nursing care for postpartum depression, part 1: Do nurses think they should offer both screening and counseling? *American Journal of Maternal/Child Nursing, 35*(4), 220–225. doi:10.1097/NMC.0b013e3181dd9d81

Segre, L. S., O'Hara, M. W., Arndt, S., & Beck, C. T. (2010). Screening and counseling for postpartum depression by nurses: The women's views. *American Journal of Maternal/Child Nursing, 35*(5), 280–285. doi:10.1097/NMC.0b013e3181e62679

Shrivastava, S. R., Shrivastava, P. S., & Ramasamy, J. (2015). Antenatal and postnatal depression: A public health perspective. *Journal of Neurosciences in Rural Practice, 6*(1), 116–119. doi:10.4103/0976-3147.143218

Soltani, H., Hutchon, D. R., & Poulose, T. A. (2010). Timing of prophylactic uterotonics for the third stage of labour after vaginal birth. *Cochrane Database of Systematic Reviews, 8,* CD006173.

Spencer, K. M. (2008). Craniosacral therapy in the midwifery model of care. *Midwifery Today: International Midwife, 87,* 14–15, 65.

Tandon, S. D., Cluxton-Keller, F., Leis, J., Le, H-N., & Perry, D. F. (2012). A comparison of three screening tools to identify perinatal depression among low-income African

American women. *Journal of Affective Disorders, 136*(0), 155–162. doi:10.1016/j.jad.2011.07.014

Terrell, M. L., Hartnett, K. P., Lim, H., Wirth, J., & Marcus, M. (2015). Maternal exposure to brominated flame retardants and infant Apgar scores. *Chemosphere, 118,* 178–186.

U.S. Environmental Protection Agency. (2013). *What you need to know about fish and mercury.* Retrieved from http://water.epa.gov/scitech/swguidance/fishshellfish/outreach/advice_index.cfm

Vejrup, K., Brantsæter, A. L., Knutsen, H. K., Magnus, P., Alexander, J., Kvalen, H., . . . Haugen, M. (2014). Prenatal mercury exposure and infant birth weight in the Norwegian Mother and Child Cohort Study. *Public Health and Nutrition, 17*(9), 2071–2080.

Viljoen, E., Visser, J., Koen, N., & Musekiwa, A. (2014). A systematic review and meta-analysis of the effect and safety of ginger in the treatment of pregnancy-associated nausea and vomiting. *Nutrition Journal, 13,* 20. doi:10.1186/1475-2891-13-20

Premature Ovarian Failure

Alramadhan, E., Hanna, M. S., Hanna, M. S., Goldstein, T. A., Avila, S. M., & Weeks, B. S. (2012). Dietary and botanical anxiolytics. *Medical Science Monitor, 18*(4), RA40–RA48. doi:10.12659/MSM.882608

Chen, Y., Fang, Y., Yang, J., Wang, F., Wang, Y., & Yang, L. (2014). Effect of acupuncture on premature ovarian failure: A pilot study. *Evidence-Based Complementary and Alternative Medicine,* 718675. doi:10.1155/2014/718675

Colafrancesco, S., Perricone, C., Tomljenovic, L., & Shoenfeld, Y. (2013). Human papilloma virus vaccine and primary ovarian failure: Another facet of the autoimmune/inflammatory syndrome induced by adjuvants. *American Journal of Reproductive Immunology, 70*(4), 309–315.

Corazza, O., Martinotti, G., Santacroce, R., Chillemi, E., Di Giannantonio, M., Schifano, F., & Cellek, S. (2014). Sexual enhancement products for sale online: Raising awareness of the psychoactive effects of yohimbine, maca, horny goat weed, and ginkgo biloba. *BioMed Research International,* 841798. doi:10.1155/2014/841798

Dording, C. M., Schettler, P. J., Dalton, E. D., Parkin, S., Walker, R., Fehling, K., . . . Mischoulon, D. (2015). A double-blind placebo-controlled trial of maca root as treatment for antidepressant-induced sexual dysfunction in women. *Evidence-Based Complementary and Alternative Medicine,* 949036. doi:10.1155/2015/949036

Jo, J., Lee, Y. J., & Lee, H. (2015). Effectiveness of acupuncture for primary ovarian insufficiency: A systematic review and meta-analysis. *Evidence-based Complementary and Alternative Medicine,* 842180. doi:10.1155/2015/842180

Johansson, J., & Stener-Victorin, E. (2013). Polycystic ovary syndrome: Effect and mechanisms of acupuncture for ovulation induction. *Evidence-Based Complementary and Alternative Medicine,* 762615. doi:10.1155/2013/762615

Kodaman, P. H. (2010). Early menopause: Primary ovarian insufficiency and surgical menopause. *Seminars in Reproductive Medicine, 28*(5), 360–369.

Lee, M. S., Shin, B. C., Yang, E. J., Lim, H. J., & Ernst, E. (2011). Maca (*Lepidium meyenii*) for treatment of menopausal symptoms: A systematic review. *Maturitas, 70*(3), 227–233.

Little, D. T., & Ward, H. R. (2014). Adolescent premature ovarian insufficiency following human papillomavirus vaccination: A case series seen in general practice. *Journal of Investigative Medicine High Impact Case Reports, 2*(4), 2324709614556129.

Pangas, S. A. (2012). Regulation of the ovarian reserve by members of the transforming growth factor beta family. *Molecular Reproduction and Development, 79*(10), 666–679. doi:10.1002/mrd.22076

Powers, C. N., & Setzer, W. N. (2015). A molecular docking study of phytochemical estrogen mimics from dietary herbal supplements. *In Silico Pharmacology, 3*, 4. doi:10.1186/s40203-015-0008-z

Qureshi, N. A., & Al-Bedah, A. M. (2013). Mood disorders and complementary and alternative medicine: A literature review. *Neuropsychiatric Disease and Treatment, 9*, 639–658. doi:10.2147/NDT.S43419

Rosenberg, S. M., & Partridge, A. H. (2013). Premature menopause in young breast cancer: Effects on quality of life and treatment interventions. *Journal of Thoracic Disease, 5*(Suppl. 1), S55–S61. doi:10.3978/j.issn.2072-1439.2013.06.20

Stojanovska, L., Law, C., Lai, B., Chung, T., Nelson, K., Day, S., . . . Hanies, C. (2015). Maca reduces blood pressure and depression in a pilot study in postmenopausal women. *Climacteric, 18*(1), 69–78.

Torrealday, S., & Pal, L. (2015). Premature menopause. *Endocrinology and Metabolism Clinics of North America, 44*(3), 543–557.

Zhen, X., Qiao, J., Li, R., Wang, L., & Liu, P. (2014). Serologic autoimmunologic parameters in women with primary ovarian insufficiency. *BMC Immunology, 15*, 11. doi:10.1186/1471-2172-15-11

Zhou, K., Jiang, J., Wu, J., & Liu, Z. (2013). Electroacupuncture modulates reproductive hormone levels in patients with primary ovarian insufficiency: Results from a prospective observational study. *Evidence-based Complementary and Alternative Medicine*, 657234. doi:10.1155/2013/657234

Premenstrual Syndrome (PMS)

Abdollahifard, S., Koshkaki, A. R., & Moazamiyanfar, R. (2014). The effects of vitamin B1 on ameliorating the premenstrual syndrome symptoms. *Global Journal of Health Science, 6*(6), 144–153. doi:10.5539/gjhs.v6n6p144

Akbarzadeh, M., Dehghani, M., Moshfeghy, Z., Emamghoreishi, M., Tavakoli, P., & Zare, N. (2015). Effect of *Melissa officinalis* capsule on the intensity of premenstrual syndrome symptoms in high school girl students. *Nursing and Midwifery Studies, 4*(2), e27001. doi:10.17795/nmsjournal27001

Ataollahi, M., Akbari, S. A. A., Mojab, F., & Alavi Majd, H. (2015). The effect of wheat germ extract on premenstrual syndrome symptoms. *Iranian Journal of Pharmaceutical Research, 14*(1), 159–166.

Bertone-Johnson, E. R., Whitcomb, B. W., Missmer, S. A., Manson, J. E., Hankinson, S. E., & Rich-Edwards, J. W. (2014). Early life emotional, physical, and sexual abuse and the development of premenstrual syndrome: A longitudinal study. *Journal of Women's Health, 23*(9), 729–739. doi:10.1089/jwh.2013.467

Bunevicius, A., Leserman, J., & Girdler, S. (2012). Hypothalamic-pituitary-thyroid axis function in women with a menstrually related mood disorder: Association with histories of sexual abuse. *Psychosomatic Medicine, 74*(8), 810–816. doi:10.1097/PSY.0b013e31826c3397

Bunevicius, A., Rubinow, D. R., Calhoun, A., Leserman, J., Richardson, E., Rozanski, K., & Girdler, S. S. (2013). The association of migraine with menstrually related mood disorders and childhood sexual abuse. *Journal of Women's Health, 22*(10), 871–876. doi:10.1089/jwh.2013.4279

Bibliography

Chen, H-Y., Huang, B-S., Lin, Y-H., Su, I-H., Yang, S., Chen, J., . . . Chen, Y-C. (2014). Identifying Chinese herbal medicine for premenstrual syndrome: Implications from a nationwide database. *BMC Complementary and Alternative Medicine, 14,* 206. doi:10.1186/1472-6882-14-206

Chocano-Bedoya, P. O., Manson, J. E., Hankinson, S. E., Willett, W. C., Johnson, S. R., Chasan-Taber, L., . . . Bertone-Johnson, E. R. (2011). Dietary B vitamin intake and incident premenstrual syndrome. *The American Journal of Clinical Nutrition, 93*(5), 1080–1086. http://doi.org/10.3945/ajcn.110.009530

Chocano-Bedoya, P. O., Manson, J. E., Hankinson, S. E., Johnson, S. R., Chasan-Taber, L., Ronnenberg, A. G., . . . Bertone-Johnson, E. R. (2013). Intake of selected minerals and risk of premenstrual syndrome. *American Journal of Epidemiology, 177*(10), 1118–1127. http://doi.org/10.1093/aje/kws363

Dante, G., & Facchinetti, F. (2011). Herbal treatments for alleviating premenstrual symptoms: A systematic review. *Journal of Psychosomatic Obstetrics and Gynecology, 32*(1), 42–51. doi:10.3109/0167482X.2010.538102

Delara, M., Ghofranipour, F., Azadfallah, P., Tavafian, S. S., Kazemnejad, A., & Montazeri, A. (2012). Health related quality of life among adolescents with premenstrual disorders: A cross-sectional study. *Health and Quality of Life Outcomes, 10,* 1. doi:10.1186/1477-7525-10-1

Die, M. V., Burger, H., Teede, H., & Bone, K. (2013). *Vitex agnus-castus* extracts for female reproductive disorders: A systematic review of clinical trials. *Planta Medica, 79*(7), 562–575. doi:10.1055/s-0032-1327831

Direkvand-Moghadam, A., Sayehmiri, K., Delpisheh, A., & Kaikhavandi, S. (2014). Epidemiology of premenstrual syndrome (PMS)—A systematic review and meta-analysis study. *Journal of Clinical and Diagnostic Research, 8*(2), 106–109. doi:10.7860/JCDR/2014/8024.4021

Ebrahimi, E., Khayati Motlagh, S., Nemati, S., & Tavakoli, Z. (2012). Effects of magnesium and vitamin B6 on the severity of premenstrual syndrome symptoms. *Journal of Caring Sciences, 1*(4), 183–189. doi:10.5681/jcs.2012.026

Fathizadeh, N., Ebrahimi, E., Valinani, M., & Yar, M. H. (2010). Evaluating the effect of magnesium and magnesium plus vitamin B6 supplement on the severity of premenstrual syndrome. *Iranian Journal of Nursery and Midwifery Research, 15*(Suppl. 1), 401–405.

Fleischman, D. S., Bunevicius, A., Leserman, J., & Girdler, S. S. (2014). Menstrually related mood disorders and a history of abuse: Moderators of pain sensitivity. *Health Psychology, 33*(2), 147–154.

Gillings, M. R. (2014). Were there evolutionary advantages to premenstrual syndrome? *Evolutionary Applications, 7*(8), 897–904. doi:10.1111/eva.12190

Grosso, G., Pajak, A., Marventano, S., Castellano, S., Galvano, F., Bucolo, C., . . . Caraci, F. (2014). Role of omega-3 fatty acids in the treatment of depressive disorders: A comprehensive meta-analysis of randomized clinical trials. *PLoS ONE, 9*(5), e96905. doi:10.1371/journal.pone.0096905

Jang, S., Kim, D., & Choi, M-S. (2014). Effects and treatment methods of acupuncture and herbal medicine for premenstrual syndrome/premenstrual dysphoric disorder: Systematic review. *BMC Complementary and Alternative Medicine, 14,* 11–11. doi:10.1186/1472-6882-14-11

Kashani, L., Saedi, N., & Akhondzadeh, S. (2010). Femicomfort in the treatment of premenstrual syndromes: A double-blind, randomized and placebo controlled trial. *Iranian Journal of Psychiatry, 5*(2), 47–50.

613

Kim, S-Y., Park, H-J., Lee, H., & Lee, H. (2011). Acupuncture for premenstrual syndrome: A systematic review and meta-analysis of randomised controlled trials. *BJOG: An International Journal of Obstetrics and Gynaecology, 8*(8), 899–915. doi:10.1111/j.1471-0528.2011.02994.x

Marjoribanks, J., Brown, J., O'brien, P. M. S., & Wyatt, K. (2013). Selective serotonin reuptake inhibitors for premenstrual syndrome. *Cochrane Database of Systematic Reviews*, CD001396. doi:10.1002/14651858

Ozgoli, G., Selselei, E. A., Mojab, F., & Majd, H. A. (2009). A randomized, placebo-controlled trial of *Ginkgo biloba* L. in treatment of premenstrual syndrome. *Journal of Alternative and Complementary Medicine, 15*(8), 845–851. doi:10.1089/acm.2008.0493

Schellenberg, R., Zimmermann, C., Drewe, J., Hoexter, G., & Zahner, C. (2012). Dose-dependent efficacy of the *Vitex agnus castus* extract Ze 440 in patients suffering from premenstrual syndrome. *Phytomedicine, 19*(14), 1325–1331. doi:10.1016/j.phymed.2012.08.006

Stolberg, M. (2000, July). The monthly malady: A history of premenstrual suffering. *Medical History, 44*(3), 301–322.

Usman, S. B., Indusekhar, R., & O'Brien, S. (2007). Hormonal management of premenstrual syndrome. *Best Practice & Research Clinical Obstetrics & Gynaecology, 22*(2), 251–260.

Zamani, M., Neghab, N., & Torabian, S. (2012). Therapeutic effect of *Vitex agnus castus* in patients with premenstrual syndrome. *Acta Medica Iranica, 50*(2), 101–106. Retrieved from http://acta.tums.ac.ir/index.php/acta/article/view/4464

Skin Disorders

Bath-Hextall, F. J., Jenkinson, C., Humphreys, R., & Williams, H. C. (2012). Dietary supplements for established atopic eczema. *Cochrane Database of Systematic Reviews, 2*, CD005205. doi:10.1002/14651858.CD005205.pub3

Cao, H., Yang, G., Wang, Y., Liu, J. P., Smith, C. A., Luo, H., & Liu, Y. (2015). Complementary therapies for acne vulgaris. *Cochrane Database of Systematic Reviews, 1*, CD009436. doi:10.1002/14651858.CD009436.pub2

Garner, S. E., Eady, A., Bennett, C., Newton, J. N., Thomas, K., & Popescu, C. M. (2012). Minocycline for acne vulgaris: Efficacy and safety. *Cochrane Database of Systematic Reviews, 8*, CD002086. doi:10.1002/14651858.CD002086.pub2

Jordan, R., Cummins, C. C. L., Burls, A., & Seukeran, D. D. C. (2001). Laser resurfacing for facial acne scars. *Cochrane Database of Systematic Reviews, 1*, CD001866. doi:10.1002/14651858.CD001866

Kraft, J., & Freiman, A. (2011). Management of acne. *Canadian Medical Association Journal, 183*(7), E430–E435. doi:10.1503/cmaj.090374

Vulvodynia

Abbott, J., & Won, H. R. (2010). Optimal management of chronic cyclical pelvic pain: An evidence-based and pragmatic approach. *International Journal of Women's Health, 2*, 263–277.

Arnold, L. D., Bachmann, G. A., Rosen, R., Kelly, S., & Rhoads, G. G. (2006). Vulvodynia: Characteristics and associations with comorbidities and quality of life. *Obstetrics and Gynecology, 107*(3), 617–624.

Bibliography

Bachmann, G. A., Rosen, R., Arnold, L. D., Burd, I., Rhoads, G. G., Leiblum, S. R., & Avis, N. (2006). Chronic vulvar and other gynecologic pain: Prevalence and characteristics in a self-reported survey. *Obstetrical and Gynecological Survey, 51*(1), 313–314.

Beco, J., Climov, D., & Bex, M. (2004). Pudendal nerve decompression in perineology: A case series. *BMC Surgery, 4*(15). doi:10.1186/1471-2482-4-15

Cohen-Sacher, B., Haefner, H. K., Dalton, V. K., & Berger, M. B. (2015). History of abuse in women with vulvar pruritus, vulvodynia, and asymptomatic controls. *Journal of Lower Genital Tract Disease, 19*(3), 248–252.

Eilati, E., Bahr, J. M., & Hales, D. B. (2013). Long-term consumption of flaxseed enriched diet decreased ovarian cancer incidence and prostaglandin E2 in hens. *Gynecologic Oncology, 130*(3). doi:10.1016/j.ygyno.2013.05.018

Falsetta, M. L., Foster, D. C., Woeller, C. F., Pollock, S. J., Bonham, A. D., Haidaris, C. G., . . . Phipps, R. P. (2015). Identification of novel mechanisms involved in generating localized vulvodynia pain. *American Journal of Obstetrics and Gynecology, 213*(1), 38.e1–38.e12. http://doi.org/10.1016/j.ajog.2015.02.002

Harlow, B. L., Kunitz, C. G., Nguyen, R. H., Rydell, S. A., Turner, R. M., & Maclehose, R. F. (2014). Prevalence of symptoms consistent with a diagnosis of vulvodynia: population-based estimates from 2 geographic regions. *American Journal of Obstetrics and Gynecology, 210*(1), 40.e1–e8.

Leclair, C. M., Goetsch, M. F., Korcheva, V. B., Anderson, R., Peters, D., & Morgan, T. K. (2011). Differences in primary compared with secondary vestibulodynia by immunohistochemistry. *Obstetrics & Gynecology, 117*(6), 1307–1313.

Smith, E. M., Ritchie, J. M., Galask, R., Pugh, E. E., Jia, J., & Ricks-McGillan, J. (2002). Case-control study of vulvar vestibulitis risk associated with genital infections. *Infectious Diseases in Obstetrics and Gynecology, 10*(4), 193–202.

Tu, F. F., Hellman, K. M., & Backonja, M. M. (2011). Gynecologic management of neuropathic pain. *American Journal of Obstetrics and Gynecology, 205*(5), 435–443.

Ventolini, G. (2011). Measuring treatment outcomes in women with vulvodynia. *Journal of Clinical Medicine Research, 3*(2), 59–64.

Woods, J. L., Hensel, D. J., & Fortenberry, J. D. (2010). Gynecological symptoms and sexual behaviors among adolescent women. *Journal of Pediatric and Adolescent Gynecology, 23*(2), 93–95.

Contraception

American College of Obstetricians and Gynecologists. (2014). *Frequently asked questions. Gynecological problems. FAQ022: Contraception.* Retrieved from http://www.acog.org/-/media/For-Patients/faq022.pdf?dmc=1&ts=20150721T1436130143

Diedrich, J., & Madden, T. (2015). *Who is at increased risk of IUD expulsion?* Retrieved from http://providers.bedsider.org/articles/who-is-at-increased-risk-of-iud-expulsion

Galea, L., Wainwright, S., Roes, M., Duarte-Guterman, P., Chow, C., & Hamson, D. (2013). Sex, hormones and neurogenesis in the hippocampus: Hormonal modulation of neurogenesis and potential functional implications. *Journal of Neuroendocrinology, 25*(11), 1039–1061. doi:10.1111/jne.12070

Institute for Reproductive Health. (2015). *TwoDay Method®.* Retrieved from http://irh.org/projects/fam_project/twoday-method/

McNeilly, A. (2001). Lactational control of reproduction. *Reproduction, Fertility, and Development, 13*(7–8), 583–590. Retrieved from http://www.ncbi.nlm.nih.gov/pubmed/11999309

McNeilly, A. (2001). Neuroendocrine changes and fertility in breast-feeding women. *Progress in Brain Research, 133,* 207–214. Retrieved from http://www.ncbi.nlm .nih.gov/pubmed/?term=Neuroendocrine+changes+and+fertility+in+breast-feeding +women

McNeilly, A., Tay, C., & Glasier, A. (1994). Physiological mechanisms underlying lactational amenorrhea. *Annals of the New York Academy of Sciences, 709*(1), 145–155. doi:10.1111/j.1749-6632.1994.tb30394

Nelson, R. (2015). *The pill has prevented 400,000 cases of endometrial cancer.* Retrieved from http://www.medscape.com/viewarticle/849065

Shih G. (2015). *Does being overweight affect your birth control?* Retrieved from http:// bedsider.org/features/164-does-being-overweight-affect-your-birth-control

Stern, L. (2015). *Talking fertility awareness methods with your patients.* Retrieved from http:// providers.bedsider.org/articles/talking-fertility-awareness-methods-with-your-patients

Health Literacy and Health-Care Access

Armstrong, K., Putt, M., Halbert, C. H., Grande, D., Schwartz, J. S., Liao, K., . . . Shea, J. A. (2013). Prior experiences of racial discrimination and racial differences in health care system distrust. *Medical Care, 51*(2), 144–150. http://doi.org/10.1097/ MLR.0b013e31827310a1

Ayis, S., Wellwood, I., Rudd, A. G., McKevitt, C., Parkin, D., & Wolfe, C. D. A. (2015). Variations in health-related quality of life (HRQoL) and survival 1 year after stroke: Five European population-based registers. *BMJ Open, 5*(6), e007101. doi:10.1136 /bmjopen-2014-007101

Barry, M. J., & Edgman-Levitan, S. (2012). Shared decision making—Pinnacle of patient-centered care. *New England Journal of Medicine, 366*(9), 780–781.

Beagan, B. L., Fredericks, E., & Goldberg, L. (2012). Nurses' work with LGBTQ patients: "They're just like everybody else, so what's the difference?" *Canadian Journal of Nursing Research, 44*(3), 44–63.

Berlin, E. A., & Fowkes, W. C. (1983). Teaching framework for cross-cultural care: Application in Family Practice. *Western Journal of Medicine, 139*(6), 934–938.

Boscardin, C. K., Grbic, D., Grumbach, K., & O'sullivan, P. (2014). Educational and individual factors associated with positive change in and reaffirmation of medical students' intention to practice in underserved areas. *Academic Medicine, 89*(11), 1490–1496.

Burke, S. E., Dovidio, J. F., Przedworski, J. M., Hardeman, R. R., Perry, S. P., Phelan, S. M., . . . van Ryn, M. (2015). Do contact and empathy mitigate bias against gay and lesbian people among heterosexual medical students? A report from Medical Student CHANGES. *Academic Medicine: Journal of the Association of American Medical Colleges, 90*(5), 645–651. http://doi.org/10.1097/ACM.0000000000000661

Dauvrin, M., & Lorant, V. (2015). Leadership and cultural competence of healthcare professionals: A social network analysis. *Nursing Research, 64*(3), 200–210. doi:10.1097 /NNR.0000000000000092

Derksen, F., Bensing, J., & Lagro-Janssen, A. (2013). Effectiveness of empathy in general practice: a systematic review. *British Journal of General Practice, 63*(606), e76–e84. doi:10.3399/bjgp13X660814

Donald, F., Martin-Misener, R., Carter, N., Donald, E., Kaasalainen, S., Wickson-Griffiths, A., . . . Dicenso, A.(2013). A systematic review of the effectiveness of advanced practice nurses in long-term care. *Journal of Advanced Nursing, 69*(10), 2148–2161.

Bibliography

Dorsen, C. (2012). An integrative review of nurse attitudes towards lesbian, gay, bisexual, and transgender patients. *Canadian Journal of Nursing Research, 44*(3), 18–43.

Esposito, C. L. (2013). Provision of culturally competent health care: An interim status review and report. *Journal of the New York State Nurses Association, 43*(2), 4–10.

Hansen, B. R., Hodgson, N. A., & Gitlin, L. N. (2015). It's a matter of trust: Older African Americans speak about their health care encounters. *Journal of Applied Gerontology, 35*(10), 1058–1076.

Hawala-Druy, S., & Hill, M. H. (2012). Interdisciplinary: Cultural competency and culturally congruent education for millennials in health professions. *Nurse Education Today, 32*(7), 772–778.

Johnson, C., Killinger, L. Z., Christensen, M. G., Hyland, J. K., Mrozek, J. P., Zuker, R. F., . . . Oyelowo, T. (2012). Multiple views to address diversity issues: An initial dialog to advance the chiropractic profession. *Journal of Chiropractic Humanities, 19*(1), 1–11. doi:10.1016/j.echu.2012.10.003

Kavanagh, K. H., & Kennedy, P. H. (1992). *Promoting cultural diversity: Strategies for health care professionals*. Newbury Park, CA: Sage.

Landrine, H., & Corral, I. (2014). Advancing research on racial–ethnic health disparities: Improving measurement equivalence in studies with diverse samples. *Frontiers in Public Health, 2,* 282. doi:10.3389/fpubh.2014.00282

Lee, S., & Schwarz, N. (2014). Question context and priming meaning of health: Effect on differences in self-rated health between Hispanics and non-Hispanic Whites. *American Journal of Public Health, 104*(1), 179–185. doi:10.2105/AJPH.2012.301055

Lie, D. A, Lee-Rey, E., Gomez, A., Bereknyei, S., & Braddock, C. H. (2011). Does cultural competency training of health professionals improve patient outcomes? A systematic review and proposed algorithm for future research. *Journal of General Internal Medicine, 26*(3), 317–325. doi:10.1007/s11606-010-1529-0

Loftin, C., Hartin, V., Branson, M., & Reyes, H. (2013). Measures of cultural competence in nurses: An integrative review. *Scientific World Journal, 289101.* doi:10.1155/2013/289101

Lyons, S. S., Specht, J. P., Karlman, S. E., & Maas, M. L. (2008). Everyday excellence: A framework for professional nursing practice in long-term care. *Research in Gerontological Nursing, 1*(3), 217–228. doi:10.3928/00220124-20091301-08

Mercer, S. W., Jani, B. D., Maxwell, M., Wong, S. Y., & Watt, G. C. (2012). Patient enablement requires physician empathy: A cross-sectional study of general practice consultations in areas of high and low socioeconomic deprivation in Scotland. *BMC Family Practice, 13,* 6. doi:10.1186/1471-2296-13-6

Truong, M., Paradies, Y., & Priest, N. (2014). Interventions to improve cultural competency in healthcare: a systematic review of reviews. *BMC Health Services Research, 14,* 99. doi:10.1186/1472-6963-14-99

U.S. Bureau of the Census. (2012). *Population projections of the United States by age, sex, race, and Hispanic origin: 1995–2050*. Retrieved from https://www.census.gov/prod/1/pop/p25-1130.pdf

Van ryn, M., Hardeman, R., Phelan, S. M., Burgess, D., Dovidio, J., Herrin, J., . . . Przedworski, J., (2015). Medical school experiences associated with change in implicit racial bias among 3547 students: A Medical Student CHANGES Study report. *Journal of General Internal Medicine, 30*(12), 1748–1756. doi:10.1007/s11606-015-3447-7

Weech-Maldonado, R., Elliott, M. N., Pradhan, R., Schiller, C., Hall, A., & Hays, R. D. (2012). Can hospital cultural competency reduce disparities in patient experiences with care? *Medical Care, 50,* S48–S55. doi:10.1097/MLR.0b013e3182610ad1

Domestic Violence/Intimate Partner Violence (IPV)

American College of Obstetricians and Gynecologists. (2012). *Intimate partner violence.* Retrieved from http://www.acog.org/Resources-And-Publications/Committee-Opinions/Committee-on-Health-Care-for-Underserved-Women/Intimate-Partner-Violence. Retrieved August 2015

Ard, K. L., & Makadon, H. J. (2011). Addressing intimate partner violence in lesbian, gay, bisexual, and transgender patients. *Journal of General Internal Medicine, 26*(8), 930–933. doi:10.1007/s11606-011-1697-6

Dutton, M. A., James, L., Langhorne, A., & Kelley, M. (2015). Coordinated public health initiatives to address violence against women and adolescents. *Journal of Women's Health, 24*(1), 80–85.

Neufeld, B. (1996). SAFE questions: Overcoming barriers to the detection of domestic violence. *American Family Physician, 53*(8), 2575–2580, 2582.

Sprague, S., Madden, K., Dosanjh, S., Godin, K., Goslings, JC, Schemitsch, E., & Bhandari, M. (2013). Intimate partner violence and musculoskeletal injury: Bridging the knowledge gap in orthopaedic fracture clinics. *BMC Musculoskeletal Disorders, 14,* 23. doi:10.1186/1471-2474-14-23

Sprague, S., Madden, K., Simunovic, N., Godin, K., Pham, N., Bhandari, M., & Goslings, J. (2012). Barriers to screening for intimate partner violence. *Women's Health, 52*(6), 587–605.

Wu, V., Huff, H., & Bhandari, M. (2010). Pattern of physical injury associated with intimate partner violence in women presenting to the emergency department: A systematic review and meta-analysis. *Trauma Violence Abuse, 11*(2), 71–82.

U.S. Department of Justice, Office of Justice Programs, Bureau of Justice Statistics. (2012). *Crime characteristics.* Retrieved from https://www.bjs.gov/index.cfm?ty=pbdetail&iid=4536

Health Literacy and Health-Care Access

Agency for Health Care Research and Quality. (2016). *Health literacy measuring tools.* Retrieved from http://www.ahrq.gov/professionals/quality-patient-safety/quality-resources/tools/literacy/index.html

Center for Disease Control and Prevention. (2016). *Evaluate skills and programs.* Retrieved from http://www.cdc.gov/healthliteracy/ResearchEvaluate/index.html

Hartzler, A., & Pratt, W. (2011). Managing the personal side of health: How patient expertise differs from the expertise of clinicians. *Journal of Medical Internet Research, 13*(3), e62. doi:10.2196/jmir.1728

Haun, J. N., Patel, N. R., French, D. D., Campbell, R. R., Bradham, D. D., & Lapcevic, W. A. (2015). Association between health literacy and medical care costs in an integrated healthcare system: A regional population based study. *BMC Health Services Research, 15,* 249. doi:10.1186/s12913-015-0887-z

Health.gov. (n.d.). *Quick guide to health literacy fact sheet.* Retrieved from http://health.gov/communication/literacy/quickguide/factsliteracy.htm

Health.gov. (2008). *Health literacy improvement.* Retrieved from http://health.gov/communication/literacy/

Mantwill, S., & Schulz, P. J. (2015, July 10). Low health literacy associated with higher medication costs in patients with type 2 diabetes mellitus: Evidence from matched survey and health insurance data. *Patient Education and Counseling, 98*(12), 1625–1630. doi:10.1016/j.pec.2015.07.006

Robinson, T., White, G., & Houchins, J. (2006, September). Improving communication with older patients: Tips from the literature. *Family Practice Management, 13*(8), 73–78.

Saroja, S. (2010). Short assessment of health literacy-Spanish and English: A comparable test of health literacy for Spanish and English- speakers. *Health Services Research, 45*(4), 1105–1120. http://doi.org/10.1111/j.1475-6773.2010.01119.x

Zheng, J., & Yu, H. (2015). Methods for linking EHR notes to education materials. *AMIA Summits on Translational Science Proceedings,* 209–215.

Disability

Taua, C., Hepworth, J., & Neville, C. (2012). Nurses' role in caring for people with a comorbidity of mental illness and intellectual disability: A literature review. *International Journal of Mental Health Nursing, 21*(2), 163–174.

Cultural Competency

Johnson, C., Killinger, L. Z., Christensen, M. G., Hyland, J. K., Mrozek, J. P., Zuker, R. F., & Oyelowo, T. (2012). Multiple views to address diversity issues: An initial dialog to advance the chiropractic profession. *Journal of Chiropractic Humanities, 19*(1), 1–11. doi:10.1016/j.echu.2012.10.003

Spiritual Health References

Clinebell, H. J. (1992). *Well being: A personal plan for exploring and enriching the seven dimensions of life: Mind, body, spirit, love, work, play, the world.* New York, NY: Harper Collins.

Cotton, S., Zebracki, K., Rosenthal, S. L., Tsevat, J., & Drotar, D. (2006). Religion/spirituality and adolescent health outcomes: A review. *Journal of Adolescent Health, 38*(4), 472–480.

Jackson, L. J., White, C. R., O'Brien, K., DiLorenzo, P., Cathcart, E., Wolf, M., . . . Cabrera, J. (2010). Exploring spirituality among youth in foster care: findings from the Casey Field Office Mental Health Study. *Child & Family Social Work, 15*(1), 107–117. http://doi.org/10.1111/j.1365-2206.2009.00649.x

King D. E., & Bushwick, B. (1994). Beliefs and attitudes of hospital inpatients about faith healing and prayer. *Journal of Family Practice, 39*(4), 349–352.

Koenig H. G. (2012). Religion, spirituality, and health: The research and clinical implications. *ISRN Psychiatry,* 278730. doi:10.5402/2012/278730

Post D. M., & Weddington, W. H. (2000). Stress and coping of the African-American physician. *Journal of the National Medical Association, 92*(2), 70–75.

Post, S. G., Puchalski, C. M., & Larson, D. B. (2000). Physicians and patient spirituality: Professional boundaries, competency, and ethics. *Annals of Internal Medicine, 132*(7), 578–583.

Salmoirago-Blotcher, E., Fitchett, G., Leung, K., Volturo, G., Boudreaux, E., Crawford, S., . . . Curlin, F. (2016). An exploration of the role of religion/spirituality in the promotion of physicians' wellbeing in Emergency Medicine. *Preventive Medicine Reports, 3,* 189–195. http://doi.org/10.1016/j.pmedr.2016.01.009

Bibliography

Shin, J. H., Yoon, J. D., Rasinski, K. A., Koenig, H. G., Meador, K. G., & Curlin, F. A. (2013). A spiritual problem? Primary care physicians' and psychiatrists' interpretations of medically unexplained symptoms. *Journal of General Internal Medicine, 28*(3), 392–398. doi:10.1007/s11606-012-2224-0

Spirituality. (2017). Retrieved from http://en.wikipedia.org/wiki/Spirituality

University of California. (2014). *Spiritual wellness.* Retrieved from https://wellness.ucr.edu/spiritual_wellness.html

Wachholtz, A., & Rogoff, M. (2013). The relationship between spirituality and burnout among medical students. *Journal of Contemporary Medical Education, 1*(2), 83–91. doi:10.5455/jcme.20130104060612

Index

Note: Page numbers followed by *f* and *t* indicate material in figures and tables respectively.

Index

Index

Index

Index

Index

Index

Index

Index

Index

Index

Index

Index

Index

Index

Index

Index

Index

Index